Care-Related Quality of Life in Old Age

Marja Vaarama
Richard Pieper
Andrew Sixsmith
Editors

Care-Related Quality of Life in Old Age

Concepts, Models and Empirical Findings

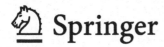 Springer

Marja Vaarama
Department of Social Work
University of Lapland, Finland
P.O. Box 122
Rovaniemi 96101
Email, personal: marja.vaarama
www.ulapland.fi/marja.vaarama

Richard Pieper
Fak. Sozial-u. Wirtschaftswiss.
Urbanistik und
Sozialplanung
University of Bamberg, Germany
21, Feldkirchenstr.
Bamberg 96045
Email, personal: richard.pieper@sowi.
uni-bamberg.de

Andrew Sixsmith
Gerontology Research Centre and
Department of Gerontology,
Simon Fraser University at Harbour Centre
2800-515 West Hastings Street
Vancouver B.C Canada V6B 5K3
Email, personal: Sixsmith@sfu.ca

ISBN 978-1-4419-2467-4   e-ISBN 978-0-387-72169-9

Printed on acid-free paper.

9 8 7 6 5 4 3 2 1

springer.com

Marja Vaarama would like to dedicate this book to her son Eetu,
Richard Pieper to his son Konrad and Andrew Sixsmith to his son Thomas.
We wish each of them many years of happiness and a good quality of life.

Foreword

The ageing of populations across the world poses a crucial challenge for the twenty-first century. Society faces three major changes: firstly, increasing numbers of active older people demanding new social structures and opportunities; secondly, increasing numbers of frail or disabled older people requiring new interventions and improved health and social care with resulting economic consequences; and finally complex economic, technological, organisational and social challenges involved in the ageing of society. If society wants to benefit from these changes, innovative social, organisational and technological responses are needed.

This book presents the findings of the Care Keys project—"Keys for Quality Performance Management of the Care of Older Persons in Europe"—and is an example of how research can respond to the challenges outlined above. Care Keys was the fruit of European Union research funding, made possible under the Quality of Life and Management of Living Resources specific programme (1998–2002) under the EC's Fifth Framework Programme for Research,[1] Technological Development and Demonstration. The activity promoting such research was Key Action 6 on the "Ageing Population and their Disabilities". This key action was established under the quality of life-specific programme to respond to the complex economic, technological, organisational and social challenges involved in the ageing of society. Community-wide cross-sectoral multidisciplinary research, combining and integrating efforts in the biological, biomedical, psychological, technological, economic and social fields, was supported with the objective of promoting healthy ageing. In the period from 1998 to 2002, over €170 million was committed to funding research in ageing relevant areas, with a total of 121 research and coordination projects being supported.

---

[1] Fifth Framework Programme for research, technological development and demonstration activities (1998–2002), Decision No 182/1999/EC of the European Parliament and of the Council of 22.12.1998, O.J. L26/1 of 01.02.1999, Council Decision No 1999/167/EC of 25.01.1999 adopting a specific programme for research, technological development and demonstration on quality of life and management of living resources (1998–2002) OJ L 64 of 12.3.1999.

Key Action 6 adopted a problem-solving approach, in which it aimed "to put research to work" to meet the challenges posed by both the ageing of individuals and the ageing of societies. It aimed to do so by taking a well-balanced holistic approach towards the challenges of ageing populations. Impressive scientific results have been already achieved by many of the projects using this "holistic approach" (http://cordis.europa.eu/life/src/conf-ageing.htm).

This book comes at an important time in the policy debate over long-term care for older persons, with questions about the level and quality of care provision, how to meet the needs of older people, how best to use scarce resources and how to ensure care-dependent older people enjoy a good quality of life all needing to be answered. The research is especially relevant to the current EU Seventh Framework Programme for Research[2] providing valuable evidence for reflecting on the needs and priorities for health and social care development. However, the theories, models and methodologies presented in this book are applicable to all welfare economies that are concerned with improving the provision of care services to enhance the lives of older people.

Kevin McCarthy
European Commission
DG Research
Health Research Directorate
Public Health Research

---

[2] Proposal for a Decision of the European Parliament and of the Council concerning the seventh framework programme of the European Community for research, technological development and demonstration activities (2007–2013), 06.04.2005 COM(2005) 119.

Preface

Quality of life (QoL) is widely recognised as an important concept and measure of outcomes in health care, and the concept is emerging more and more often also in connection with long-term care (LTC). However, although improving or maximising the QoL of the clients seems to be increasingly mentioned in care policies and development programmes of LTC of older people, it less often is a goal pursued in actual care practices. In our view, among the reasons for this are underdeveloped concepts, structures and processes of evaluation of care outcomes in the LTC of older people. Although considerable progress has been achieved in research and practice in recent years, there still are no common definitions or standards for quality available in LTC and no "golden rules" on how to care for the frail and vulnerable clients well and based on best gerontological knowledge. The quality of documentation in LTC tends to be poor and narrowly focused on clinical information, and standards for documentation are lacking, let alone the development of information technologies tailored for this purpose. Although examples of "good practice" are becoming available from all over Europe and can guide the improvement of practices, systematic quality management in LTC is underdeveloped. In addition, even if quality evaluation and care documentation are in place, the voices of older clients themselves as well as those of their informal carers tend to be neglected as they are not regularly involved in setting goals and evaluating results of care. A client orientation in care management and performance evaluation needs to be strengthened, since it is not possible to evaluate the effectiveness or efficiency of care if the experiences and evaluations of persons whose needs are to be met and whose life qualities are to be improved are not heard.

These issues are guiding this book, and to address these problems we have developed a concept of "care-related quality of life", which highlights the important role of care as a resource to improve the life quality of the clients and integrates the concepts of QoL, quality of care and care management. We have taken steps towards the specification of measures and tools to support client-oriented evaluation. The concept of care-related quality of life (crQoL) is presented here as a basis for applied research within social gerontology and as a framework for quality assurance, evaluation and performance measurement within health and social care services for older people. We examine the relationship between LTC and QoL of frail older people from theoretical, methodological and empirical perspectives. The book presents the research undertaken within the European Care Keys project[3] during the years 2003–2006, which involved partners in Finland, Estonia, Germany, Sweden and UK.

The motivation for the research is based on awareness that issues of well-being and QoL are particularly relevant in the study of older people, especially those who are vulnerable, frail or disabled. The changes in personal capacities, abilities and circumstances that often accompany old age may fundamentally challenge the basis of a person's well-being and may undermine the ability to cope with everyday life as well as the ability to secure adequate care. However, for those people who rely on regular support from health and social care services, care has a major impact on their overall QoL. For example, the social relations, the care regime and the physical environment of residential and nursing homes will play a major part in determining the QoL of residents in almost every respect. In home care, old people need not only home nursing, but also concrete help in daily living and emotional and social support to maintain the lifestyles they like even under conditions of frailty. Health and social care are not just a matter of extending life, but of enhancing QoL, and this should be a major consideration in how we assess the value and impact of the services provided and consumed. The book addresses these issues more specifically by pursuing the following questions:

1. What are the determinants of crQoL in old age?
2. How can care contribute to and support the QoL of older clients?
3. How should care be managed to facilitate good quality and effective care?

Obviously, we can only hope to make a contribution to answering these questions, but the Care Keys project was rather ambitious in combining a wide scope of approaches and objectives. The research was multidisciplinary, involving social gerontology, medical and nursing sciences, psychology, sociology, economics, management sciences, mathematics and statistics. Besides contributing to current theories, methods and empirical knowledge, also first instruments for a practical "Care Keys Toolkit" have been developed for the evaluation and management of care. This toolkit is intended to integrate the evaluation from the client's perspective with that from the professional and managerial perspective in a way that can be readily accommodated within care management practices as experience in the course of the project suggested.

At the initial stage of the project, it became clear that there are few theories, measures and knowledge available on QoL of old, care-dependent people.

---

[3] The work reported in this book has been carried out as part of the Care Keys project funded under the European Union's Quality of Life Research and Development programme, project number QLK6-CT-2002-02525, see http://www.carekeys.net

Also, definitions and concepts of quality of LTC and management of quality are scarce. There is a wealth of definitions on QoL, quality of nursing care and quality management available, but they rarely address frail old people, social care and home care or management of the quality of LTC of older people. Therefore, we had to orient our research to first conducting theoretical research establishing the necessary scientific base for our research, and then proceed to selecting and developing instrumentation, and to conduct an empirical research for validation of our concepts, models and instruments. Actually, after establishment of the general theoretical framework, the theoretical work continued, and theoretical and empirical research were developing in parallel, supporting each other, but also pursuing own priorities and interests, and in this way constituting a very rewarding iterative process along the course of the research.

Reflecting the different objectives and tasks, the book is structured into four sections:

1. Part I describes the general theoretical framework, key concepts and methodology, and demonstrates the complexity of the topic of crQoL, highlighting the need for appropriate theory, methods and instruments.
2. Part II presents the results of theoretical research within the Care Keys project, discussing three theoretical frameworks relevant for crQoL in old age: (i) The concept of the crQoL; (ii) An integrated theory of quality of LTC, trying to bridge between the social and health care, and between homecare and institutional care and (iii) A framework for management of the quality of LTC, which approaches the challenges of quality management taking the special conditions of LTC into account.
3. Part III reports and discusses empirical results of the Care Keys research as a collection of independent articles: cross-national comparisons of QoL, QoL in home care, QoL in institutional care, QoL of cognitively impaired older people, the target efficiency of care, the management of quality of LTC and a brief introduction to the Care Keys Toolkit.
4. In Part IV, a concluding chapter summarises the key themes of research cross-cutting the special themes of the chapters, with a special focus on the differences of home care and institutional care, and highlighting the results with reference to the research questions and theoretical models, and evaluates the implications for further research.

Care Keys was a complex and challenging project and demanded a high level of commitment from all who participated in it; partners, researchers from different disciplines, national user groups and our external evaluators. This book is a reflection of the commitment of all of us. It also demonstrates how we shared a common research framework and theoretical approach, but also took the liberty to employ them in our sub-studies differently. We have not tried to even out these differences in this book as we think this is a richness of our research and demonstrates the strengths of a multidisciplinary research undertaken under a common theoretical umbrella, which has been at the same time providing a common framework to guide the research, and been flexible enough to allow approaching the research problems from diverse scientific paradigms and perspectives.

The scope of the book is wide, from social theory to empirical studies, from methodological instruments to practical applications and dissemination of results. Therefore, guidance on how to read the book may be helpful. Those readers not interested in the theoretical discussions of Part II may read Part I and then proceed to the empirical chapters in Part III, according to their interests. Each empirical chapter ends with a brief summary, so a very busy reader can also first concentrate on them. Some may like to look first at the summarising chapter at the end of the book, but we should point out that the chapter is not repeating the results of other chapters, but concentrates on the discussion of cross-cutting results in view of our key research objectives and points out some challenges for future research. For those interested in the theoretical discussion and the development of theoretical models of QoL, quality of care and care management, Part II may offer new insights and a framework for own research. The practical results are only briefly described in Part II and are not the focus of this report on the Care Keys project. We have to refer the interested reader to publications in preparation and to the Care Keys website (www.carekeys.net).

We hope this book contributes to the ongoing discussion on the concept of QoL in old age, its theories and research methodology. The book also aims to give a new stimulus to the study of the effectiveness and efficiency of care, to encourage further research on the topic of crQoL and to implement strategies of quality management that promote an evaluation in the light of the preferences and needs of older people themselves.

Marja Vaarama, Richard Pieper and Andrew Sixsmith

Contents

PART III: EMPIRICAL RESULTS

PART IV: SUMMARY

Part I
Research Framework

1
The General Framework and Methods of the Care Keys Research

Marja Vaarama, Richard Pieper and Andrew Sixsmith

Introduction

Initially, there were four major research objectives in the Care Keys research:

1. What are the determinants of quality of life (QoL) of care-dependent old people; and what is the role of care in the production of it?
2. What are the determinants of quality of care from the perspectives of the clients and professional carers, and how are they inter-related?
3. How should care be managed to provide positive care outcomes?
4. Development of a Toolkit, comprising models and instrumentation for evaluating care outcomes within applied research and care management practice.

Care Keys has focused on older people who require help to cope with many aspects of daily life and are often dependent on care provided to them, either at home or in institutional settings, such as nursing homes. For many of these people, the possibilities, choices and opportunities in their everyday lives are more limited because of increasing frailty and loss of independence, with an inevitable impact on their QoL. The aim of the research was to find out how long-term care (LTC) provided to people in their homes or institutional settings impacts on their QoL and how LTC could be improved to support and enhance the well-being of the clients. A particular emphasis was on the "voice" of the clients. An initial literature review revealed that this type of research approach was rare, and the availability of appropriate models and instruments appropriate for use within Care Keys was very limited. Therefore, two further research tasks were defined:

1. To develop a theoretical model of care-related quality of life (crQoL) that also includes concepts of quality of care and management of quality of care.
2. To select, develop and validate instrumentation for research on crQoL.

Hence, the Care Keys project involved both theoretical and empirical research. This chapter outlines the general theoretical framework of the Care Keys research, and in Part II, the results of our theoretical research are discussed.

3

There were a number of themes underlying the research:

1. Quality of Life: We were interested in exploring the various theoretical definitions of QoL for different client groups, and from these derive criteria of QoL as an outcome of care for these groups, as well as validated indicators and measures.
2. Quality of Long-Term Care (QoC): We were similarly interested in theoretical definitions of Quality of Long-Term Community and Institutional Care, and the criteria and professional standards of (long-term) care for older persons, as well as indicators and measures.
3. Quality management of Long-Term Community and Institutional Care and its effects on quality of care and QoL of clients.

Bringing these ideas together was fundamental to the development of the concept of crQoL, requiring the synthesis of several theoretical perspectives, which we call the "Four Pillars of Care-Related QoL" (Fig. 1.1):

1. Production of Welfare (PoW) Theory examining the relationship between care inputs and care outcomes (e.g. QoL).
2. Theories and models of QoL, both in a general sense and more specifically those that relate to frail older people.
3. Multi-dimensional evaluation model of quality of care, emphasising multiple stakeholder perspectives in relation to care inputs, processes and outcomes.
4. Concept of target efficiency of care (TEFF), looking at the allocative efficiency of the relationship between care needs and care provision.

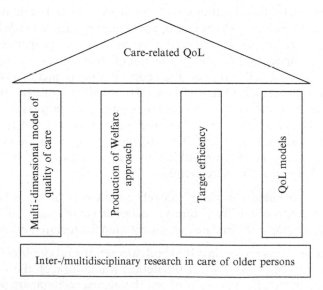

FIG. 1.1. The four "pillars" of crQoL.

The following sections in this chapter discuss each of these "pillars" in turn, which are then summarised within a "meta-model" of crQoL that guided the Care Keys research.

Pillar 1: The Production of Welfare Approach

The Care Keys project was originally inspired by the PoW approach (Davies, Bebbington, & Charnley, 1990; Davies & Knapp, 1981; Knapp, 1984; Sefton, Byford, McDaid, Hills, & Knapp, 2003). The PoW approach applies an economic framework to the realm of social and health care and has been especially developed for research and evaluation in the field of care of older people. As a general framework, it is also useful for integrating perspectives from different disciplines, such as the social, psychological, nursing, medical and management sciences represented in the Care Keys project. The basic message of the PoW is that care and services play an intermediate role, that is their task is to "produce" well-being for clients. In the QoL production process, the material (e.g. amount and qualification of staff) and non-material (e.g. courtesy of personnel) resources are combined to provide quantity (types and intensity) and quality of care, aiming at improving or supporting the well-being (in our case QoL of older) clients. The important message is to see the *intermediate role of services*, that is it is not sufficient just to look at the quality or quantity or costs of care as ends in their own right, but to see all these as inputs for QoL.

As the name indicates, the key issue is about the PoW and how outcomes (in this case QoL) are determined by the care provided. The Care Keys research was restricted in terms of data availability (especially on costs of care) and cross-sectional design, which made it impossible to implement the PoW approach in full in such a way as for example in the studies of Davies et al. (1990), Davies, Fernández, and Nomer (2000), Mozley, Sutchiffe, Bagley, Cordingley, Challis, Hukley, & Burns (2004). Nevertheless, the PoW approach served as a fruitful framework for thinking within Car Keys (QoL as the care outcome). Although, on the one hand, costs and cost-effectiveness of care were beyond the scope of the present research, preferences of the clients and their perceptions of the quality of care, as well as structures and processes of good quality care, on the other hand, had a more prominent place in the approach developed within the Care Keys project. Central concepts were client needs and preferences, care processes and care documentation, as well as care management, and their interplay with care outcomes. The PoW approach provided a framework for searching and exploring the role of care in production of well-being among care-dependent older people and for identification of models of "good care" in terms of their impact on client well-being. The research also examined how type of care, and management inputs were connected to the good care outcomes.

It is also important to recognise the contribution of informal carers and families in the PoW of older people, especially in care at home (Netten, 2004). The PoW is fundamentally a co-production and is "relational" in character, that is deeply rooted in the personal interactions and relationships between the client and the carer. Moreover, there is no such thing as "good quality care", without the involvement of the client and the informal caregiver in the care process. The PoW approach developed within Care Keys combines a research perspective on the relevant factors (variables) within the PoW with a more practical perspective, focusing on aspects and conditions that can be influenced by the professional care and by management of LTC. PoW is considered also as "co-production", not only because clients have to participate in their care in order to make it successful, but they also have to participate in the very definition of the care they need.

Pillar 2: Multi-Dimensional QoL

The final outcome of the PoW process can be conceived as regained, retained or enhanced QoL of the client. QoL should be a central concern for researchers and practitioners working in the area of LTC. However, research on the QoL of frail older people has been surprisingly limited. Considerable attention has been given to issues of health-related QoL (Bowling, 1995, 2004), for example in respect to particular illnesses or conditions (e.g. Bordereau, Szalai, Ennis, Leszcz, Speca, & Sela, 2003; Carod-Artal, Egido, González, & Varela de Seijas, 2000; Hays, Cunningham, Sherbourne, Wilson, Wu, & Clearly, 2000). Attention has been given to QoL for people, especially the elderly, who are suffering from chronic, long-term conditions, such as congestive heart failure, stroke and arthritis. Rather less attention has been given to older people who are described as "frail", or who experience multiple low-level conditions that have an influence on their QoL. Many of these people are dependent on the care and support they receive from formal (e.g. health and social care) and informal (family, neighbours, etc.) sources, and their well-being is inevitably bound up in these care relationships (Birren, Lubben, Rowe, & Deutschmann, 1991). If care is fundamental to well-being of frail older people, then a framework that specifically incorporates the role of care in the production of well-being is needed, rather than a more general concept of well-being.

In this context, a key aim in the Care Keys research was to develop a framework for crQoL and to present some empirical explorations to demonstrate its potential usefulness for research and service evaluation. The perspective emphasised the need for an interdisciplinary, or at least multidisciplinary, approach that attempted to bring together ideas about quality of care provision, the QoL of the users of services and more general ideas about the way care should be managed to improve the lives of frail older people. These issues are specifically addressed in Part II, where the results of theoretical research of the Care Keys are presented.

The literature on the concept of QoL ranges from rather narrow concepts of subjective life satisfaction to comprehensive concepts including both subjective and objective elements, both of the individual and the social and physical environments (see e.g. Bowling, 1991; Diener, 2000; Hughes, 1990;

Renwick, Brown, & Nagler, 1996). Today, QoL is most often understood as a dynamic multi-dimensional concept, which may differ between individuals and also within a person's life course. It is widely agreed that QoL has both objective (e.g. income, housing, health and mobility) and subjective (e.g. life satisfaction and happiness) elements:

QoL is a multi-dimensional evaluation, by both intra-personal and socio-economic criteria of the person-environment -system of the individual. (Lawton, 1991).

QoL is the concept to "encompass in the broad sense the social, psychological and physical domains of life, incorporating a subjective assessment of important life domains in relation to achieving satisfaction" (Bowling, 1991).

Although no single theory defines the field, the model of four domains of QoL in old age (functional competence, psychological well-being, social relations and environmental support) suggested by Lawton (1991) and the idea of "successful ageing" (Baltes & Baltes, 1990) are widely used within gerontological QoL research. In addition, Felce and Perry (1997) provide a useful framework for exploring QoL in terms of subjective and objective evaluation of five dimensions: physical, material, social, emotional and productive well-being. The WHOQOL Group (1998) (Skevington, Lotfy, & O'Connell, 2004) approaches QoL as a combination of factors: satisfaction with physical, psychological, social and environmental dimensions of QoL; perceived health; general evaluation of own QoL. Taken together, these studies suggest that

1. QoL is multi-dimensional.
2. QoL has objective and subjective dimensions.
3. QoL seems to encompass four key areas: (1) physical health and functional abilities; (2) psychological health, subjective well-being and life satisfaction; (3) social networks, activities (leisure and productive) and participation; (4) socio-economic conditions and living environment.

How well these apply also to frail older people is less clear. Tester, Hubbard, Downs, MacDonald, and Murphy (2003) have commented on research on QoL in old age by saying: "...where frail older people are concerned, the results of such work remain unsatisfactory, both theoretically and methodologically", and "...it is doubtful that a generic definition of QoL will be useful for all research purposes. Instead, QoL models specific to particular groups of older people are being developed, for example dementia-specific QoL models". We took this as a challenge for Care Keys, and defined as the first task of our research the task of trying to develop a more generic model of crQoL to be differentiated for specific target groups to see whether this approach would be more fruitful.

Besides the specific question regarding older people with dementia, it was necessary to deal with a more general question of what are the dimensions and determinants of QoL of dependent older persons. Lawton (1991) in his comprehensive model covers broadly the above-mentioned domains, and his idea of "person-environment fit" also includes the role of care as a major element of environmental support in frail older people. In addition, Frytak (2000) suggests that Lawton's model fits well with research on QoL of older people in need of external help and care. From the literature on QoL of frail old people, we found nine dimensions or factors that were considered relevant for the QoL of frail older persons living at home and in the institutions:

1. Demography
2. Socio-economic situation
3. Physical health
4. Psychological health
5. Social networks
6. Living environment
7. Lifestyle and activities
8. Traumatic life events
9. Care

These nine domains of QoL were taken as a starting point for the model of crQoL, and then refined further in terms of the four basic dimensions, following Lawton's approach, along with a preliminary definition of the measures for testing and refining the model. An initial empirical exploration of the model of crQoL was encouraging (Vaarama, Pieper, & Sixsmith, 2007), supporting its use as a "meta-model" for guiding the Care Keys research (see later).

Pillar 3: Multi-Dimensional and Multi-Actoral Evaluation of Quality of Care

Care Keys approached QoL as the final or highest level outcome of care, and quality of care and management of care as means to achieve this goal. This implies a management orientation towards clearly defined goals and the evaluation of their achievement. Goal attainment is implicit in some of the key concepts, such as target efficiency (described later), but there was a need to make this more explicit, because the orientation towards clear goals, specified interventions and criteria for achievement remained weak in the discussion of the LTC of older people. The "rationality" of this approach is often seen to be in conflict with the more "human" and "social" approach required in care. As will be discussed in Chapter 6, this is a misunderstanding of the role of rationality in care management.

The PoW approach applied in Care Keys contains an explicit commitment to a multi-dimensional conceptualisation of goals or outcomes. Too often, issues of quality are reduced to one dimension, the most frequent being money or costs. Within general management science it is already accepted that quality management has to consider a more comprehensive set of objectives and it is clear that the quality concept in social and health care must be multi-dimensional in order to capture the many aspects of quality of care and QoL. Additionally, it is recognised that concepts of quality require a consideration of both subjective and objective dimensions and cannot be simply reduced to some measure of satisfaction among the different stakeholders. Since the interests of individual clients or staff do not necessarily agree with more collective goals such as economy and equity, quality management has to represent both individual and collective goals and must therefore employ multi-dimensional concepts and instruments.

Taking these considerations into account, the well-established theory of care quality by Donabedian (1969) and its extension into three quality perspectives by Øvretveit (1998) offered a fruitful starting point for the introduction of quality considerations into the Care Keys research. This model of evaluating quality closely matches the PoW approach, as it defines care provision in terms of inputs, processes and outcomes to be evaluated from the perspectives of the clients, professionals and managers. These three perspectives refer to the three central stakeholders in care production and allow for the distinction of quality from

1. The point of view of a client considering his/her material and non-material inputs (needs and resources), the contribution to the care process, the perception of the quality of care and the outcomes in terms of QoL regained, retained or enhanced.
2. The point of view of the professionals considering care inputs as provided by professional dispositions, the process and the outcome in terms of achieving a targeted state.
3. The point of view of management considering the inputs, the process of support and the comprehensive and integrated goals of care provision, including efficiency and equity criteria.

Client Perspective

A key issue is the extent to which measurement of service performance is relevant to the people who receive care. As Baldock and Hadlow (2002) note, there is a wealth of research on quality and effectiveness of care from the managerial perspective, but rarely with more differentiated outcome measures (e.g. beyond costs) and even less measuring how well the care meets the expectations and needs of the clients. In addition, Bowling (1997) raises the same question:

...few indicators attempt to measure patients' perceptions of improvement or satisfaction with level of performance; yet it is this element which is largely responsible for predicting whether individuals seek care, accept treatment and consider themselves to be well and 'recovered'.

A move to a more client-centred view means that more attention should be paid to their personal perspectives on what their problems are, what services they want and what they think of the services that they receive. Measures of service quality from the client perspective could therefore include information, control, choice, client perceptions of their needs, client preferences regarding care and their expectations of, and satisfaction with, the services they receive. Another important aspect relating to the client perspective was the idea of QoL and the extent to which care contributes to (adds to or detracts from) the clients' well-being and participation within society. This issue will be a major focus of many of the chapters in this book.

Professional Perspective

The professional perspective on evaluation of quality of care involves the evaluation of the structures and resources for quality as well as the quality of the care interventions and care processes that directly involve clients. The intermediate outputs of care are the quantities and qualities of care, and the final outcome is the well-being of the client. The outcomes guiding care from a professional perspective need not and do not always coincide with the outcomes as desired or expected by clients, since professional standards and socio-political goals will introduce their own perspective.

In LTC, it is possible to distinguish between clinical outcomes, psychological outcomes, social outcomes and environmental outcomes for the client, and between medical, nursing and social care. Important and perhaps one of the most critical parts of professional care is needs-assessment and diagnosis, which should be comprehensive in scope in order to adequately cover the needs of the client and to be able to define appropriate interventions to meet those needs. It is therefore necessary to recognise the importance of not only physical and instrumental needs, but also psychosocial needs and needs in areas such as adaptations and improvements in the client's living environment. It is also important to recognise that care should encourage and empower clients in respect to the competencies and potentials the clients still have. For the LTC of older people, the professional perspective is vital to the discussion, as criteria for defining care quality are largely absent or "home made".

Management Perspective

If a positive impact on client's QoL is seen as the final goal of the care, the task of management is to try to ensure this for all clients within the care system. For this to be done in a systematic and equitable way, management procedures need to be in place that provide the right service of good quality for each client. These procedures include:

1. needs assessment procedures that clearly specify the care requirements of the client,
2. care planning procedures that map out an appropriate package of care for the client,
3. care delivery where the care is provided to the client and where the interaction with client takes place,
4. evaluation processes where the care outcomes, efficiency of resource use and equity of distribution are evaluated,

5. quality management processes relating to quality concepts for the service, work organisation, resource management, personnel management and cooperation in integrated care systems.

These perspectives were included in the Care Keys research framework by embedding them in the "meta-model" and by drafting a higher level matrix-model to identify relevant determinants for each dimension.

Pillar 4: The Concept of TEFF

The fourth pillar of Care Keys research is the concept of TEFF (target efficiency) of care (Bebbington & Davies, 1983; Davies et al., 1990; Kavanagh & Stewart, 1995) and the model Vaarama, Mattila, Laaksonen, and Valtonen (1997) developed for use in the evaluation of care performance at the aggregated care level. This model was evaluated and further developed in the Care Keys project. The basic idea of TEFF is that people should receive the service and care that they are in need of, and the resources should be allocated efficiently according to these needs. In addition, the distribution should be equitable. The idea is illustrated in Fig. 1.2, where N = peoples' needs, S = care supply and A is the correct allocation.

The model defines the following concepts that are important for different levels of care management, namely

1. the degree of needs-responsiveness of care (horizontal target efficiency: $H = A/N$),
2. the efficiency of resource use according to the given need (vertical target efficiency: $V = A/S$),
3. the resource availability, given by the ratio of $H/V = S/N$, degree of over- and under-targeting of resources,
4. the equity of distribution of care resources, given by the variability of H/V or of the utility produced by care.

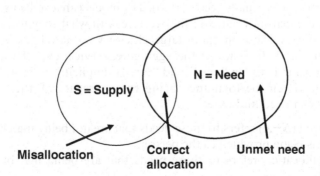

FIG. 1.2. The need-supply-comparison: correct allocation, misallocation and unmet need (Bebbington & Davies, 1983; Davies et al., 1990; Kavanagh & Stewart, 1995; Vaarama et al., 1997).

Horizontal target efficiency is the proportion of the people in need who receive the service or the extent to which those deemed to be in need of a particular service actually receive it. Thus, it is also a measure of unmet need, as suggested e.g. by Davies et al. (1990). Vertical target efficiency is the proportion of recipients of a service who satisfy the criteria of a priority need or the extent to which the available care resources are received by those deemed to be in need. Thus, it measures the efficiency of resource allocation against the need being satisfied (Bebbington & Davies, 1983; Davies et al.; Vaarama et al., 1997).

The ratio H/V measures the sufficiency of resources and the allocative efficiency of the resource use. It can be seen describing the extent to which the care needs as defined in care plans for a client or for a client group *are* satisfied, and *could* be satisfied, on the condition that all resources would be allocated correctly. At the same time, the potential for improvement of the target efficiency under the given resources can be seen. H/V varies between 0 and ∞. When $H/V = 1$, the optimal situation occurs, where the amount of resources and need are equal, and if targeted correctly, the resources are sufficient to meet the priority need. Over-targeting is shown, when $H/V > 1$. The amount of resources is higher than the need. By reallocation all the need can be met, and rest of the resources can be saved, transferred to some other purpose or the number of recipients can be increased. An unfavourable situation is when $H/V < 1$, where even if all the resources were optimally targeted, they would not be sufficient to meet the priority need (Vaarama et al., 1997).

In general, if H/V is unequal to 1, there is an imbalance between the resources and priority need (see Bebbington & Davies, 1983). As H/V describes the resources delivered to a client relative to his/her need ($H/V = S/N$), it can be also the base of equity measures that aim towards a fairer or more equal distribution of resources, relative to the clients needs.

The basic model is very flexible and can be used in different ways, for example as an objective measure, looking at what a person needs and comparing it with what care they actually receive (Ho). The model can also be used subjectively (Hs), comparing what care they receive with what they feel they need (i.e. perceived need). The concept of target efficiency was developed to measure service equity and efficiency at the aggregate, service level. However, the basic relationship between "need" and "care" is implicitly an individual one, with overall system performance being the aggregate of the individual match between need and care:

1. Unmet need ($N-A$) refers to those needs that are not being matched by the care that is being provided to the person.
2. Correct allocation refers to those needs that are being met by the care provided.
3. Incorrect allocation is any care provided that the person does not actually need.

The value of the TEFF measures is that they provide an important set of indicators for quality and performance management. The basic theoretical approach underlying the TEFF concept is the PoW approach. However, the identification of needs and supply must also draw more specifically on frameworks describing needs and supply within LTC. As the development and empirical testing of the Care Keys TEFF model will demonstrate, the application of the TEFF requires appropriate instruments to measure needs and supply, accompanied with accurate care documentation. In trying to develop new instruments for measuring need and supply within the Care Keys project, care documentation proved to be a major obstacle. Care documentations (assessments, care plans and documentations of actual supply) varied considerably between and within countries, and the correspondence between categories of needs and the services to satisfy these needs was generally unclear. Furthermore, the theoretical background of existing classifications or documentation systems was either unclear or not suited for the purposes of Care Keys. Thus, theoretical and methodological approaches had to be combined to specify a new classification system (see Chapter 11).

Summary—The Theoretical Framework of the Care Keys Research

In this chapter, we have briefly introduced the four key concepts or "pillars" underlying the research presented in this book. In this final section, we will integrate these concepts, firstly, within a meta-model of crQoL and, secondly, within a multi-actor model for the evaluation of care outcomes.

A Meta-Model of crQoL

Figure 1.3 illustrates how the "four pillars" described earlier were incorporated within a "meta-model of crQoL", which guided the Care Keys research and was tested and empirically verified in the research. The overarching perspective is that of PoW and the relationships between inputs, outputs and outcomes of care. The "meta-model" combines the PoW approach, Øvretveit's model and the ideas about QoL into a single comprehensive model of crQoL.

In this model, we assume:

1. Client-specific circumstances result in a need for care, and for care to be efficient it must respond to the individual needs and circumstances of a client, and respect their preferences (individual inputs).
2. Professional care uses diverse care inputs and processes to produce care that meets the client needs and preferences, and given quality standards (care inputs).
3. Management uses diverse inputs and processes to facilitate provision of good quality care and efficient use of resources (care inputs).

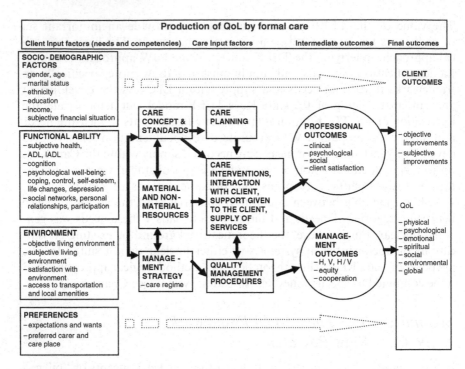

Fɪɢ. 1.3. The Care Keys "meta-model".

4. We differentiate between two types of intermediate care outcomes: professional and management outcomes; they are means to achieve client outcomes.
5. Client outcomes are considered as multi-dimensional and as final outcomes of care.
6. This model assumes a connection between care and QoL, and examines how care could be provided to maximise the desired outcomes.

A Multi-Actor and Multi-Dimensional Framework for Evaluation of the Quality of Care

As described earlier, the quality matrix from Øvretveit (1998) was used as a starting point to develop an evaluation scheme that was suitable for the purposes of practical quality management in the LTC of older people (Table 1.1). This way of simultaneously combining the perspectives of the client, professional and management within a single framework opens a new and more comprehensive view on the evaluation of care. The model provides for multidisciplinary, multi-actoral, multi-dimensional and multi-methodological quality evaluation, and

TABLE 1.1. The Care Keys matrix for multi-dimensional and multi-actor evaluation of long-term care (adapted from Øvretveit 1998; see also Vaarama & Pieper, 2005).

Evaluation perspectives	Inputs	Process	Outcomes
Client quality	Client needs, resources and expectations	Dignity, interaction, empowerment, choice, control	Improved well-being, LS, subjective QoL (profile, global), morale
Professional quality	Staff qualification, motivation, quality standards	Good professional care, continuity, courtesy	Meeting professional standards, no mistakes, client satisfaction
Management quality	Sufficient resources, structures for quality, legal framework	Needs-led supply, efficient resource use, conflict resolution	Good horizontal and vertical TEFF, H/V, equity of distribution

puts the client at the centre of the evaluation, not as an object but as an active participant.

Placing the three perspectives in the framework of PoW, the input–process–outcome dimension received a more specific theoretical background for interpretation. At the same time, the PoW approach was further differentiated by introducing explicitly the perspectives of different stakeholders in the production process. This makes explicit the need to consider the clients' perspective throughout the whole process of production. Furthermore, an additional focus is introduced by considering the informational base of care and looking in more detail into the process of care production by professionals, considering care as professional outcome and not only as intermediate output to provide client outcomes.

The distinction of subjective and objective factors had to be made more clear and explicit. Therefore, whenever appropriate, the Care Keys research differentiated in each "box" between subjective and objective indicators. The original matrix distinguishes between perspectives in the sense that certain indicators are important from the point of view of certain stakeholders, but it does not systematically differentiate between subjective and objective indicators. In Care Keys, client-specific indicators are located in the client "row", and client outcome is considered to be a general goal of professional care, differentiated in the client outcome "box". Professional care indicators are located in the second "row", and professional care outcomes are seen as targeted care outcomes in this "row". Management indicators are combined in the third "row" specifying also outcomes that may reach beyond the client or staff perspective (e.g. equity, target efficiency of the services).

To include a multi-dimensional concept of quality in the quality matrix it was necessary to develop a dimensional framework that would allow to order the relevant factors of QoL, quality of care and quality of management within the matrix. Here a general theoretical approach drawing on social system theory proved to be fruitful, both on the conceptual level by providing a dimensional order and on the empirical level, since the dimensional structure could also be reproduced inductively from the pilot studies.

As the theoretical and empirical analyses of the Care Keys research will demonstrate, a contribution to a better understanding of quality of care in relation to QoL of clients is achievable. Still, the concept of crQoL remains at an early stage of development. There is not yet an established and agreed understanding of the term and no single recognised definition or measurement. Therefore, crQoL in the context of the present research is approached pragmatically and should be understood within the context of the research aims and objectives to guide the search for objective and subjective measures of quality within LTC.

References

Baldock, J. C., & Hadlow, J. (2002). Self-talk versus needs-talk: An exploration of the priorities of housebound older people. *Quality in Ageing, 3*(1), 42–48.

Baltes, P. B., & Baltes, M. M. (1990). Psychological perspectives on successful aging: The model of selective optimization with compensation. In P. B. Baltes, & M. Baltes (Eds.), *Successful aging. Perspectives from the behavioural sciences.* Cambridge, MA: Cambridge University Press.

Bebbington, A., & Davies, B. (1983). Equity and efficiency in the allocation of the personal social services. *Journal of Social Policy, 12*, 309–330.

Birren, J. E., Lubben, J. E., Rowe, J. C., & Deutschmann, D. E. (Eds.). (1991). *The concept and measurement of QoL in frail elderly.* New York: Academic Press.

Bordereau, L., Szalai, J. P., Ennis, M., Leszcz, M., Speca, M., Sela, R., et al. (2003). QoL in a randomized trial of group psychosocial support in metastatic breast cancer: Overall effects of the intervention and an exploration of missing data. *Journal of Clinical Oncology, 21*, 1944–1951.

Bowling, A. (1991). *Measuring health. A review of QoL measurement scales.* Philadelphia, PA: Open University Press.

Bowling, A. (1995). *Measuring disease; a review of disease-specific QoL measurement scales.* Buckingham: Open University Press.

Bowling, A. (1997). *Measuring health: A review of QoL measurement scales* (2nd ed.). Buckingham: Open University Press.

Bowling, A. (2004). *Measuring health: A review of QoL Measurement Scales* (3rd ed.). Buckingham: Open University Press.

Carod-Artal, J., Egido, J. A., González, J. L., & Varela de Seijas, E. (2000). QoL among stroke survivors evaluated 1 year after stroke: Experience of a stroke unit. *Stroke, 31*, 2995–3000.

Davies, B., Bebbington, A., Charnley, H., et al. (1990). Resources, needs and outcomes in community-based care. A comparative study of the production of welfare for elderly people in ten local authorities in England and Wales. Canterbury: PSSRU University of Kent at Canterbury.

Davies, B., Fernández, J., & Nomer, B. (2000). *Equity and efficiency policy in community care. Needs, service productivities, efficiencies and their implications.* England: Ashgate.

Davies, B., & Knapp, M. (1981). *Old people's homes and the production of welfare.* London: Routledge & Kegan Paul.

Diener, E. (2000). Subjective well-being. *American Psychologist, 55*, 34–43.

Donabedian, A. (1969). Some issues in evaluation the quality of nursing care. *American Journal of Public Health, 59*, 1833–36.

Felce, D., & Perry, J. (1997). QoL: The scope of the term and its breadth of measurement. In R. I. Brown (Ed.), *QoL for people with disabilities. Models, research and practice*. Cheltenham: Stanley Thornes.

Frytak, J. (2000). Assessment of QoL. In R. Kane, & R. Kane (Eds.), *Assessing older persons. measures, meaning and practical applications*. New York: Oxford University Press.

Hays, R. D., Cunningham, W. E., Sherbourne, C. D., Wilson, I. B., Wu, A. W., Cleary, P. D., et al. (2000). Health-related QoL in patients with human immunodeficiency virus infection in the United States: Results from the HIV Cost and Services Utilization Study. *American Journal of Medicine, 108*, 714–722.

Hughes, B. (1990). QoL. In S. Peace (Ed.), *Researching social gerontology*. London: Sage.

Kavanagh, S., & Stewart, A. (1995). Economic evaluations of mental health care. In M. Knapp (Ed.), *The economic evaluation of mental health care* (pp. 27–60). PSSRU. CEMH. Arena. Aldershot.

Knapp, M. (1984). *The economics of social care. Studies in social policy*. Hong Kong: MacMillan Education.

Lawton, M. P. (1991). A multidimensional view of QoL in frail elders. In J. Birren, J. Lubben, J. Rowe, & D. Deutchman (Eds.), *The concept of measurement of QoL in frail elders* (pp. 3–27). San Diego, CA: Academic Press.

Mozley, C., Sutcliffe, C., Bagley, H., Cordingley, L., Challis, D., Huxley, P., et al. (2004). *Towards quality care. Outcomes for older people in care homes*. Aldershot: Ashgate.

Netten, A. (2004). The social production of welfare. In M. Knapp, D. Challis, J.-L. Fernandez, & A. Netten (Eds.), *Long-term care: Matching resources and needs*. Aldershot: Ashgate.

Øvretveit, J. (1998). *Evaluating health interventions. An introduction to evaluation of health treatments, services, policies and organizational interventions*. Buckingham: Open University Press.

Renwick, R., Brown, I., & Nagler, M. (Eds.). (1996). *QoL in health promotion and rehabilitation*. Thousand Oaks, CA: Sage.

Sefton, T., Byford, S., McDaid, D., Hills, J., & Knapp, M. (2003). *Making the most of it. Economic evaluation in the social welfare field*. Layerthorpe: Joseph Rowntree Foundation.

Skevington, S. M., Lotfy, M., & O'Connell, K. A. (2004). The World Health Organization's WHOQOL-Bref QoL assessment: Psychometric properties and results of the international field trial. A report from the WHOQOL Group. *Quality Life Research, 13*(2), 299–310.

Tester, S., Hubbard, G., Downs, M., MacDonald, C., & Murphy, J. (2003). Exploring perceptions of QoL of frail older people during and after their transition to institutional care. Research Findings 24, Growing Older Project. <http://www.shef.ac.uk/uni/projects/gop/GOFindings24.pdf>

Vaarama, M., Mattila, V., Laaksonen, S., & Valtonen, H. (1997). *Target efficiency—report on development and piloting of the target efficiency indicators and model*. Helsinki: Stakes.

Vaarama, M., & Pieper, R. (2005). *Managing integrated care for older persons. Stakes and the European Health Management Association*. Saarijärvi: Gummerus Printing.

Vaarama, M., Pieper, R., & Sixsmith, A. (2007). Care-related QoL in old age. Conceptual and empirical exploration. In H. Mollenkopf, & A. Walker (Ed.). *Quality of Life in Old Age. International and Multi-Disciplinary Perspectives*. Dordrecht, The Netherlands: Springer, pp. 215–32.

WHOQOL Group (1998). Development of the World Health Organization WHO-QOL-Bref QoL assessment. The WHOQOL Group. *Psychological Medicine, 28*(3), 551–558.

2
Instrumentation of the Care Keys Research

Marja Vaarama, Ene-Margit Tiit, Seija Muurinen, Richard Pieper, Kai Saks, Andrew Sixsmith and Margaret Hammond

Introduction

Research on care-related quality of life (crQoL) focuses mainly on the interaction between the quality of care (QoC) and the quality of life (QoL). However, the conditions for a good QoC are also important, that is the resources, structures and processes which facilitate good care outcomes. For comprehensive evaluation of care-related QoL, all the perspectives that have been included in the multi-dimensional and multi-actoral evaluation model developed in the Care Keys project are important. Hence, the instrumentation of the research carried out within Care Keys was designed to cover all the different elements within the meta-model and quality matrix that guided the project:

1. Subjective QoL in old persons receiving home care or care in institutional settings, and determinants of it.
2. Objective (assessed) QoL in old persons, and determinants of it.
3. QoL in old persons with dementia.
4. Subjective QoC in old persons using home care or care in institutional settings, and determinants of it.
5. Professional quality of home care and care in institutional settings, and determinants of it.
6. Quality management of home care and care in institutional settings, and determinants of it.

It followed from this, firstly, that instruments were needed for carrying out interviews with clients to access their subjective perceptions about their QoL and the QoC they received. Secondly, instruments had to describe the QoL as professionally assessed and documented including professional (e.g. clinical) care outcomes. Thirdly, instruments were required for the evaluation of the QoL of older persons with dementia, who may be unable to provide the information themselves. Fourthly, a standardised instrument was needed for the collection of information on professional QoC, covering key components within the meta-model. Fifthly, an instrument was required to collect all the information needed from the perspective of management. Besides quality management information, the instrument also had to collect information at the organisational level on such issues as material resources, costs and organisational structures for quality management. The information sources for this information were the care managers at different management levels.

For the selection of the instruments, the following five criteria were agreed on within the Care Keys project:

1. Items must cover all the areas of theoretical framework and be reflected in the meta-model.
2. Items should be based on instruments validated in previous research (if available).
3. The structure of the validated instruments should be maintained.
4. For those items that have no validated scales, validated single-item questions should be used.
5. Instruments should be appropriate for use with frail, older people and should be easy to answer and administer.

Developing instrumentation that fulfilled these criteria presented a major methodological challenge and the process for developing the instrumentation followed a number of stages:

1. Literature reviews of instrumentation relating to the key domains within the theoretical framework.
2. Examination of data available and instruments used in care evaluation by service providers in the participating countries.
3. Initial empirical investigations on existing representative databases of key research areas, such as QoL and QoC.
4. Based on the initial work, iterative process of defining, testing and refining instrumentation for piloting in the participating countries.
5. Finalisation of the Care Keys instrumentation.

This chapter details the process behind the selection of instrumentation, together with a description of the various instruments examined and selected. The chapter on data and statistical methods (see Chapter 3) presents the Care Keys pooled database that was collected by using the common instrumentation and common data collection procedure.

Development of the Instrument for Client Interviews (CLINT)

Measuring QoL and its Determinants

To provide an overview of the available validated instruments for use in the interviews with older persons who regularly use care services, we examined the instrumentation used in a number of major projects on QoL in old age that also involved aspects of care in the study design:

1. OASIS (Old Age and Autonomy: the Role of Service Systems and Intergenerational Family Solidarity) (Löwenstein, 2001; Löwenstein, Katz, Mehlhausen-Hassoen, & Prilutzky, 2002).
2. norLAG (The Norwegian Life Course, Ageing and Generation Study) (Solem, 2003).
3. BASE (The Berlin Ageing Study) (Baltes & Mayer, 1999).
4. LASA (Longitudinal Ageing Study Amsterdam) (http://ssg.scw.vu.nl/lasa).
5. Growing Older (GO) Project of the University of Sheffield, UK (http://www.shef.ac.uk/uni/projectss/gop/).
6. Finnish national studies (Vaarama, 2004; Vaarama, Hakkarainen, & Laaksonen, 1999; Vaarama & Kaitsaari, 2002).
7. WHOQOL measure (WHOQOL Group, 1998).

The review grouped the instrumentation within the following nine domains:

1. Subjective QoL
2. Personal resources affecting QoL
3. Physical health and functional ability
4. Social relationships
5. Home and environment
6. Use of help and services
7. Socio-economic and demographical factors
8. Preferences for care
9. Life changes

Measures of Subjective QoL

Life Satisfaction (LS)

Satisfaction with life is a measure that can be used as a single question, or it can be divided to sub-dimensions. It has often been measured with a single-item question: "how satisfied are you with your (quality of) life"? This type of question is also included in the WHOQOL-Bref instrument (WHOQOL Group, 1998) and in the Philadelphia Geriatric Centre Morale Scale (PGCMS) (Lawton, 1975). WHOQOL-Bref additionally covers several specific dimensions of life (e.g. health, environment), and these types of more specific satisfaction questions usually complement the general question (in LASA, OASIS, norLAG). A general "life satisfaction" question has been included in OASIS, BASE, LASA and norLAG and seems to be an essential part of measuring subjective well-being. There are also different indices for measuring LS such as the five-item Satisfaction with Life Scale (Pavot, Diener, Colvin, & Sandvik, 1991), which was used in BASE and norLAG. This scale also measures the cognitive or evaluative aspect of QoL.

Morale

PGCMS (Lawton, 1975) has been validated on frail older persons and can be used also in institutional care where clients' state of health is usually poor. The idea of the PGCMS is to cover several dimensions of QoL of older persons in a single general tool. The 17 items are answered only with "yes" or "no" and a total score is calculated. PGCMS can be divided into three factors: agitation, attitude towards own aging and lonely dissatisfaction. According to Lawton, the agitation dimension can be used as a scale for assessing an older person's anxiety. Attitude towards own aging captures the individual's perception of changes taking place in his life and his or her evaluation of those changes. Items on the lonely dissatisfaction factor represent the older person's satisfaction with the amount of social interaction he or she is experiencing. This instrument was available in all the project countries' languages, except Estonian. The use of PGCMS does not require any permission and is free of charge. Both interview- and self-administered versions are available, but oral administration is recommended, because the frailest older people may not be able to mark their answers themselves. Single items of the PGCMS were used in BASE and norLAG. The GO project also used PGCMS.

Affect

In addition to the intellectual evaluation of one's life, researchers have suggested that there are two other higher-order dimensions of subjective well-being: positive affect (PA) and negative affect (NA) (e.g. Watson, Clark, & Tellegen, 1988). In contrast to the intellectual evaluations of one's life in general, NA and PA are emotional responses consisting of moods such as zest and interest (for PA) and distress and anxiety (for NA) (Kercher, 1992). The Positive/Negative Affect Scale (PANAS, Watson, Clark & Tellegen, 1988) is widely used for measuring PA and NA by gerontologists. A shorter, 10-item version of the original 20-item scale is often used for older people (e.g. OASIS, SNAC, Kercher, 1992), but longer versions have also been used (e.g. BASE, norLAG).

Happiness (H)

No specific happiness scale was used in any of the reviewed studies, but several instruments described here and included in the survey instruments (e.g. depression scales) also include items on happiness. A happiness question is also included in the PGCMS. Following Veenhoven (2002), we may interpret happiness to be a more general concept on a similar level as QoL.

Multi-Dimensional QoL

WHOQOL-Bref (WHOQOL Group, 1998) is an instrument developed by the World Health Organisation for measuring QoL multi-dimensionally, although it is not specifically designed for older people. The WHOQOL Group sees QoL as a multi-dimensional construct that includes an evaluation of physical health, psychological well-being, social relationships and physical environment. The strength of the WHOQOL-Bref is that it has been developed in cross-cultural settings. WHOQOL-Bref includes many important dimensions that would otherwise need to be asked separately (e.g. feeling safe, pain, subjective financial situation, satisfaction with personal relationships). In addition, a single-item question on global QoL is included. WHOQOL-Bref was used in OASIS study, and also in the British GO project (http://www. shef.ac.uk/uni/projects/gop/). In norLAG, WHOQOL-Bref was not used, but instead a shorter scale was developed, which seems to be based extensively on WHOQOL items. WHOQOL-Bref was used in the Care Keys piloting stage by Estonia, UK and Sweden. WHOQOL-Bref was available in all project languages except Finnish, but permission was given to translate this instrument into Finnish. WHOQOL-OLD (Power, Quinn, Schmidt, & WHOQOL-OLD Group, 2005) is an instrument specifically developed for older people, but was not available at the initial stage of the Care Keys research.

Measures of Personal Resources Affecting QoL

Although QoL is generally seen as an outcome, there are several other scales that often also appear in QoL studies that address the person's physical, psychological, social, financial and environmental resources that may affect on QoL. Instruments that measure the person's psychological resources are perhaps the most closely connected to the concept of QoL.

Depression

Depression significantly affects QoL, and is associated with health, pain, perceived health and satisfaction with services, and therefore it was necessary to include some measure of depression. The Centre for Epidemiologic Studies Depression Scale (CES-D, Radloff, 1977) is widely used, and there is also a revised version available, at least in English. CES-D has been used in large European studies on the QoL of older persons: norLAG, BASE and LASA. OASIS did not include any specific depression scale. CES-D is available in multiple languages and does not require any permission for use. The Hamilton Depression Scale (Hamilton, 1967) was used in BASE in addition to CES-D. Use of this instrument requires interviewer training.

Anxiety

Anxiety seems to be measured less often than depression in the recent QoL studies. In LASA, the anxiety dimension of the Hospital Anxiety and Depression Scale (HADS) (Zigmund & Snaith, 1983) was used. This subscale consists of seven items. The HAD scale is not derived from factor analysis but from clinical experience. None of the four reviewed studies used the depression subscale of HADS. PGCMS also includes a dimension of anxiety. In norLAG, five items from the Hopkins Symptoms Check List were used (Derogatis, Lipman, Rickels, Uhlenhuth, & Covi, 1974).

Cognition

The Mini Mental State Examination (Folstein, Folstein, & McHugh, 1975) was used in LASA and BASE; norLAG and OASIS did not include an assessment of cognitive status.

Coherence

Antonovsky's (1993) Sense of Coherence scale was used by Vaarama and Kaitsaari (2002) to measure psychological resources of cognitively well old Finns. Antonovsky's scale was also used in the Finnish pilot study of the European Excelsa project and the piloting stage of Care Keys.

Coping

Selective Optimization with Compensation, based on the theory of success-ful ageing (Baltes & Baltes, 1990), was used in BASE and norLAG. The scales used by Baltes included 12–48 items, but for norLAG the scale was short-ened to 9 items. The scale consists of pairs of statements and the respond-ent is asked to mark which statement describes a person that is most like himself or herself. Unfortunately, this scale was not available in English for this review. In OASIS, coping style was measured with a five-item Tenacious Goal Pursuit (TGP) and Flexible Goal Adjustment (FGA) scale (Brand-stätter & Renner, 1990). Responses are given along a five-point scale. TGP measures the tendency to persist with old priorities and styles even when they are no longer functional, and the FGA dimension measures readiness to adjust goals to changes in situations.

Control

The Mastery Scale (Locus of Control) (Pearlin & Schooler, 1978) consisted originally of seven statements that measure the sense of mastery. This scale was used in LASA and norLAG and is probably the most widely used mastery scale. The 14-item Control BASE scale (Kunzmann, Little, & Smith, 2002) was developed in BASE, and a shorter version (six items) was used also in norLAG. This scale differentiates between control over negative and positive events. In the version used by norLAG, two items measured internal control over positive events, two measured internal control over negative events, one measured external control over positive events and one measured external control over negative events. This scale was not available in English for this review. In norLAG and BASE self-efficacy was measured with only one item. The NorLAG team also piloted Schwarzer's seven-item scale, and there was a strong correlation between this scale and the chosen one item (Solem, 2003).

Self-Esteem

NorLAG measured self-esteem using the ten-item self-esteem scale (Rosenberg, 1965). According to Rosenberg, self-esteem is self-acceptance or a basic feeling of self-worth. There is evidence that this scale is suitable for use with older people. Among older people, attitudes towards old age predict self-esteem (Bowling, 1991).

Purpose of Life

NorLAG used one of the subscales of the Psychological Well-Being Scale (Ryff & Keyes, 1995) to measure purpose of life. The shortest version of the scale includes three items. The other dimensions of the Psychological Well-Being Scale measure self-acceptance, autonomy, environmental mastery, positive relations with others and personal growth.

Loneliness

In LASA, the 11-item and in norLAG, the 3-item Loneliness scale (de Jong-Gierveld & van Tilburg, 1999) was used, together with the loneliness question from CES-D. PGCMS also includes one question on loneliness. A general question on the frequency of feeling lonely is also often used (e.g. SNAC, OASIS). In LASA, parts of the UCLA Loneliness Scale (Russell, Peplau, & Cutrona, 1980) were used as this is the most well-known measure of loneliness and seems to be a quite common scale if loneliness is measured with a relatively broad instrument.

Measures of Physical Health and Functional Ability

Subjective Health

Subjective health is sometimes used as a proxy for QoL. Perceived health is usually measured with a simple question that asks the person to evaluate his or her current health status, or as satisfaction with health. A satisfaction with health question is included in the WHOQOL-Bref.

Functional Ability

Various activities of daily living (ADL) and instrumental activities of daily living (IADL) scales can be used to measure physical ability and functioning. These scales are usually complemented with subjective evaluations of physical health and information on diagnosed diseases, medication and healthy lifestyle (regular exercise, smoking, alcohol consumption). When more extensive data collection is possible, physical tests are often added to this toolkit. Both nor-LAG and OASIS (and also the Swedish SNAC) used SF-12 (Ware, Kosinski, & Keller, 1996) for measuring ADL, IADL and perceived health. This instrument is a shorter version of SF-36 and consists of 12 items. In addition to activities of daily living, SF-12 includes two questions on perceived health in general. NorLAG additionally calculated Body Mass Index and posed specific questions on diseases and use of medication. LASA created its own survey on health issues, consisting of perceived health and different ADL and IADL questions. The same kinds of ADL and IADL questions were included in norLAG, BASE and SNAC. LASA and norLAG also included specific questions on vision and hearing. WHOQOL-Bref (used in OASIS) includes one question on pain and one on the need of medical treatment in daily life. Use of medication was also asked in norLAG.

Measures of Social Relationships

There are three basic dimensions in measuring social relationships: quantity, quality and satisfaction. In many studies, it has been noted that the person's satisfaction with his or her social contacts is more important than the actual number of these contacts. However, quantity of contacts is usually still measured. OASIS research had a specific emphasis on family solidarity and therefore social networks were mapped extensively. This included very detailed information on children (including e.g. their marital status, received and given help). The quality of the relationship with children was also explored with 12 questions. Relationships with parents and other family members were also studied in great detail. A shortened 54-item version of the Intergenerational Family Solidarity and Conflict Measures for Survey Assessment (Bengtson & Roberts, 1991) was used in OASIS, and parts of the same scale were included also in norLAG. In WHOQOL-Bref and in PGCMS an item on the satisfaction with social relationships is included.

Measures of Home and Environment

In almost all studies, basic background information covers at least ownership of housing, type of housing and living alone/with others. In addition, satisfaction with housing was asked in OASIS and in norLAG. OASIS also covered problems and shortcomings of housing and the living environment, as also the Finnish studies of Vaarama. In norLAG and in Vaarama, also questions on distance to local services and amenities (shop, GP, public transport stop) were included. WHOQOL-Bref includes a question on satisfaction with transport. LASA, norLAG and OASIS all asked about the person's attachment to his living area; the simplest way was to ask how many years the respondent had been living in the same area.

Measures of Use of Help and Services

In the studies reviewed here, the use of care and support services was mostly not the main focus, and therefore this dimension was generally covered quite briefly and no commonly used instruments are available. OASIS, NorLAG and Vaarama asked three dimensions of help intensity, provider (informal/ formal) and type (in OASIS: household chores, transport and shopping, personal care). NorLAG and Vaarama also combined register information on service use with the interview data. None of the available research questionnaires included questions on satisfaction with services, and only Vaarama asked the adequacy of help and unmet needs. These questions are, however, very relevant in the Care Keys framework.

Measures of Demographic and Socio-Economic Factors, Preferences and Life Changes

Most QoL studies include some kind of measure relating to the person's background:

1. gender (also included in WHOQOL-Bref),
2. age (also included in WHOQOL-Bref),
3. marital status (also included in WHOQOL-Bref),
4. education (also included in WHOQOL-Bref),
5. economic situation (subjective and objective) (subjective also included in WHOQOL-Bref),
6. preferences (OASIS used five-item scale, Daatland, 1990),
7. life changes and traumatic life experiences (in norLAG, SNAC, LASA, Vaarama et al., 1999).

Measuring Subjective QoC

As demonstrated later in this chapter, from the range of instruments reviewed earlier, the WHOQOL-Bref and PGCMS were selected to measure QoL, and a number of validated single-item questions to measure other determinants of QoL. However, the review revealed that few scales had been used to measure care-related issues, especially from the client perspective, that is, their subjective evaluations on how well the care they receive meets their needs and preferences. To capture this area, another literature review was employed as a part of the development of QoC instrumentation, and the results were then evaluated by the research team and with care managers and professionals participating in the local user groups.

For quality of home care, there was no single, validated, commonly used European scale available. A crosswalk exercise was carried out using a broad range of sources to address the domains and indicators of quality of established importance within home care, nursing care and residential care. Sources included the Picker Institute (www.pickereurope. org), SERVQUAL (Parasuraman, Zeithaml, & Berry, 1985, 1986, 1994; Parasuraman, Berry, & Zeithaml, 1988), home care satisfaction measures (Geron, Smith, Tennstedt, Sette, Chassler, & Kasten, 2000; Raynes, Temple, Glenister, & Coulthard, 2001), the CUES model (Lelliot, Beevor, Hogman, Hyslop, Lathlean, & Ward, 2001), QUOTE methodology (Sixma, van Campen, Kerssens, & Peters, 2000), Lawton's indicators of quality for dementia care services (Lawton, 2001), Urman and Urman's nursing home satisfaction indicators (1997), Duffy's study of long-term care satisfaction (Duffy, Duffy, & Kilbourne, 1997), RAI (Morris et al., 1994) and the American Health Consumer Association state consumer questions on long-term care (Tellis-Nayak, 2001).

It was difficult to find validated measures for subjective quality of institutional care. Therefore, instruments also used in the project countries were mapped, including some practice-validated measures that were accepted for testing in the Care Keys research. The first selection was done by choosing scales and single-item questions that were free to use and at least practice validated. The following client assessments were found as important:

1. Living conditions in the care home, including the physical environment and the socio-emotional atmosphere of the institution.
2. Care procedures, describing how the clients evaluate the wellness of the procedures carried out by staff, especially how the staff assisted or supported the clients in ADL, IADL functions and in psychological, spiritual and social needs.
3. Care principles and ethics, described as clients' experiences of their treatment (human dignity, equality, privacy, autonomy and empathy).
4. Interpersonal communication and relationships.
5. Social relationships.
6. Physical, psychological, spiritual and social well-being of the client.

A set of questions about subjective QoC was developed and included in the client interview instruments (CLINT) developed in the CareKeys research and based mainly on the approach of Paljärvi, Rissanen, and Sinkkonen (2003). The measurement covered the following eight domains (see also Chapter 5):

1. Appropriateness of care, operationalised as the subjective evaluation of the sufficiency of care, in terms of received help and duration.
2. Continuity of care, operationalised as having a person in charge of care, the client usually seeing the same care workers, and care workers keeping to the agreed timetable.
3. The professional and interactional skills of the care workers, operationalised as the client's experiences of his or her treatment and of the kindness, honesty and trustworthiness of the care workers, as well as the client's evaluation of the professional skills of the care workers.
4. The quality of interaction between the client and the care workers, operationalised by the client's subjective evaluations of these issues.
5. The autonomy and control of the client, operationalised by the client's evaluations of how well the care plan is followed up, whether he or she gets enough information on his or her own care, and the possibilities for the client to plan his or her own day.
6. Safety of living at home, operationalised by client's access to necessary home adaptations and safety devices, and as client's own feeling of safety at home.
7. Care-quality outcomes, operationalised in terms of clinical outcomes (usage of sleeping pills, unintended loss of weight, falls, pressure ulcers, pain) and personal outcomes (cleanliness of home, state of personal hygiene, satisfaction with own dressing and the quality of meals).
8. General satisfaction with care, operationalised by client's general satisfaction with care and readiness to recommend the service to the other people in need.

A second version of the set of these questions (RELINFO) was developed for clients with dementia. Since they cannot respond themselves the questions were slightly rephrased to be completed by relatives as questionnaires.

The Care Keys research team then constructed our new scales using the following criteria:

1. Interview format
2. Simple phrasing
3. 2–5-Point response scales
4. Both negatively and positively phrased items
5. Inclusion of both general satisfaction and specific items
6. Inclusion of items about information availability, choice and control

Draft scales were evaluated by the project team and national user groups, and for testing the instruments, backward and forward translations were carried out, along with focus group discussion of professionals within each partner country. The final version of the survey for institutional care used in the pilot study consisted of 52 closed questions, mainly using a three-point response scale, including two questions of overall satisfaction. The home care survey was shorter, consisting of 34 questions. Finally, both surveys included open questions regarding the best aspects of care and service and the areas for improvement, to identify previously unconsidered areas of importance.

Selecting the Instrumentation to Evaluate the QoL in Clients with Dementia

A key aim of the client interview (CLINT) in Care Keys is to provide a client perspective on QoL and satisfaction with services. However, people with communication difficulties, including people with cognitive impairment, are a significant group of clients who are often unable to respond to the interview format of instruments such as the PGCMS and the WHOQOL-Bref. In a study by Balcombe, Ferry, and Saweirs (2001), 46% of patients admitted to an acute care of the elderly hospital ward were excluded from taking part in a study using the PGCMS because of cognitive impairment or communication difficulties, effectively making them "voiceless" within the research process. Deficits in attention, orientation, memory, judgement, insight and communication may affect their ability to understand or respond to questions, or to communicate subjective states. As the Care Keys project did not want to exclude the clients with dementia, there was a need to determine valid measures to give them also a voice in our study.

The evaluation and piloting of the instruments for clients with dementia was undertaken in participating project countries. A number of instruments to assess well-being were considered and it was seen as important to cover the same domains, as far as possible, as those covered by the WHOQOL-Bref and the PGCMS. We did not want to assume a qualitative difference in the important areas for QoL in people with dementia, in what is generally a progressive but individually variable condition. Some instruments, such as QOL-AD (Logsdon, Gibbons, McCurry, & Teri, 2002) and DQoL (Brod, Stewart, Sands, & Walton, 1999), are only suitable for people with mild to moderate impairment and/or people living at home; indications were that people with mild to moderate impairment could respond to the items in the WHOQOL-Bref and the PGCMS, and there would be no particular advantage in substituting another scale. Some scales, although designated as QoL scales, rely primarily on the presence or absence of symptoms of depression. Depression is an important issue and needed to be included in the assessment of people with dementia, but we also wanted a broader assessment of well-being.

The two QoL scales for clients with moderate to severe dementia were piloted: the Quality of Life in Late Dementia scale (QUALID, Weiner, Martin-Cook, Svetlik, Sainem, Foster, & Fontaine, 2000); and the Well-Being Profile (WBP, Bruce, 2000), based on dementia care mapping and the theory of well-being of Kitwood and Bredin (1992). Possible depression scales included the Cornell Scale for Depression in Dementia (Alexopoulos, Abrams, Young, & Shamoian, 1988) and the Depressive Signs Scale (Katona & Aldridge, 1985).

Ultimately, the instruments chosen were the QUALID and the Cornell Scale for Depression in Dementia. QUALID was developed in the Department of Psychiatry at the University of Texas Southwestern Medical Center to assess the effects of treatment on QoL in people with severe dementia. It consists of 11 observable behaviours rated for the previous week on a five-point Likert scale by interview with a caregiver. It also includes two questions for the interviewer to rate the quality of the information. A sum score of responses indicates relative well-being in a range 11–55, with lower scores representing higher QoL. Although relatively new and untested, the scale was appropriate for our use and was well received during the pilot testing. The Cornell Scale for Depression in Dementia is completed by an interviewer and includes both the responses of the client and a relative or care person who knows the client well, and based on the week prior to interview. Responses use a three-point scale (symptom absent, mild or intermittent or severe). The scale includes 19 items covering mood-related signs (anxiety, sadness, lack of reactivity to pleasant events, irritability); behavioural disturbance (agitation, retardation, multiple physical complaints, loss of interest); physical signs (appetite loss, weight loss, lack of energy); cyclic functions (diurnal variation of mood, difficulty falling asleep, multiple awakenings during sleep, early morning awakening); ideational disturbance (suicidal, poor self-esteem, pessimism, mood congruent delusions). A sum score indicates overall depression with scores also for the different sub-components.

For the empirical testing and reporting of results, it was necessary to be able to describe the respondents' cognitive functioning. Either the Cognitive Performance score (CPS, Morris et al., 1994) from a current RAI assessment, where available, or the standardised Mini Mental State Exam (Folstein et al., 1975) were used to categorise respondents according to cognitive function into one of the three groups, using the following scores (Hartmaier et al., 1995):

1. The cognitively intact, borderline or mildly impaired, who have MMSE scores >18, or CPS scores of 0, 1 or 2.
2. The moderately impaired, who have MMSE scores of 16, 17 or 18; or CPS score of 3.
3. The severely impaired, who have MMSE scores of 15 or less, or CPS scores of 4, 5 or 6.

Developing Instruments for Extracting Data on Quality of Professional Care from the Care Documentation (InDEX)

To measure the quality of professional care as reflected in care documentation, common measures of quality of professional care and a common instrument were necessary. Again it was important to use instruments based on scientific research and those that were freely available. The criteria for selection of the professional QoC measures were similar to those for the QoL, but some additional criteria were also to be met:

1. Items should cover the areas defined in the meta-model and in the theoretical framework of QoC.
2. Items should cover the areas in the multi-actoral model of care quality applied, that is harmonised with the client interview and management instruments.
3. The instruments should have established validity.
4. The measures shall be free for use in research and practice.
5. The measures should be compatible with existing care documentation systems and assessment tools as far as possible to avoid extra data collection.

The literature review revealed that there was no single universal definition of QoC. As with the concept of QoL, QoC is a complex and multi-dimensional concept. In spite of this, there are plenty of instruments to evaluate the professional quality of nursing care, although only a few were available for free use in research. In respect to social care, we did not find any validated measures. The validity of the instruments in free use was not always clear, and some areas in which Care Keys was interested were not covered by previous research at all. To be able to define a set of measures that would allow the study of all the relevant areas, it was decided to accept practice-validated instruments and test their validity within the Care Keys project. To ensure compatibility with other instruments, crosswalks between Care Keys instrumentation and certain assessment tools were also done. An additional problem was that the project countries represented different care cultures, and reported negative attitudes among nursing and social care staff towards the enquiries and evaluations. It was a great challenge to specify an instrument that could meet these challenges and be usable in all project countries.

Developing the InDEX measure for extracting data from care documentation had several phases, from a literature review through piloting and testing to the completion of the instruments. During the literature review it was possible to find some previously developed data extraction instruments such as Senior Monitor (Goldstone & Maselino-Okai, 1986), but this was not available for free use. In addition, some measures developed by Muurinen (2003) could be exploited in the development of the CareKeys instrumentation, and, additionally, the selection of indicators and the design of the instruments was guided by care theories and the CK quality matrix (see Chapters 5 and 6).

At the beginning, InDEX consisted of different data collection methods, such as data extraction, observation and client interview. The final instrument comprised only data extraction from client documents. The pilot version of InDEX included many of the same domains and care dimensions as the final instrument, but the number of questions was much bigger than in the final version.

The pilot instruments included background information of the client, measures of functional status such as ADL, IADL, cognition (MMSE, Folstein et al., 1975), depression scales and dependency scoring using instruments such as the Barthel scale (Mahoney & Barthel, 1965). For the calculations of target efficiency indicators (TEFF, see Chapter 11), need and supply were to be collected in a way that made it possible to compare needs with responsiveness of care. This was a difficult problem to solve as there were many models of care, many classifications of needs and supply and the supply was often poorly documented. The solution was found in dividing needs and supply into 11 care tasks, including the prophylaxis of complications of care, representing four dimensions of care (see Chapters 5 and 11).

As care theories suggested, the assessment of documentation of the care planning and care interventions was an important part of the InDEX instrument. In the first phase of InDEX development this was based on phases of the care process. The variables covered needs assessment, goal setting, selection of care interventions, assessing the needs responsiveness of care and the degree of goal achievement and the quality of the interventions. To start with, questions were developed using the Handbook for documentation of City of Helsinki as a basis (City of Helsinki, 2002). In the later phases of the instrument development, the results of the crosswalk between the care theories were used to bring the assessment into agreement with the four dimensions of care and the CK quality matrix (Chapter 5).

Developing the Instrument for Quality of Management (ManDEX)

To be able to realise the multi-actoral approach to the evaluation of care and care outcomes, in addition to instruments for client interviews and collection of data on professional care quality, an instrument for collection of data from care management was also necessary. As well as the challenge of cross-national and -cultural differences, it was important to bear in mind that the management perspective not only refers to the specific tasks of management, but also includes a consideration of the client perspective and the professional perspective in terms of specifying the final outcome (QoL) and the provision of quality care (QoC). Therefore, the ManDEX instrument needed to be harmonised with other instruments (CLINT and InDEX).

The literature review highlighted a wealth of quality management principles for services in general (see e.g. Bruhn, 2003; Zeithaml, Berry, & Parasuraman, 1988), but references to quality standards and indicators in social and health care for older persons are still rare (Blonski & Stausberg, 2003; Currie, Harvey, West, McKenna, & Keeney, 2005; Department of Health, 2003; Donabedian, 1969; Gebert, 2001; Görres, 1999; Haubrock & Gohlke, 2003; Kane, 1998; Øvretveit, 1998; Porell & Caro, 1998; Spector & Mukamel, 1998). Based on the review, QoM instrumentation was to cover the following items:

1. *QoM inputs*: concept quality, work organisation, financial resources, concept for cooperation.
2. *QoM process*: concept application, documentation quality, quality management activities (e.g. care ward rounds, quality circles), utilisation of staff and resources (e.g. overtime hours, changes in staff roster), actual cooperation.
3. *QoM outcome*: target efficiency of care, equity of distribution, availability of resources, cooperation quality and the subjective satisfaction of the manager (with equity, effectiveness, efficiency, resource availability and cooperation).

Developing the set of management indicators within the framework of the CK quality matrix with four quality dimensions, we achieved also a correspondence with the balanced scorecard approach (see Chapter 6 and 12). Thus, a cross-check with indicators used in this approach could be used (Eskola & Valvanne, 2000; Friedag & Schmidt, 2004; Kaplan & Norton, 1996; Niven, 2003; Valvanne, 2005).

The literature review did not offer validated instruments that directly fitted the Care Keys scheme, so a new instrument was developed and piloted by the Care Keys team. As the professional perspective and management perspective partially overlap, the quality of management is also ultimately measured by care outcomes for the clients. Thus, the starting points for development of the ManDEX instrument were the indicators specified for QoL and QoC. The instrument was also to address all the information to be collected at the level of the care providing organisation, rather than at the client level.

The structure of the items for evaluation of the quality of management of care and the three instruments for data collection are summarised in Table 2.1. The organisation of the data in the CK quality matrix for practical purposes is described elsewhere (Chapters 6 and 13). In addition, QUALID and Cornell Scale for Depression in Dementia were used with cognitively impaired clients.

TABLE 2.1. Summary of the instrumentation developed in Care Keys.

Instrument	Description	Comments
CLINT	Instrument for the collection of data by interview from the client and/or informal carer and/or formal carer in cases of incapacity of the client. Data include: basic identification information on home/life situation subjective IADL, ADL and need of help social networks, activities and participation subjective QoC subjective QoL scales: WHOQOL-Bref, PGCMS	Research procedures need to consider: criteria for selection of respondent(s) ethical procedures description of interview situation description of home care situation training of interviewers
InDEX	Instrument for the extraction of data from the individual care documentation including: identification information background information on client status and resources assessment of functional abilities and needs care plan professional QoC scales clinical outcomes	Research procedures need to consider: data quality missing cases confidentiality ethical rules interpretation guides
RELINFO	Instrument for collection of data from relatives or informal carer of client, also in cases of incapacity of the client	Comparable with CLINT
ManDEX	Management survey instrument for the collection of data from the care managers and from administration. Data include: basic information on the service organisation staff and resources information management concept/ quality management evaluation (subjective) of management performance (last 6 months) cost information	Management data are collected from the documentation of the institution and from the manager. It is assumed that the manager will also participate in the analyses of the documentation to clarify uncertainties and give subjective opinions

Piloting the CLINT, InDEX and ManDEX Instruments

Piloting of the instruments employed both qualitative and quantitative methods, and was done in two stages, both of which involved several iteration rounds:

1. *Preparation stage* (March 2003–December 2003), when earlier gathered national data sets were used to test the initial model of crQoL and to cover some areas of further research.

2. *Piloting* (January 2004–August 2004), when a fairly limited data set was gathered from participant countries with the special aim to check the instruments (both earlier introduced and new, original ones) for use within Care Keys project, and to select and design the most suitable and efficient instruments for the given population and purposes of the project.

Preparation Stage

In the preparation stage, Estonia used a nationally representative database of 806 persons over 65 years of age (Saks, Tiit, & Käärik, 2000), and applied the model of four qualities of life from Veenhoven (2000) on this data. The groups of variables, consisting of 15–35 variables, were used to define integrated factors (components of QOL) using exploratory factor analysis. Variables of different aspects of QoL, measured by various scales and questions, were successfully integrated into standardised factors describing the main components of QoL. Between all the components of QoL there were significant empirical correlations. A number of significant models were able to forecast the components of QoL according to living conditions, environment, social network, etc. It was also possible to build a meta-model using structural equations methodology (Maruyama, 1986) integrating all factors influencing the QoL and all components QoL created (Saks, Tiit, & Vähi, 2003).

The Finnish research team used a production of welfare research design on a random database of 281 face-to-face interviews of Finns over 75 years of age (average age 84). The database covered the requirements of the initial Care Keys meta-model quite well, and made it also possible to test some instruments, such as an application of the PGCMS, Life-satisfaction and Happiness. Factor analyses organised the QoL outcome measures and determinants as clear factors, and suggested a direct connection between care and QoL, and that the QoL in old age is also connected to the physical living environment and housing conditions, acute illness and traumatic life events. The results are published in Vaarama, Pieper, and Sixsmith (2007).

In addition, the group level pilot TEFF model (Vaarama & Hertto, 2003; Vaarama, Mattila, Laaksonen, & Valtonen, 1997) was tested analysing care need and care supply data in the partner countries using different national data. The experiences with existing data sets demonstrated the usability and efficiency of TEFF models in all project countries, but also highlighted the QoC documentation in the project countries, which was too poor to allow readily the use of TEFF analyses at the group level. From this it followed that there was a need to develop client level TEFF models as well (see Chapter 11).

The preparation stage gave support to the model of crQoL on which Care Keys was based, and the results guided the first definition of the Care Keys instrumentation.

The Piloting Stage

Results of Piloting CLINT

The pilot CLINT instrument used validated single items to cover the following areas: background information, housing and environment, social relationships, hobbies and participation; functional ability; QoC, using specially developed questionnaires on satisfaction with Home Care (34 closed and 4 open questions) and satisfaction with nursing home care (52 closed and 3 open questions) covering also depression, life events and spiritual well-being. In addition, Estonia, Sweden and UK piloted the following instruments: WHOQOL-BREF, The Sense of Coherence scale, CESD-R Depression Scale, The Cornell-Brown Scale for Quality of Life in Dementia (Ready, Ott, Grace, & Fernandez, 2002), Personal mastery Scale. In addition, the RAI questionnaires (Morris et al., 1994, 1997) were checked but not used in analyses. In total, there were 167 questions (numeric variables) for analysis.

Scales that were not available in all project languages were translated, back-translated, checked for meaning and adjusted and piloted before use. For example, Antonovsky's Sense of Coherence Scale was translated from English into Estonian, reviewed by an expert group (four persons), translated back into English by an independent translator, back-translation checked by an English expert and corrected on the basis of comments. The WHOQOL-Bref was translated by an independent translator from English into Finnish on approval of the WHO, reviewed by a group of experts (five persons) and by a group of five older Finns aged 75–87 in the City of Helsinki, translated back into English by another independent translator, back-translation checked by an English expert and corrected on the basis of comments.

Experiences of piloting and evaluation of instruments were received from all partners, and in addition, expert evaluations were received from a collaborating team in Spain. The total number of interviewed pilot cases was 26 for IC (Finland 5; UK 5; Sweden 5; Estonia 6; Germany 5) and 21 for HC (Finland 5; UK 3; Sweden 5; Estonia 4; Germany 4). Interviews with CLINT-IC took from 45 to 180 min, with CLINT-HC from 45 to 140 min, and the average time with both was about 1 h. For each pilot case, a completed InDEX was also received, and the average time for completion of the instrument was similar to CLINT.

Testing results on the pooled test-database of Estonia, Sweden and UK suggested the following results:

1. Most of the variables (test questions) worked in the sense that the answers were not concentrated to any single point of scale.
2. The distribution of answers was similar in different countries and/or care types. In many cases, there were no significant differences between the distributions/mean values of variables given by clients from different countries/service groups. This fact confirmed the regularity and acceptability of results.

3. The correlations between the variables from the same instrument had values in range 0.1–0.5, and higher correlations were very exceptional. The average values of correlations were in the range 0.2–0.25. Most of the variables from all the instruments turned out to be correlated.
4. The most reliable results for measuring QoL were given by the WHOQOL-Bref.

Based on feedback from clients and interviewers, refinements were made for the final CLINT instrumentation:

1. There were many negative comments from respondents concerning the Sense of Coherence Scale, and interviewers found the scale too difficult and unsuitable for older clients. Non-response rate was high compared with the other scales we used. The decision was made to omit this from the final instrumentation.
2. The CES-D was not well received by interviewers, many of whom were uncomfortable with the generally negative phrasing of the scale; asking nurses and other caregivers to administer a depression screening scale can be problematic if the scale is perceived to be too negative. Caregivers were reluctant to engage with these distressing topics. Instead, the PGCMS was used to assess morale as a proxy for depression.
3. The Personal Mastery Scale was rejected as it was too complicated for use with the study population.
4. The wording of difficult or confusing items was changed, unless they were part of validated scales.
5. Response scales were harmonised.
6. Interviewers found the WHOQOL-Bref was generally easy to use and quite easy for people to understand and respond to. The scale was not too long or taxing, and the five-point scale was easy to use, and was thus retained.
7. Single items were selected for measurement of person, context and situational factors.
8. The structure of the instrument was improved.

Results of Piloting InDEX and ManDEX

The goal of piloting the InDEX was, in addition to the testing of statistical power of the instrument, to find out how elements of InDEX could be extracted, and more precisely to get answers to the following three questions:

1. Where was the information extracted from (care documents, client, care personnel, informal caregiver, additional assessing of client, something else).
2. How was the information extracted (browsing care documentation—what documentation specifically, asked from client, asked from staff, asked from informal caregiver, additional test performed, etc.).
3. What items of InDEX were not possible to fill in? What was the reason?

The feedback on InDEX highlighted a number of specific changes required for the final version of the instrument to

1. Improve usability
2. Harmonise the home care and institutional care versions
3. Harmonise with ManDEX
4. Eliminate redundancies
5. Simplify scoring
6. Shorten the instrument

The content of the management instrument ManDEX were developed in parallel with InDEX, and, in addition, a substantial part of the indicators of management outcomes were also specified already by the module based on the needs and supply data obtained by InDEX. ManDEX was evaluated qualitatively in a four-step iterative process using expert evaluation. The national user groups offered a valuable source of expertise as they were designed to be representative of the care management systems in each country, and as such, participants included care managers from diverse management levels and both from social and health sectors and mixed organisations of providers. The CK quality matrix was discussed in user groups to assure that the ManDEX instrument was comprehensive.

The feedback on ManDEX reflected the somewhat different situations of management in the partner countries, and it was necessary to harmonise the instrument to be usable in all countries. The feedback of the experts suggested also that the standards of care and the goal attainment logic of the professional and management perspective should be reflected better in the indicators of QoM. As a consequence, a list of 13 care-quality standards and a list of 7 risk prevention procedures were included in the ManDEX to cover compliance with standards by professionals and by management. The set of questions in ManDEX could be reduced, on the one hand, by systematically checking whether variables could be extracted and constructed from InDEX. On the other hand, additions had to be made:

1. Information was needed on the client groupings that were used in practice by management and by professionals. A distinction of "administrative client groups" (e.g. categories of financing) and "special client groups" (e.g. risk groups for special treatments) was introduced and a description requested from managers in ManDEX.
2. The suggestions for the elaboration of the goal attainment logic and the inclusion of a subjective dimension of self-evaluation by management led to the inclusion of additional variables and questions on goals and their achievement, especially in the part on management outcomes.
3. The sub-dimension of cooperation with other institutions and services was expanded with more differentiated items in the part on management concept and outcomes.

The final HC-CLINT included 191 + 35, IC-CLINT 170 + 32, HC-InDEX 207 + 4, IC-InDEX 208 + 4, HC-ManDEX 112 + 10 and IC-ManDEX 114 + 10 questions (here the first number shows the number of contextual questions, while the second number refers to questions about the interviewing process). Based on the experiences of their use in the Care Keys empirical research, all instruments were reduced to cover only the key information to be collected to evaluate the crQoL and the quality of professional care and care management.

Summary of the Care Keys Instrumentation

A year-long procedure to define and test the instruments for empirical research resulted in a final set of instruments comprising various scales and measures drawing on a range of data sources (Table 2.1):

1. CLINT is an instrument for client interviews, including internationally validated instruments also such as WHOQOL-Bref and PGCMS.
2. InDEX is used for extraction of data from care documents, and includes both scientifically and practice-validated instruments to measure quality of professional care.
3. ManDEX collects data from care manager's perceptions of the institution, care processes in the institution or service, perception of the quality of the cooperation with other services and evaluations of goal attainment using instruments developed in Care Keys.
4. QUALID and Cornell Scale for Depression in Dementia are internationally validated scales to collect data from third-party observers on QoL of persons with dementia.
5. With the decision to include dementia clients, the pilot research highlighted the need to collect information from relatives, and the RELINFO instrument was created for this.

The instruments were developed, on the one hand, as research instruments to collect the information required for empirical research on care as determining the QoL of frail older persons. On the other hand, there was continuously a focus on the development of tools that can be used in practice. Therefore, one aim in the design of the instrument and of the research analyses was to find a set of indicators that would allow to reduce the instruments to practical tools collecting the information for quality management in long-term care and in correspondence to existing care documentations.

References

Alexopoulos, G. S., Abrams, R. C., Young, R. C., & Shamoian, C. A. (1988). Cornell scale for depression in dementia. *Biological Psychiatry, 23*, 271–284.

Antonovsky, A. (1993). The structure and properties of the sense of coherence scale. *Social Science and Medicine, 36*, 725–733.

Balcombe, N. R., Ferry, P. G., & Saweirs, W. M. (2001). Nutritional status and well being. Is there a relationship between body mass index and the well-being of older people? *Current Medical Research and Opinion, 17*(1), 1–7.

Baltes, P. B., & Baltes, M. M. (1990). Psychological perspectives on successful aging: The model of selective optimization with compensation. In P. B. Baltes, & M. Baltes (Eds.), *Successful aging. Perspectives from the behavioural sciences.* Cambridge, MA: Cambridge University Press.

Baltes, P. B., & Mayer, K. U. (Eds.). (1999). *The Berlin Aging Study, aging from 70 to 100.* Cambridge, MA: Cambridge University Press.

Bengtson, V. L., & Roberts, R. E. L. (1991). Intergenerational solidarity in aging families. In P. Benner, Ch. A. Tanner, & C. A. Chesla *Pflegeexperten, Pflegekompetenz, klinisches Wissen und alltägliche Ethik.* Bern: Hans Huber, 2000.

Blonski, H., & Stausberg, M. (Eds.). (2003). *Prozessmanagement in Pflegeorganisationen.* Hannover: Schlütersche Verlag.

Bowling, A. (1991). *Measuring health. A review of quality of life measurement scales.* Glasgow: Open University Press.

Brandstätter, J., & Renner, G. (1990). Tenacious goal pursuit and flexible goal adjustment. Explication and age-related analysis of assimilative and accommodative strategies of coping. *Psychology and Aging, 5*(1), 58–67.

Brod, M., Stewart, A. L., Sands, L., & Walton, P. (1999). Conceptualization and measurement of quality of life in dementia: The dementia quality of life instrument (DQoL). *The Gerontologist, 39*, 25–35.

Bruce, E. (2000). Looking after well-being: A tool for evaluation. *Journal of Dementia Care, 8*(6), 25–27.

Bruhn, M. (2003). *Qualitätsmanagement für Dienstleistungen. Grundlagen, Konzepte, Methoden. 4., verbesserte.* Auflage: Springer.

City of Helsinki (2002). Social Services Department. Handbook for documentation. Unpublished, in internal use only, updated 2005.

Currie, V., Harvey, G., West, E., McKenna, H., & Keeney, S. (2005). Relationships between quality of care, staffing levels, skill mix and nurse autonomy: Literature review. *Journal of Advanced Nursing, 51*, 73–82.

Daatland, S. O. (1990). What are families for? On family solidarity and preferences for help. *Ageing and Society, 10*, 1–15.

de Jong-Gierveld, J., & van Tilburg, T. (1999). *Manual of the loneliness scale.* Amsterdam: Vrije Universiteit.

Department of Health (UK). (2003), Domiciliary Care: National Minimum Standards.

Derogatis, L. R., Lipman, R. S., Rickels, K., Uhlenhuth, E. H., & Covi, L. (1974). The Hopkins Symptom Checklist (HSCL): A self-report symptom inventory. *Behavioral Science, 19*, 1–15.

Donabedian, A. (1969). Some issues in evaluation the quality of nursing care. *American Journal of Public Health, 59*, 1833–1836.

Duffy, J. A., Duffy, M., & Kilbourne, W. (1997). Cross national study of perceived service quality in long-term care facilities. *Journal of Aging Studies, 11*(4), 327–336.

Eskola, I., & Valvanne, J. (2000). *Kotihoidon kehittäminen Helsingissä* (Home Care Programme for Helsinki City) Sosiaaliviraston julkaisusarja A 7/2000. City of Helsinki, Social Services Department, Helsingin kaupungin sosiaalivirasto.

Folstein, M., Folstein, S., & McHugh, P. (1975). Mini mental state, a practical method for grading the cognitive state of patients for the clinician. *Journal of Psychiatry Research, 12*, 187–198.

Friedag, H. R., & Schmidt, W. (2004). *Balanced scorecard.* Planegg bei München.

Gebert, A. (2001). *Qualitätsbeurteilung und Evaluation in der Qualitätssicherung in Pflegeheimen* (Quality assessment and evaluation in quality assurance in nursing homes). Bern: Huber Publisher.

Geron, S. M., Smith, K., Tennstedt, S., Jette, A., Chassler, D., & Kasten, L. (2000). The home care satisfaction measure: A client-centred approach to assessing the satisfaction of frail older adults with home care services. *Journal of Gerontology (B): Psychological Sciences and Social Sciences, 55*, S259–S270.

Goldstone, L., & Maselino-Okai, C. (1986). Senior Monitor. An index of the quality of nursing care for senior citizens on hospital wards. Newcastle upon Tyne: Newcastle upon Tyne Polytechnic Products Ltd.

Growing Older Project. <http://www.shef.ac.uk/uni/projects/gop>

Görres, St. (1999). *Qualitätssicherung in Pflege und Medizin* (Quality assurance in care and medicine). Bern: Huber Publisher.

Hamilton, M. (1967). A rating scale for depression. *Journal of Neurology Neurosurgery and Psychiatry, 23*, 56–62.

Hartmaier, S. L., Sloane, P. D., Guess, H. A., Koch, G. G., Mitchell, C. M., & Phillips, C. D. (1995). Validation of the minimum data set cognitive performance scale: Agreement with the mini-mental state examination. *The Journals of Gerontology. Series A, Biological Sciences and Medical Sciences, 50*(2), M128–M133.

Haubrock, M., & Gohlke, S. (2001). *Benchmarking in der Pflege* (Benchmarking in care. A benchmarking study of home care services). Bern: Huber Publisher.

Kane, R. L. (1998). Assuring quality in nursing home care. *Journal of the American Geriatrics Society, 46*, 232–237.

Kaplan, R. S., & Norton, D. P. (1996). *Translating strategy into action. The balanced scorecard.* Boston, MA: Harvard Business School Press.

Katona, C. L., & Aldridge, C. R. (1985). The dexamethasone suppression test and depressive signs in dementia. *Journal of Affective Disorders, 8*, 83–89.

Kercher, K. (1992). Assessing subjective well-being in the old-age. *Research on Ageing, 14*, 131–168.

Kitwood, T., & Bredin, K. (1992). A new approach to the evaluation of dementia care. *Journal of Advances in Health and Nursing Care, 1*(5), 41–60.

Kunzmann, U., Little, T., & Smith, J. (2002). Perceiving control: A double-edged sword in old age. *Journal of Gerontology. Psychological Sciences, 57B*(6), 484–491.

Lawton, M. P. (1975). The Philadelphia Geriatric Center Morale Scale: A revision. *Journal of Gerontology, 30*, 85–89.

Lawton, M. P. (2001). Quality of care and quality of life in dementia care units. In L. S. Noelker, & Z. Harel (Eds.), *Linking Quality of Long-Term Care and Quality of Life* (pp. 148). New York: Springer.

Lelliott, P., Beevor, A., Hogman, G., Hyslop, J., Lathlean, J., & Ward, M. (2001). Carers' and users' expectations of services—user version (CUES-U): A new instrument to measure the experience of users of mental health services. *British Journal of Psychiatry, 179*, 67–72.

Logsdon, R. G., Gibbons, L. E., McCurry, S. M., & Teri, L. (2002). Assessing quality of life in older adults with cognitive impairment. *Psychosomatic Medicine, 64*, 510–519.

Löwenstein, A., Katz, R., Mehlhausen-Hassoen, D., & Prilutzky, D. (2002). The Research Instruments in the OASIS Project – Old Age and Autonomy: The Role of Service Systems and Intergenerational Family Solidarity. Haifa, The Center for Research and Study of Ageing – The Faculty for Welfare and Health Studies, University of Haifa.

Mahoney, F., & Barthel, D. (1965). Functional evaluation: The Barthel index. *Maryland State Medical Journal, 14*, 61–65.

Maruyama, G. M. (1986). *Basics of structural equation modeling.* Thousand Oaks, CA: SAGE Publications.

Morris, J. N., Fries, B. E., Mehr, D. R., Hawes, C., Phillips, C., Mor, V., et al. (1994). MDS cognitive performance scale. *Journal of Gerontology, 49M*, 174–182.

Morris, J., Fries, B. E., Steel, K., Ikegami, N., Bernabei, R., Carpenter, G. I., et al. (1997). Comprehensive Clinical Assessment in Community Settings: Applicability of the MDS-HC. *Journal of the American Geriatrics Society, 45*, 1017–1024.

Muurinen, S. (2003). Hoitotyö ja hoitohenkilöstön rakenne vanhusten lyhytaikaisessa laitoshoidossa (Care and staff-mix in institutional respite care for elderly). *Academic Dissertation. Acta Universitatis Tamperensis, 936*. Tampere University Press. Tampere.

Niven, P. R. (2003). *Balanced scorecard – Schritt für Schritt*. Einführung, Anpassung und Aktualisierung. Weinheim: Wiley GmbH & Co. KG&A.

Øvretveit, J. (1998). *Evaluating health interventions. An introduction to evaluation of health treatments, services, policies and organizational interventions*. Buckingham, Philadelphia, PA: Open University Press.

Paljärvi, S., Rissanen, S., & Sinkkonen, S. (2003). Kotihoidon sisältö ja laatu vanhusasiakkaiden, omaisten ja työntekijöiden arvioimana - Seurantatutkimus Kuopion kotihoidosta. *Gerontologia, 2*, 85–97.

Parasuraman, A., Berry, L. L., & Zeithaml, V. A. (1988). 'SERVQUAL: A multiple-item scale for measuring customer perceptions of service quality'. *Journal of Retailing, 64*, 12–40.

Parasuraman, A., Zeithaml, V. A., & Berry, L. L. (1985). A conceptual model of service quality and its implications for future research. *Journal of Marketing, 49*, 41–50.

Parasuraman, A., Zeithaml, V. A., & Berry, L. L. (1986). *SERVQUAL: A Multiple-Item Scale for Measuring Customer Perceptions of Service Quality*. Cambridge, MA: Marketing Science Institute.

Parasuraman, A., Zeithaml, V. A., & Berry, L. L. (1994). Reassessment of expectations as a comparison standard in measuring service quality: Implications for future research. *Journal of Marketing, 58*, 111–124.

Pavot, W., Diener, E., Colvin, C. R., & Sandvik, E. (1991). Further validation of the satisfaction with life scale: Evidence for the cross-method convergence of well-being. *Journal of Personality Assessment, 57*, 149–161.

Pearlin, L. I., & Schooler, C. (1978). The structure of coping. *Journal of Health and Social Behaviour, 19*, 2–21.

Porell, F., & Caro, F. G. (1998). Facility-level outcome performance measures for nursing homes. *The Gerontologist, 38*, 665.

Power, M., Quinn, K., Schmidt, S., & WHOQOL-OLD Group (2005). Development of the WHOQOL-Old module. *Quality of Life Research, 14*, 2197–214.

Radloff, L. S. (1977). The CES-D scale: A self-report depression scale for research in the general population. *Applied Psychological Measurement, 1*, 385–401.

Raynes, N., Temple, B., Glenister, C., & Coulthard, L. (2001). *Quality at home for older people: Involving service users in defining home care specifications*. Bristol: The Policy Press. Published in association with Joseph Rowntree Foundation.

Ready, R. E., Ott, B. R., Grace, J., & Fernandez, I. (2002). The Cornell-Brown Scale for Quality of Life in Dementia. *Alzheimer Dis. Assoc. Disord, 16*(2), 109–15.

Rosenberg, M. (1965). *Society and the adolescent self-image*. Princeton, NJ: Princeton University Press.

Russell, D., Peplau, L. A., & Cutrona, C. E. (1980). The revised UCLA loneliness scale: Concurrent and discriminant validity evidence. *Journal of Personality and Social Psychology, 39*, 472–480.

Ryff, C. D., & Keyes, C. L. M. (1995). The structure of psychological well-being revisited. *Journal of Personality and Social Psychology, 69*, 719–27.

Saks, K., Tiit, E.-M., & Käärik, E. (2000). *Health and coping of older Estonians.* University of Tartu.

Saks, K., Tiit, E.-M., & Vähi, M. (2003). Measuring and modelling the quality of life of older Estonians. The 7th Tartu Conference on Multivariate Statistics. Abstracts.

Sixma, H. J., van Campen, C., Kerssens, J. J., & Peters, L. (2000). Quality of care from the perspective of elderly people: The QUOTE-elderly instrument. *Age and Ageing, 29*, 173–178.

Solem, P. E. (2003). *Forskningsinstrumentene i norLAG* (Research instruments in norLAG). norLAG. Den norske studien av livsløp, aldring og generasjon. Oslo: NOVA.

Spector, W. D., & Mukamel, D. B. (1998). Using outcomes to make inference about nursing home quality. *Evaluation & The Health Professions, 21*, 291–315.

Tellis-Nayak, V. (2001). In search of a universal satisfaction survey tool: An analysis of satisfaction-survey instruments for nursing home residents, families and staff. A report submitted to the American Health Care Association.

Urman, G. C., & Urman, H. N. (1997). Measuring consumer satisfaction in nursing home residents. *Nutrition, 13*, 705–707.

Vaarama, M. (2004). Ikääntyneiden toimintakyky ja hoivapalvelut. Nykytila ja vuosi 2015 (Independent living and QoL in Old Age, and the role of care. State of the Art in Finland and prospects up to the year 2015). In *Ikääntyminen voimavarana. Tulevaisuusselonteon liiteraportti 5* (Ageing as a resource). Valtioneuvoston kanslian julkaisusarja 33/2004. Helsinki: Edita Prima Oy. <www.vnk.fi/julkaisut>

Vaarama, M., Hakkarainen, A., & Laaksonen, S. (1999). Vanhusbarometri 1998 (Old Age Barometer 1998). Sosiaali- ja terveysministeriön selvityksiä 1999:3. Helsinki.

Vaarama, M., & Hertto, P. (2003). Efficiency and equity of the care of older persons—exploring an evaluation model. *Revista Española de Geriatría y Gerontología.* <http://www.stakes.fi/carekeys/presentations.html>

Vaarama, M., & Kaitsaari, T. (2002). Ikääntyneiden toimintakyky ja koettu hyvinvointi (Functional ability in old age and subjective well-being). In M. Heikkilä, & M. Kautto (Eds.), *Suomalaisten hyvinvointi* (Well-being of Finns). Jyväskylä: Gummerus.

Vaarama, M., Mattila, V., Laaksonen, S., & Valtonen, H. (1997), Target efficiency. Report on development and piloting of the target efficiency indicators and model, STAKES.

Vaarama, M., Pieper, R., & Sixsmith, A. (2006). Care-related quality of life. The concept and empirical exploration. In H. Mollenkopf, & A. Walker (Eds.), *Quality of life in old age.* International and Multi-Disciplinary Perspectives. New York: Springer Science and Business Media.

Valvanne, J. (2005). Integrating social and health care in practice—A Finnish example. In M. Vaarama, & R. Pieper. *Managing integrated care for older persons.* Stakes and the European Health Management Association, Gummerus Printing.

Veenhoven, R. (1996). Happy life-expectancy. A comprehensive measure of quality-of-life in nations. *Social Indicators Research, 39*, 1–58.

Veenhoven, R. (2000). The four qualities of life. Ordering concepts and measures of the good life. *Journal of Happiness Studies, 1*, 1–39.

Ware, J. E., Kosinski, M., & Keller, S. D. (1996). A 12-item Short Form Health Survey: Construction of scales and preliminary tests of reliability and validity. *Medical Care, 34*(3), 220–233.

Watson, D., Clark, L., & Tellegen, A. (1988). Development and validation of brief measures of positive and negative affect: The PANAS scales. *Journal of Personality and Social Psychology, 54*(6), 1063–1070.

Weiner, M. F., Martin-Cook, K., Svetlik, D. A., Sainem, K., Foster, B., & Fontaine, C. S. (2000). The quality of life in late-stage dementia (QUALID) scale. *Journal of the American Medical Directors Association, 1*, 114–116.

WHOQOL Group (1998). Development of the World Health Organization WHO-QOL-Bref quality of life assessment. The WHOQOL Group. *Psychological Medicine, 28*(3), 551–558.

Zeithaml, V. A., Berry, L. L., & Parasuraman, A. (1988). Communication and control processes in the delivery of service quality. *Journal of Marketing, 52*(4), s.35–48.

Zigmund, A. S., & Snaith, R. P. (1983). The hospital anxiety and depression scale. *Acta Psychiatrica Scandinavica, 67*, 361–370.

Websites

http://www.emoryhealthcare.org/departments/fuqua/CornellScale.pdf, 28:551–558.
http://www.pickerinstitute.org, accessed July 2006
http://www.shef.ac.uk/uni/projects/gop/
http://ssg.scw.vu.nl/lasa/

3
Care Keys Data and Statistical Methods

Ene-Margit Tiit, Kai Saks and Marja Vaarama

Introduction

In order to elaborate the instruments, test the Care Keys methodology and build models, it was necessary to have different databases, covering all relevant client groups in all participant countries and containing measurements of all variables that might influence the crQoL of clients. The first databases were developed to test and pilot the various instruments for final data collection (see Chapter 2). After the instrumentation was finalised, national data collection took place during November 2004–March 2005, using common tools and a common data collection procedure. The national data sets were then combined to create a pooled database for empirical research that covered all the areas necessary for checking hypotheses and model building.

The Care Keys pooled database (CKPD) contained data on about 1,500 clients from 5 European countries, with an average more than 500 measured variables per case. The structure of data was quite complicated, with the data being drawn from interviews with clients, caregivers (in some cases also relatives), extracted from the care documentation and from managers of services. The overall response rate was moderate, mainly because of the health of clients and lack of information within care documentation. The following data processing tasks were required to create the pooled database:

1. Merging national data sets, cleaning, handling missing values, making imputations (where necessary and possible).
2. Exploratory analysis of data (on national and integrated, conditionally European level) to find the leading tendencies and estimate the distributions of variables, checking working hypotheses.
3. Compressing the data, calculating new variables (indexes).
4. Finding key-indicators with the aim of optimising the list of variables that would be measured in future.
5. Measuring dependencies and building models describing the factors influencing quality of life (QoL).

6. Creating meta-models to follow the multilevel structure of factors influencing the QoL of clients via quality of care (QoC) and other factors.

Mainly classical multivariate statistical methods were used in the data analysis, using the SPSS and SAS packages.

Designing the Care Keys Pooled Database

Aims of Creating Care Keys Pooled Database

The pooled Database was created using the Care Keys instruments. The aim of this database was:

1. To check the usability of all questions of the original Care Keys instruments.
2. To define the Key Indicators, the most useful variables to be used in future in the Care Keys toolkit.
3. To test the Care Keys theoretical concepts and methodology.
4. To build the models describing the influence of different variables (background, life experiences, management, professional and perceived QoC, etc.) on the subjective QoL of frail old clients of home and institutional care.
5. To integrate all different level models within meta-models describing the QoL.

The new database needed to be large enough to allow the different methods and models to be implemented. In order to get solid and reliable data from the various participating countries, with their different cultural backgrounds and situations, a robust framework was imposed for sampling and collecting data.

Design of Care Keys Pooled Database

For client interviews, each country had a target sample of 300 clients over 65 years of age, to give a total sample of 1,500 cases. These samples were either random or total samples. As a high non-response was expected for frail old persons, especially those receiving home care (in the Helsinki pilot study this was 70%), a master sample was required that was to be at least 50% larger than the intended net sample. The net sampling scheme is presented in Table 3.1.

TABLE 3.1. Target samples (65+) by country.

Country	Home care	Nursing homes	Sheltered housing
Estonia	150	150	
Finland	150	150	
Germany	150	150	
Sweden	150	150	
UK		150	150
Total	600	750	150

The cognition level of respondents in the master sample was determined by the Mini Mental State Examination (MMSE; Folstein, Folstein, & McHugh, 1975) or the Cognitive Performance Scale (CPS; Revised Long-Term Care Resident Assessment Instrument, 2002) to select the appropriate data collection instruments, so that clients with impaired cognition could be included in the survey. A client in the master sample who could not be interviewed because of acute sickness, death or moving to an institution from home care was to be replaced with the next similar case in the master sample. Successfully completed interviews formed the net sample, and sampling was terminated when 150 interviews of HC clients and 150 interviews of IC clients were completed. After a complete client interview (CLINT), other necessary data were extracted from his care documents (InDEX). If any additional assessment information was required, this was not to be older than 6 months prior to the interview. Each partner was responsible for getting the necessary ethical approval for collection of data from the clients and care documents. All client data was handled in a manner that ensured confidentiality. National data sets were encrypted before being sent for pooling to ensure the anonymity of the interviewees.

Data Collection Procedure

All partners used the common instruments CLINT, InDEX, QUALID and Cornell scales and ManDEX, which were translated into the various project languages (see Chapter 2). The instruments were used in a similar way, no national modifications were allowed and all partners had to present the questions in the same order. Finland and Germany also used the RELINFO to gather data from close relatives.

In order that the appropriate instrument was used for interviewing, each client was classified according to their cognition level, and the following rules were accepted for the use of instruments:

1. GROUP 1 (CPS 0–2 or MMSE 19–30)—CLINT + InDEX.
2. GROUP 2 (CPS 3 or MMSE 15–18)—CLINT + InDEX. If client interview was not possible then the same procedure as for group 3.
3. GROUP 3 (CPS 4–6 or MMSE 0–14)—Parts "Background information" and "Observations on care home" of CLINT + InDEX, QUALID + Cornell, voluntarily also RELINFO.

Interviewers were trained using a common protocol. To avoid useless data collection, the InDEX, ManDEX and RELINFO instruments were only completed after the CLINT had been successfully completed with the client in the first instance. All data had to be saved and imputed as SPSS (or Excel) files, using specially designed common templates, and sent to the Estonian partner for pooling. The final scheme for data collection is presented in Table 3.2.

Although the data collected in the various countries cannot be seen as "representative" of the target populations as whole in those countries,

TABLE 3.2. Plan for data collection.

Instrument to be used	Who measures	Source of information
CLINT	Researcher/interviewer	Client interview
InDEX	Researcher or nurse + ward manager	Client documents
ManDEX	Researcher or managers by self-completion	Manager
QUALID + Cornell	Nurse or researcher	Client observation, interview of relative
RELINFO[a]	To be delivered to relative by nurse	Questionnaire for relatives

[a]Use of the instrument was voluntary.

the service providers participating in the research were not untypical of those countries and the pooled data can be seen as broadly reflecting the national situations. The selection of provider organisations and clients utilised different methods of random sampling in the different countries (cluster-sampling in UK, master sampling in Finland and Sweden, random + total sampling in Germany and simple + master sampling in Estonia); the only nonrandom (convenience) sampling was HC in Sweden (about 3% of total sample size).

Care Keys Pooled Database

The Preliminary Set of Collected Data

Data collection was carried out between November 2004 and April 2005. The total amount of measurements was about 650,000 units. A total of 48 data files were created, identified by unique client identification numbers:

1. 13 InDEX files (1,496 cases),
2. 17 CLINT files (1,406 cases),
3. 9 Dementia QoL files (409 cases),
4. 9 ManDEX files (68 cases).

For all clients there were both completed InDEX and either CLINT or QUALID/Cornell scales, but in some cases (especially in moderately impaired clients) both CLINT and QUALID/Cornell were completed—at least partly (see Table 3.3).

Altogether more than 1,500 individuals were included in the pooled database, although the contribution of the different countries varied somewhat (Fig. 3.1). The final number of individual clients does not follow on exactly from Table 3.3, as some clients (moderately impaired) had been included more than once and some small files (including HC data from Espoo, Finland) were not included in the pooled data set. Additionally, the number of cases was reduced during the data-cleaning process.

TABLE 3.3. Preliminary Care Keys full data set (April 2005).

Country	IC			HC				
	CLINT	InDEX	Merged	CLINT	InDEX	Merged	Dementia	ManDEX
Finland	179	154	181	229[a]	124	229	97	27
Sweden	52	158	168	55	50	55	120	6
Estonia	153	152	152	149	149	150	45	15
UK	89	60	91	156	100	135	8	1
Germany	131	131	131	91	91	91	107	19
Merged	604	655	723	680	514	660	377	68

[a] Contains also an extra control database of home care clients in Espoo ($n = 80$), which is not included in the pooled database.

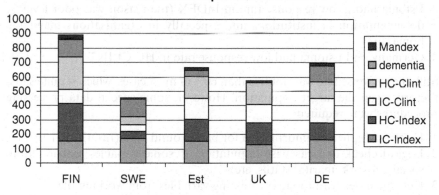

FIG. 3.1. The preliminary set of collected data.

TABLE 3.4. The response rate by instruments.

Instrument	InDEX IC	InDEX HC	CLINT-IC	CLINT-HC	Dementia	ManDEX
Response rate (%)	52.7	45.21	63.7	67.0	65.4	74.7

Quality of Raw Data: Response Rates

A number of problems were found in the data:

1. Low response rate, especially with InDEX, demonstrating that the care documentation of the participating providers and institutions did not contain the necessary information (see Table 3.4).
2. Cognition scores were not measured in all cases. Some instruments for measuring cognition were used for which there were no grouping rules.
3. The differentiation between the clients with normal and lowered cognition was not made in all cases according to the data collection protocol, and in some cases the use of instruments did not correspond to the clients' cognition score.

4. In the UK, a number of variables were redesigned and renamed specifically for people living in sheltered housing. Adding them to pooled database was technically very laborious. For this reason this group was excluded from some analyses.
5. The additional information collected for clients using the QUALID and Cornell instruments varied somewhat (in some cases background and observations were missing) and RELINFO was used only in Finland and Germany.

The response rate for the various instruments varied between 45 and 75 (Table 3.4).

The biggest problems with response rate were the following:

1. UK had a low response rate in ManDEX (only one filled-in form).
2. Estonia had a low response rate in InDEX (the reason was poor level of documentation in institutions and especially in organisations managing home care).
3. Germany and Estonia had low response rate in HC CLINT.

Still, the response rate was not less than 60% in most cases, which is quite satisfactory, given the target population. However, some special data processing procedures were required:

1. Deleting duplicated information for background data (InDEX, CLINT).
2. Logical check and casewise imputation of some variables (cohabitation, social network, marital status, etc).
3. Deleting cases with too many missing variables from working files.
4. EM imputation of numerical variables (using special software).

Identification and Merging of Data

As a first step, the files were merged using the identification numbers. The following identification numbers were in use:

1. Service provider/institution identification code: *aaabbb*, where *aaa* forms the country code and *bbb* the institution's code.
2. Interviewer/extractor code *aaadd*, where *aaa* forms the country code and *dd* the interviewer's or extractor's code.
3. Client identification code: *aaabbbccc*, where *aaa* forms the country code, *bbb* the institution's code and *ccc* the client's code.

Interviewer numbers were used only for initial data checking and were dropped from pooled data files. Client identification numbers were used for merging client data from the different instruments (InDEX and CLINT and/or DementiaQoL). These codes worked well, and in the whole data set there were only very few coding mistakes. Institution codes were used to integrate ManDEX data with client's individual data. There were some problems here: institution names had been used instead of codes in the data input, requiring some recoding.

The merging of the data files required that all sub-files containing data from different countries should have the same variable descriptions: codes, types, codes of missing values and also lengths (textual variables). All these conditions were fulfilled in using the templates, but there were some problems:

1. The length of textual variables varied, as in some countries very long comments were written in the documents.
2. Some random mistakes in the variable codes were discovered.
3. Some special variables were added, among them variables describing clients of sheltered housing.

As a first step, two files saving the whole initial data (including all textual comments in their full size) were created—these were HCArchive (containing the data of clients of Home Care, 735 clients and 708 variables) and ICArchive (containing the data of clients of Institutional Care, 785 clients and 619 variables). In these data sets, no transformations of initial variables were made; the HC data set also contained 48 special variables for Sheltered Housing. These files were saved and sent for analysis by the German team.

Allocating Clients to Cognition Groups

An important task was to differentiate between cognitively and non-cognitively impaired clients. Unfortunately, the cognition score was not measured in all cases and in almost half the cases it was not possible to divide the clients into groups using the initially created rules (see Table 3.5). An alternative was to divide the clients by the instruments used in measuring QoL. Here the situation was somewhat better (Table 3.6).

TABLE 3.5. Tools used for measuring the cognition score of clients.

Tool	Home care Frequency	%	Institutional care Frequency	%	Total Frequency	%
CPS/RAI	21	2.9	115	14.6	136	8.9
MMSE	317	43.1	280	35.7	597	39.3
RAI	1	0.1	117	14.9	118	7.8
0–6			5	0.6	5	0.3
Berger_Scale			14	1.8	14	0.9
Missing	396	53.9	254	32.4	650	42.8
Total	735		785		1,520	

TABLE 3.6. The distribution of clients by QoL instruments answered.

		Institutional care Norm QoL				Home care Norm QoL		
		Yes	No	Total		Yes	No	Total
Dem QoL	Yes	46	284	330	Yes	6	71	77
	No	388	67	455	No	477	181	658
	Total	434	351	785		483	252	735

Table 3.6 indicates that 407 clients had a completed Dementia QoL measure (at least partly) and 917 clients had (at least partly) at least one of the instruments measuring QoL of people with normal cognition. These instruments were not completed, or inadequately completed for 248 clients (16.7%) and both were completed for 52 clients (3.4%). Subsequently, all cases were divided into three files: Normal HC, Normal IC and Dementia based on instruments used:

1. Normal HC—CLINT-HC, InDEX-HC and ManDEX.
2. Normal IC—CLINT-IC, InDEX-IC and ManDEX.
3. Dementia—InDEX (IC or HC), DementiaQL, ManDEX.

Cleaning the Data and Creating Working Files

In the data-cleaning process, the following steps were followed:

1. Any case who belonged to Group 3 (MMSE < 15 or CPS > 3) was deleted from Normal HC and Normal IC files.
2. Any case belonging to Group 1 (MMSE > 18 or CPS < 4) was excluded from the Dementia group.
3. Any case with no information from QoL questions and with more than 50% missing values in the CLINT and InDEX was deleted.

After this three working data files were created:

1. Home care—435 cases.
2. Institutional care—513 cases.
3. Dementia—394 cases.

A total of 178 cases (11.7%) from the initial data files were excluded from the final data files, but the original data were saved in archive files.

Calculation of Initially Defined New Variables and QoL Components

The following actions were carried out:

1. Variable identifying country was created.
2. Background data from CLINT and Index were integrated to minimise missing values.
3. Age of the client at 1.01.2005 was calculated.
4. Virtually all text string variables and all variables characterising the interviewing process were deleted.

All the QoL instruments had specific rules for calculating integrated QoL scores. The only change from the original instrument was made in WHOQOL-Bref. Here the question (belonging to the social domain) "How satisfied you are with your sexual life" was substituted by the question "Do you feel alone?" from WHOQOL-100, having the opposite scale (1—not at all, ..., 5—extremely). The reason of this substitution was that in piloting stage the question about sexual life was offensive to many clients (with poor health, widowed or lacking partners). Before the calculation of QoL scores, the concordance of variables belonging to this component was measured (using Cronbach α and correlation analysis). As a result, a minor mistake (from translation or questionnaire design) was found in the PGCMS component "Loneliness", where in some countries the direction of scale was different from others. This fact was discovered and corrected before calculation of the QoL scores.

To calculate the integrated QoL scores the following steps were followed:

1. For all clients, the number of missing values in QoL variables was counted.
2. For all cases, where number of missing values was less than 40%, the missing values of QoL variables were imputed, using EM procedure, where for forecasting the missing values other QoL variables and some background variables were used.
3. Using the imputed data, the integrated QoL scores (in the case of WHO-QOL-Bref domains) were calculated by original rules, taking also into account the direction of scales of all variables.
4. To make the results comparative, all variables were scaled on a 0–100 scale (0—minimum possible and 100—maximum possible value, the higher values corresponding to better values).

All EM-imputed QoL variables and Integrated values (scaled and simply summarised) were merged into working data files, in which all the original data were also saved.

List of Care Keys Pooled Data files

Table 3.7 presents the most useful Care Keys data files:

1. The first files, containing only original data, are two archive files.
2. The files IC-all, HC-all and Dem-all differentiate cases according to instruments completed. No data cleaning was carried out, but textual variables were deleted.
3. The files HC-working, IC-working and Dem-working include the data after cleaning and EM imputing.
4. The files HC-min and IC-min include TEFF variables (see Chapter 11), and all initial variables were substituted by EM-imputed ones.

The final file listed in Table 3.7 contains moderately demented people (Group 2) from all files, which is why the number of variables is the largest. All these data sets were made available for analysis by partners within the Care Keys project.

TABLE 3.7. Care Keys data files (EM-use: 0—no, 1—partly, 2—totally).

| Name | Date | Inclusion (0—no, 1—yes) | | | | | | EM use | Number of | |
		HC	IC	Dem	InDEX	CLINT	ManDEX		Cases	Variables
HC_Archive	10.04.05	1	0	1	1	1	1	0	735	708
IC_Archive	10.04.05	0	1	1	1	1	1	0	785	619
HC_all	13.04.05	1	0	1	1	1	1	0	735	540
IC_all	12.04.05	0	1	1	1	1	1	0	785	456
Dem_all	10.05.05	0	0	1	1	0	0	0	407	370
Dem_working	31.01.06	0	0	1	1	0	1	1	394	457
HC_working	31.01.06	1	0	0	1	1	1	2	513	829
IC_working	31.01.06	0	1	0	1	1	1	2	435	760
HC_min	3.03.06	1	0	0	1	1	1	2	513	365
IC_min	28.02.06	0	1	0	1	1	1	2	435	411
mod_dem	8.03.06	1	1	1	1	1	1	1	165	1,205

Statistical Methods Used in Care Keys Project

Data processing was primarily carried out using SPSS. For some additional procedures SAS was also used and some special procedures were programmed using Excel software.

Data Handling, Checking the Quality, Data Cleaning

As usual in the case of large and complex data sets, the data cleaning and quality control process was quite challenging. The following procedures were carried out.

Checking for Technical Errors and Scales, Completing Information

The data from the various countries, using a range of instruments with different client groups had to be merged to create working data files. For this there were some necessary technical checks: uniqueness of indicators, fit of clients' and institutions' indicators, types, lengths and names of variables, etc., codes of missing values. Values outside the ranges of variables were checked and either substituted with the most probable value or deleted. In cases where systematic errors in scales were discovered, the distributions of variables by countries were checked. Some variables were interpreted in different ways in some countries and these errors were corrected.

Before building integrated indexes/components, the correlations between variables were calculated and compared countrywise. Where large differences occurred (opposite signs of correlations) the values were scrutinised and converted if required. Similarly, the Cronbach alpha-coefficients of all variables included within the indexes/domains were checked and compared countrywise. Background data were collected in two documents (one filled-in by client, the other by careworker) and some values were missing in both of these. Comparing both documents, the number of missing values was minimised using the following rules in cases of discrepancies: for birth date, gender and education the *InDEX* (documented value) had higher priority; for first language, marital status and cohabitation the *CLINT* (answers of client) has higher priority.

Creating New Variables

Several nominal variables (marital status, country) were coded as a set of *dummy variables* for use in models. Some other new variables were created using *logical operations*, for example from "first language" the variable "is the first language common for given country" was created. A series of *indexes* were created for QoL following the definitions given in literature; to make all indexes/domains comparable, standardised versions (scale 0–100) were calculated. In analysing process several *linear combinations* of initial variables were used to compress the information, also using factors analysis to create indexes. A General QoL measure was created as a linear combination of QoL domains and standardised (0–100). Original TEFF variables, including "met needs", were calculated as new variables and added to the files. Variables were used also to create several *subsets of data*, notably national data sets used in country specific analysis, and data sets specifically for creating hypotheses for subsequent testing using the pooled data.

Imputation

The data had quite high non-response rate, but in many cases this appeared to be random. For instance, the distribution of answers to QoL questions (PGCMS and WHOQOL-Bref) for clients of IC is given in Fig. 3.2. Nevertheless, the number of persons answering all questions (and usable in analysis) was only 200 (13% of the sample). To avoid major losses of valuable information,

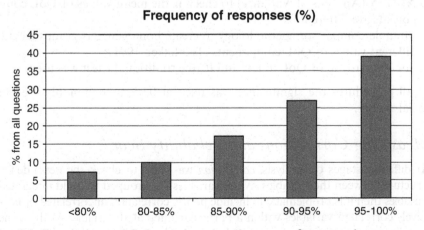

FIG. 3.2. Completeness of QoL questionnaires (frequency of responses).

especially in multivariate procedures, it was decided that for cases with at least half of the data present, the imputation of variables having numeric or order scale would be carried out. The EM-imputation method (Little & Rubin, 1987) was used as one of the most effective methods, allowing control of bias in means, variance and correlations. All indexes were calculated after imputations.

Checking Statistical Assumptions

For model building it is necessary to check the distribution of dependent variables. In most models the dependent variables are calculated as linear combinations of initially measured variables (domains of QoL or factors of QoC). The proximity of their distributions to normal distribution was checked (using Kolmogoroff statistics, χ^2-statistics or higher moments).

Explanatory Data Analysis

Descriptive Analysis

The descriptive analysis (estimation of means and variances, description of the distribution of variables, characterisation of the situation and resources of care clients) was mainly carried out separately by the participating national research teams.

Testing Hypotheses

In analysing the QoL in different countries, it was necessary to compare the QoL components by countries and also by care types. With this aim the following methods were used:

1. ANOVA (Analysis of Variance) to check if the mean values of QoL components are different.
2. Multiple comparison methodology to create homogeneous groups having different values of QoL components (Toothaker, 1991).
3. For comparison of QoL in HC and IC the traditional t-test was used.

In all procedures the significance was fixed at 0.05, as commonly used in social studies.

Measuring Correlations and Reliability Scores

At different stages of analysis, *correlation* was used to check the dependency structure between the variables. When variables are grouped to build integrated variables then it is problematic to include poorly correlated, uncorrelated or negatively correlated variables within a particular integrated variable. At the same time, linear combinations of very highly correlated variables add little information compared with initial variables. Both of these can be checked using the *Cronbach α coefficient*. Not only too low, but also too high values of α-coefficient indicate that the variables to be combined have not been chosen effectively.

In model building, especially in the case of large numbers of potential explanatory variables, it is important to avoid high correlations (multiple partial correlations) between explanatory variables, which cause *multicollinearity* and interpretation problems.

In some cases, correlation analysis between blocks of variables (canonical correlations) may help in model building. This approach was used to find connections between objective (measured by caregivers) and subjective (assessed by clients) QoC.

In the main, *linear correlations* were used to test the dependences between variables, but in some cases *nonparametric correlations* (Spearman ρ, Kendall τ) were also used. As the scales were generally short and correlations rather weak, there were practically no differences between Pearson and nonparametric correlations. This was also the case with binary variables. Following this, there is no reason to believe that the use of linear correlations (technically easier and fitting logically with the model-building approach) would produce biased or incorrect conclusions.

Factor Analysis

Explanatory factor analysis (mainly using the Principal Components' procedure with units on main diagonal) was one of the main data analysis methods used. The number of factors was defined either by the usual criterion (eigenvalues > 1) or using the description rate (usually >50%). In most cases, Varimax (or Quartimax) rotation was used to get better interpretable factors. Factor analysis was used with different aims: to analyse the dependence structure in blocks of originally created Care Keys' variables; to compress the information measured by blocks of variables; to check the effectiveness of indexes given by adapted instruments; and to define original indices. In meta-modelling, *confirmatory factor analysis* was also used to define latent variables.

Defining Key Variables

As the initial number of variables measured was very large, a major task was to reduce the number of *measured variables* (with a view to the future application of the Care Keys instruments). For this, the following procedure was elaborated. Starting with several dependent variables $Y_1, Y_2, \ldots, Y_k$ forming a vector Y and a large number of potential explanatory variables $X_1, X_2, \ldots, X_m$, the aim was to find the best subset of Xs to model the dependent variables in the best way. For this, the descriptive power of each X was defined for the vector Y in the following way:

Let us have a stepwise linear model for Y_i,

$$Y_i = \sum_{j=0}^{m_i} b_j X_j, \tag{3.1}$$

where the independent variables X_j are ordered by decreasing the change $\delta(i,j)$ of the determination coefficient R^2 caused by X_j. Then $\delta(i,j)$ is the descriptive power of variable X_j for the dependent variable Y_i. The descriptive power of the model (1) is evidently $R^2 = \sum_{j=1}^{m} \delta(i,j)$, and the descriptive power of variable X_j for the vector Y is:

$$D_j = \sum_{i=1}^{k} \delta(i, j), \tag{3.2}$$

Now it is possible to order all explanatory variables by their descriptive power and select, among all potential explanatory variables, the subvector X^* with components $X_1^*, \ldots X_q^*$ (q much less than k) that have the highest descriptive power for given vector Y of dependent variables.

In practice, some additional checks were added:

1. The factor analysis of data set X was carried out and checked that for each significant factor at least one variable is represented in the set (subvector) X^*.
2. Correlations between the variables x_j^* must not be too high (in our case the critical level $r \leq 0.6$ was taken).

If the choice of variables agrees with the theoretical concepts, then the set of variables $X_1^* \ldots X_q^*$ was taken as the key variables.

On average, we had $q = 0.2k$, meaning that the number of explanatory variables can be shortened about 5 times, while preserving about 70–80% of the descriptive power of initial set of variables.

Model Building

Linear Models

The final step of most empirical research is model building. When the dependent variable can be considered as numeric, with a distribution close to normal, then the most effective approach is to use linear regression. This is the situation in building models for QoL components. In all cases, the stepwise procedure was used to select the best subset of explanatory variables and determination was measured using the square multiple correlation coefficient R^2. As the sample sizes are, in general, quite big (about 500 cases in all models), the selection methods work without problems and quite big models (containing up to 25–30 explanatory variables) may be statistically significant (on the level 0.05).

Linear models were built relating QoL components to clients' background and life experiences, subjective and objective QoC, met needs and many other factors. The best models describe up to 60–70% of variability of QoL components and general QoL. Using only the key variables, the scale of the models drops substantially, whereas the descriptive power is maintained almost at the optimal level. Similar models were also built for indices characterising the subjective QoC defined by documented QoC, environment and management. The results were similar, but the models had somewhat lower description rate.

Logistic Models

If the dependent variable is the probability of an event, then logistic regression is the most effective tool for model building. The same method can also be used in the case of arbitrary binary (or, in more advanced form—discrete non-numeric) variables. In some cases, the numeric variable (especially when its distribution differs substantially from normal) was transformed to a binary or ordinary variable and then logistic modelling was used. In the Care Keys project most of the main models were built in two ways, using both linear and logistic models, but only the best solution is given. In practically all cases the quality of the models (measured by R^2 in linear and by Nagelkerke's R^2 in logistic models) was very similar, but in most cases linear models were somewhat preferable. In addition, the number, list and impact of explanatory variables were similar in both models.

Structural Equations Modelling

Structural Equation Modelling (initially LISREL method; Joreskog, 1969) is a very general and powerful multivariate analysis technique that includes specialised versions of a number of other analytical methods as special cases (Maruyama, 1998). One of the fundamental ideas in multivariate analysis is the idea of statistical (linear or non-linear) dependence. The rules become more complex if the dependence structure is multilevel and number of variables is large, but the basic message remains the same: it is possible to test whether *variables are interrelated through a set of linear relationships by examining the variances and covariances of the variables*. SEM models, characterising the directions of influences, can also describe and check hypotheses about *causal* dependencies. Causal models were created for QoL in Estonia (Saks, Tiit, & Vähi, 2003) and the results appeared quite informative. Several causal models were built within the Care Keys project, integrating all measured groups of variables and having QoL as outcome (latent) variables.

Conclusions

The process of compiling and developing the CKPD demonstrated that it is possible to create a common working data set compiled from very different sources, provided and completed by persons with very different background and education, in the following complicating conditions:

1. The research instruments were in five languages.
2. The cultural background and conditions (institutions, care organisations) were different in different countries.
3. The target group consisted of frail old people, part of them being cognitively impaired.
4. The data contained sensitive questions.
5. The documentation used was of extremely poor quality in some countries.
6. The time for completing the work was restricted.

Despite these problems the data generated by the Care Keys project was of high quality, with all important conditions formulated by European Statistical system (Brancato, 2006) being met. The database offered the Care Keys researchers the possibility to carry out a range of statistical analyses, check working hypotheses and create the models and meta-models. The preconditions for achieving good quality data were:

1. carefully created, translated and unified instruments,
2. common rules for data collection process and templates for data input,
3. use of effective imputation procedure in creating working data files.

However, some problematic issues remain:

1. The sampling scheme did not standardise the choice of institutions, hence it is possible that effect of the selection of institutions is amalgamated with the country effect.
2. In some cases, the client instrument that was used did not correspond with the client's group (by cognition score), leading to some cases being dropped from the working files.

To conclude, the CKPD allowed the research team to test several scientifically important hypotheses and build empirical models confirming the theoretical concepts and new findings in the area of crQoL of frail old persons. Even though care institutions were not randomised and some countries used total samples of a single provider, the data remains valid for modelling and for drawing preliminary conclusions as the basis for further research.

References

Brancato, G. (2006). Recommended practises for questionnaire design and testing in the European Statistical System. <http://www.statistics.gov.uk/events/q2006/>

Folstein, M., Folstein, S., & McHugh, P. (1975). Mini mental state, a practical method for grading the cognitive state of patients for the clinician. *Journal of Psychiatric Research, 12*, 187–198.

Joreskog, K. G. (1969). A general approach to confirmatory maximum likelihood factor analysis. *Psychometrika, 34*, 183–202.

Little, R. J. A., & Rubin, D. B. (1987). *Statistical analysis with missing data*. New York: John Wiley.

Maruyama, G. M. (1998). *Basics of structural equation modeling*. Thousand Oaks, CA: SAGE Publications.

Revised Long-Term Care Resident Assessment Instrument User's Manual. Version 2.0. (2002). Centers For Medicare & Medicaide Services.

Saks, K., Tiit, E.-M., & Vähi, M. (2003). Measuring and modelling the quality of life of older Estonians. The 7th Tartu Conference on Multivariate Statistics. Abstracts.

Toothaker, L. E. (1991). *Multiple comparisons for researchers*. Newbury Park, CA: Sage Publications, Inc.

Part II
Theoretical Results

4

The Concept of Care-Related Quality of Life

Richard Pieper and Marja Vaarama

Introduction

In gerontology, there is a substantial and increasing body of theoretical and empirical research on quality of life (QoL) in old age, especially in psychology and health-related research. However, a specific focus on QoL of frail older persons or older persons with permanent need of external help is rare, and even more neglected is the role of care for their QoL. In addition, the question of how much the existing definitions really reflect the opinions of older people themselves has got too little attention (Bowling, Gabriel, Banister, & Sutton, 2002). These notions motivated the Care Keys research to search for a better understanding of the role of homecare and institutional care for the QoL of frail older persons. Applying the production of welfare approach (see Chapter 1), the aim was to produce information on the specific life situations of these older persons, and on the linkages between care and QoL. By providing a model of care-related QoL we aimed at a concept that would allow for the evaluation of care practices in view of their outcomes for frail older persons, thus supporting development of care practices as well as quality management of (long-term) care.

Searching for a theoretical model of QoL of frail older persons we found suitable starting points, but also encountered unresolved issues and open questions. This situation prompted the Care Keys research to proceed in two directions. First, we selected concepts and instruments that were available in the literature, introduced some preliminary adaptations to the life circumstances of frail older persons receiving care, and investigated the relation of care quality to QoL as an outcome. Second, we took a closer look at the theoretical issues and their relevance for a concept of care-related QoL. While the empirical research is reported elsewhere (see Part III), the results of the theoretical reflections on QoL are presented and discussed in this chapter.

Three issues, or bundles of questions, were identified as relevant for a theory-grounded concept of care-related QoL. First, a number of existing models can offer valuable starting points for the development of a concept of care-related QoL, but the problem is that they contain many different dimensions or domains of life, and typically there is little or no theoretical background provided to evaluate if these dimensions are *comprehensive* enough to cover all relevant aspects of life. Moreover, we find arguments for the development of concepts of QoL specific to certain groups such as persons with specific age, gender, health problems, disabilities or socio-economic conditions. Thus, the issue is whether we should adopt a general or a specific model of QoL, and if we choose a general model, how we should make it more specific to capture the special life situation and the experiences by a certain group. In the present case of care-dependent older persons, care is an important element of the life situation which has to be included in the concept. Second, there is a discussion distinguishing between conditions or determinants of QoL, and factors of QoL. In the present context, we might conceive of care as an external condition of life quality provided by care services, or consider care as an integral part of the life situation of the person "filling in the gaps" opened up by impairments or by lack of social support (see Chapter 10). The production of welfare approach conceives care primarily as an intermediate output that is "delivered" and produces the "final outcome" of QoL. But not only has the role of *care* to be clarified, but also the role of the *client* in the production of QoL, since the client appears as a co-producer in care, and his or her capacities of self-help and of utilising care support have a great impact on the effects of care. Thus (features of) the clients appear also in the role of a condition of their own QoL. Third, there is an agreement in the literature on QoL that issues of evaluation are inherent in the concept of quality requiring reference to criteria of "goodness", but it is not always clear which criteria are to be employed and how. Such normative issues raise, for instance, the question whether asking the client's own subjective evaluations is sufficient to solve normative problems, or whether the evaluation has to include processes of communication and "negotiation of order" (Strauss, Schatzmann, Bucher, Erlich & Sabshin, 1963, pp. 147–68) involving other persons (e.g. the carer) or agencies (e.g. socio-political decision-makers), and how the client is empowered to participate in care decisions.

To further clarify the concept of QoL and, more specifically, of care-related QoL we want in this contribution to

1. Review research approaches and empirical findings on the impact of care for QoL of frail older persons;
2. Discuss three theoretical models of QoL by Brown & Brown (2003), Lawton (1983, 1991) and Veenhoven (1996, 2000) and
3. Combine the main components of these models into a model of care-related QoL in frail or care-dependent older persons.

This contribution should be seen in the context of the theoretical analyses on quality of care (QoC) and quality of management (QoM) (Chapters 5 and 6). We will propose a general, four-dimensional model, which may contain different specifications of life domains and indicators for different groups *within* its dimensional framework depending on, for example individual living conditions, lifestyles, personalities, subjective evaluations of life circumstances and—as in the present case—availability of care services. To address the issues indicated earlier, we will distinguish three different sub-models that combine objective circumstances and subjective interpretations (structural model), ask for the role of the client and the role of care (production model) and reflect on the "negotiation of order" in care processes (normative model).

Care-Related QoL Research: Approaches and Findings

Following the three issues identified earlier, we may distinguish approaches to the study of QoL according to their focus on (1) the *specific life situation* of frail or care-dependent older persons, (2) the *role of care* and other determining factors of QoL and (3) the participation of older persons in the *"negotiation of order"* in the care process.

The Specific Life Situation of Older Persons and the Effects of Care

Considering the specific life situation of older persons and the effects of care, an extensive review was conducted in the Care Keys project. Although considerable attention has been given to issues of health-related QoL, research on QoL of older people who can be described as "frail" has been neglected. Gerritsen, Steverink, Ooms, & Ribbe (2004) provide a useful review of a number of conceptual models of QoL of older people receiving care, notably Faulk (1988), Hughes (1990), Lawton (1983, 1991, 1994) and Ormel, Lindenberg, Steverink, & Vonkorff (1997). However, a specific focus on frail older people is rare (Birren, Lubben, Rowe, & Deutchman, 1991; Tester, Hubbard, Downs, MacDonald, & Murphy, 2003; Chapter 1). Analysing the research results we found at least eight dimensions or factors that were generally considered relevant for the QoL of frail older persons living at home and in the institutions: demographic and socio-economic factors; physical-functional abilities and mental health; personal and psychological factors; life satisfaction; social networks and participation; living environment; life changes and events; and care. The factors are also represented in the theoretical framework of the Care Keys research (Fig. 1.3).

Such a list of factors relevant for a "good life" can only be a starting point, and researchers have proceeded in different ways. Searching for a theoretical model of QoL, the diverse aspects of a person's life and environment are grouped into: (i) an empirical model to include all relevant *domains*, or (ii) theoretically with reference to some model of the "good" or "productive" life with the *dimensions* depending on the theoretical approach. Whereas these approaches will result in some taxonomy or structural model, other approaches assume a causal order and (iii) identify a causal model with *variables* specifying conditions, causes and QoL as effect, or (iv) distinguish—in a more practice oriented perspective—a production model with conditions and input *factors*, processes and interventions, and outcome factors combined in strategies of planned change or the production of welfare (see e.g. Vaarama, Pieper, & Sixsmith, 2007). These approaches are not mutually exclusive and are combined in research, and the suggested distinction of domains, dimensions, variables and factors is also not followed, but only suggested in the present context to indicate the differences of approaches.

Empirical models may draw on the disciplines involved (e.g. medical, psychological, social) or identify life domains such as physical well-being, material well-being, social well-being, emotional well-being and productive well-being (see Cummins, 1997; Felce & Perry, 1997). Diverse aspects of the person's life and the environment may be included without specification of the relation they do have to (the theory of) the person, and often theories are regarded as unnecessary for the tasks at hand (practical empiricism), or even as essentially impossible because of the individuality of life situations (phenomenological approaches) (see Bengtson, Putney, & Johnson, 2005). A problem with this strategy is that it offers no clear scheme to evaluate the *completeness* of the domains and the *adequate weight* of elements. Completeness is intended by the comprehensiveness and richness of the empirical base reaching from statistical data, survey data, observations, tests and interviews, to document analyses and personal narratives of older persons. Still, aspects frequently appear in different domains of the same scheme receiving implicitly a higher weight (Cummins, 1997). An example is "counting" medical aspects twice by including them first in their own right, and implicitly again in categories of functional (dis-) ability. The problem is typically addressed by submitting the list to a factor analysis, which provides an inside into the dimensional structure and allows giving more adequate weights to particular items. The issue of completeness is not solved this way, since aspects missing in the list do not appear in the dimensional structure. An example of this approach is the QoL-assessment instruments developed by the WHOQOL Group (Power, Quinn, Schmidt, & WHOQOL-OLD Group, 2005; Skevington, Lofty, & O'Connell, 2004).

A theoretical approach will specify dimensions of the structural model, and the framework might be quite general, for example drawing on a theory of systems (Freund, Li, & Baltes, 1999; Veenhoven, 2000), or more specific like the model of QoL of older persons with frailty or dementia by Lawton (1991) employing environmental psychology, or the model for older persons in transition from home to institution by Tester et al. (2003) using a gerontological framework. In this approach, we may distinguish between theoretical frameworks focusing on objectively measurable and quantitative phenomena typically including conditions of the social and physical environments (e.g. Lawton, 1991); frameworks focusing on QoL as a "social construction" generated by communication and interaction and socio-culturally determined (e.g. Adams & Gardiner, 2005) and frameworks focusing on the subjective experiences of older persons and their personal life histories (e.g. Gubrium, 1993).

A problem with theoretical models can be their intimate linkage to certain basic theoretical frameworks and discussions that influence the concept of

QoL and can make it difficult to establish a theoretical base. As recent accounts of positions in the theory of ageing demonstrate, even established reviewers in gerontological theory have doubts about the role of theory beyond the role of a "sensitizing scheme" or a "heuristic" strategy (Bengtson et al., 2005; Marshall, 1999). Especially the importance of individual experience, the social construction of meaningful life histories and a critical post-modern position are interpreted as incompatible with what is seen as established positivistic science (Bengtson et al., 2005; Kenyon, Ruth, & Mader, 1999). The discussion of theoretical positions is beyond the scope of the present contribution, but an adequate concept of QoL will have to integrate these approaches—or fail to capture the many facets of quality of "life". A step in this direction is made in Care Keys by distinguishing different sub-models.

As stated earlier, structural models try to describe the specific life situation of a certain group, and often the application of a general model of QoL is questioned. The problem can be seen even within the narrower concept of care-related QoL concerning, for instance, the question whether concepts of homecare and institutional care can use the same model. As Netten (2004) observes, QoL of persons needing care is primarily a result of a social production in the household by the older person and other household members since most older persons live at home. We might add that under changing household structures also persons not actually living in the household might contribute to the production (e.g. the children living in the neighbourhood). Therefore, QoL will be determined by the household situation with homecare making a certain contribution. The content of care-related QoL changes drastically with institutionalisation. Although in homecare we can conceive services as additional support to social household production, in residential care the household itself is essentially substituted. This clearly has—often discussed—consequences for the autonomy of the client and his or her control over the (remaining) activities of daily living. But it also means that the physical and socio-emotional environments constitute important aspects of the overall QoL (and of the quality of care). Moreover, the social and psychological needs are dependent on the institution as a *social* environment, not only a *professional care* environment (see also Tester et al., 2003). Lawton (1994) has been a pioneer in researching the influence of the physical and social environments, and he has also noted that the social dimension is important even in the case of institutional dementia care.

A range of more specific factors appear in the literature (e.g. Baldock & Hadlow, 2002; Bowling, Gabriel, Banister, & Sutton, 2002; Birren et al., 1991; Faulk, 1988; Gerritsen, Steverink, Ooma, & Ribbe, 2004; Hughes, 1990; Tester et al., 2003; Vaarama, Pieper, & Sixsmith, 2007). First, QoL in *homecare* apparently has to be differentiated. When the environment has been diminished to the home, similar features as in institutional care may apply, but those not yet housebound but dependent on other's help appear to have different QoL determinants. Especially self-efficacy, mobility and loneliness turn out to be important factors, and material resources have a substantial influence.

In general, the scope of reasons of variation in QoL can be expected to be larger among the homecare clients than clients living in the institution. Second, QoL of old people in *institutional care* seems to have some very specific determinants. Being able to "be oneself" in terms of gender, ethnicity and cultural values is important. The living environment has to satisfy subjective needs such as having personal objects at the care home, and the spiritual, socio-emotional, cultural and organisational contexts of the institution has to fit to the personal lifestyle. Relationships between staff and residents, continuity of care relations, and being able to communicate verbally or nonverbally are essential, as are responsiveness to frailty (practical help in daily activities) and to emotional needs. Food (variety, choice, proper preparation, good service) has a special importance, and so have the cleanliness of the staff and facilities, but safety and security also play a role in the institutions. Material resources seem not to be as important for persons in the institutions as for those living at home—apparently these are perceived as taken care of in the institution. Subjective QoL in the institutions seems to encompass relational and emotional features of *care* more than that at home—when the environment has been diminished to the institution, one's actual world is also there, and the expectations focus on what happens within its four walls, and how one can express oneself there. This poses a big challenge for the careworkers in the institutions, as well as for care regimes and care concepts. It also has an impact on the concept of care-related QoL, since the literature review has shown that care enters into the life situation quite differently in homecare and institutional care, which is also confirmed by the empirical analyses in Care Keys (see Part III). Still we would argue that the solution should not be to conceptualise a new QoL model for each target group, but rather to develop a generic multi-dimensional model, which allows for the adaptation of domain specifications to the circumstances of particular groups of persons.

The Role of Care and Other Determining Factors

Considering the focus on the role of care and other determining factors raises some issues both in the case of causal models and in the case of the production of welfare models. First, regarding the role of *care*, the previous research gives unstable results: in some studies care has a direct impact on QoL; in others, care has an indirect impact on QoL; and in still others care seems not to have any impact at all. Often the impact seems to be somewhat underlying as statistical analysis does not always reveal it but qualitative analyses do. The Care Keys project based its research on an adaptation of a production of welfare model, where care was seen as an intermediating factor for the QoL of clients, and the target efficiency of care was considered as a method to ensure responsive care and relative equity in distribution of resources (see Chapters 1 and 11). The decision was based on the evidence for the applicability of this type of approach in previous, similar type of research (Vaarama, 2004; Vaarama & Kaitsaari, 2002) and in the model explorations at an early stage of the Care Keys project (Vaarama & Hertto, 2003; Vaarama et al., 2007). The evidence demonstrated a direct connection between care and subjective QoL, but showed also that the subjective QoL was lowest with persons with low economic status, who had deficits in their indoor and outdoor living environments and poor subjective target efficiency of care, that is their expectations were not met.

The standards and requirements for *quality* of care which are assumed for care to have positive effects, and which correspond also to the expectations of the clients are a neglected issue in research. It is care of a certain quality that makes the contribution to the client's QoL, and care quality can vary a lot, and have varying impact on autonomy, competence, self-identity and social and psychological well-being of the client (see Chapter 5). Not only the objective satisfaction of assessed needs by care is important for care-related QoL, but also the degree to which the preferences and expectations of clients are met, thus, measuring also the subjective relevance of a service for the client. In addition, the information the client gets about the services is essential for the client's evaluation of the contribution of care to his or her QoL. Again we might assume here a difference in the expectations in homecare and in institutional care. Among the other determining factors, especially the impact of *life events* seems to be recognized as risk factor for good QoL, and traumatic or negative life events receive more attention in the literature than positive events. This might be due to the prevailing "deficit model" of aging, which neglects the fact that personal growth under the impact of favourable conditions is a possibility in old age (Baltes & Baltes, 1990). It also signals the difficulties of conceptualising and assessing unique events and unexpected changes in the description of QoL. Among the events often experienced as traumatic is the transition from own home to residential care (Tester et al., 2003).

Whereas the systematic role of life events as determining *external* factors may be unproblematic, this is not so clear for the role of care, which may have, as stated earlier, a quite immediate role in the conceptualisation of care-related QoL. The problem can be observed also regarding the role of the client in care as a co-producer of care outcomes. There is a substantial literature on the role of psychological resources in determining the ability to cope with problems and situations. For example, psychological factors such as "resilience" (Staudinger, Freund, Linden, & Maas, 1999), "self-control" (Abeles, 1991) or "perceived control" (Pearlin, Lieberman, Menaghan, & Mullen, 1981) have been introduced to explain why some people appear better able to cope and adapt to everyday life changes. In this case, the *internal* dynamics of the client, and his or her contribution and responsibility for care outcomes are analysed in the causal model. There is a wealth of research on causal models in this perspective (Baltes & Mayer, 1999; Brandstätter & Lerner, 1999; Renwick, Brown, & Nagler, 1996; Schalock & Siperstein, 1996; Vaarama et al., 2007). Actually, we should distinguish two causal approaches: (i) an approach focusing on *objective structural conditions* of certain QoL measures, making a distinction between individual or subjective QoL measurements and socio-economic, cultural, educational and health conditions and standards of living (e.g. social indicators research, Atkinson, Cantillon, Marlier, & Nolan, 2002; Veenhoven, 1996) and (ii) an approach typically focusing on *subjective* QoL and analysing also *intermediate variables*, that is properties of the person mediating QoL as described earlier (e.g. neuroticism, resilience, sense of control). Both approaches tend to adopt narrower concepts of QoL. The objective social indicator and "standard-of-living" approaches usually exclude subjective accounts (at least beyond standardised surveys); the subjective "quality-of-life" approach treats QoL measures as "final outcome" limited to life satisfaction or subjective well-being (Diener, 1994). These causal approaches have the advantage that objective factors and subjective outcomes are measured independently and interpreted in a causal order. But, as we will see, the distinction objective versus subjective qualities of life can create a lot of conceptual confusion. Although it is widely accepted that subjective well-being as reflected in self-reports of a person is an important indicator of QoL, it is not generally agreed that such reports on life satisfaction should have an exclusive status in measuring QoL, or should even be equated with QoL as "final" outcome (see also Davies & Knapp, 1981). Additionally, the theoretical role of intermediate factors as parts of, or conditions of QoL becomes a problem since important properties of the person and his or her life situation (such as the competence to act and make choices, the ownership of the home or being embedded in social relations) do appear only in their subjective perception in the concept of subjective QoL.

A similar problem arises in intervention and production models. This perspective introduces—explicitly or implicitly—a change agency conducting the production which in more reflecting schemes may encompass the client as co-producer. Generally, QoL will appear as a complex product encompassing subjective and objective aspects, which will be analysed with reference to goals and interventions, and, indeed, other goals or products may be intended, for example benefits for informal carers, equity of distribution or other collective social benefits in the production of welfare (Brown & Brown, 2003; Davies & Knapp, 1981; Knapp, 1984, 1995). Domain-specific concepts often have this perspective, like health-related QoL or, in the present case, care-related QoL as a strategy for care quality management. A problem of this approach is connected to the concept of a service. Typically, a service is considered to be external to the (the concept of) QoL; it is an intermediate output in the production of welfare. But in services in general, especially in care services, we have to assume a co-production of care which implies that the services are part of the ongoing daily activities of the client, and the experience of the quality of *care* is an important factor in the quality of *life* of the older person. Actually, this problem is plaguing the application of the very *definition* of quality to QoL. As defined by international standards (ISO), quality is defined as the property of something to satisfy given needs. This applies to services, but QoL is an *end* in itself, and it is not meaningful to speak of life as a *means* to satisfy needs. A concept of QoL of frail older persons will, therefore, have to recognise the role of care as a product or service *and* as an integral feature of the client's life situation. Moreover, current theory and practice emphasise the need for a "holistic" client-centred approach: the professional carers will try to enhance the autonomy and competence of the client (e.g. rehabilitation, support of self-help), they will act as social partners contributing to the social relations (e.g. substituting for missing relatives in giving orientation and meaning), and will influence the psychological well-being of the client (e.g. by taking care of anxieties and depression). Thus, care-related QoL must reflect also the positive and negative effects of care on other dimensions of QoL.

Communication and Negotiation of Care Content and Goals

Considering the meaning of care relatedness as referring to the processes of communication and negotiation of care content and goals, there is a growing body of literature emphasising the importance of the autonomy of the client of strengthening his or her capacities for self-help, and of involvement in the decision-making process in care, even in the case of dementia care (Adams & Gardiner, 2005; Kitwood & Bredin, 1992; Owen & NCHRDF, 2006; Secker, Hill, Villencau, & Parkman, 2003; Tanner, 2001). The person's involvement in the decision-making process on the level of care, on the management level and even on a social policy level (if only through representatives) can have a major impact on the way services are evaluated by the person (satisfaction with services) and in terms of a sense of well-being (Owen & NCHRDF, 2006). Although much of the policy on older people emphasises the promotion of independence, research literature suggests that older people are less likely than other groups to have a say in the care decision process (Hardy, Young, & Wistow, 1999; Secker et al., 2003; Tanner, 2001). Good care and care management need to involve clients in order to make those decisions responsive to perceived needs and to engender a sense of personal involvement, commitment and control over one's own life (Chapters 5 and 6).

Revisiting Three Models of Quality of Life

Lawton's Model of Four Sectors of Good Life

A basic concept in Lawton's theory of QoL (Lawton & Nahemow, 1973) is the idea of a person–environment fit, which assumes that increasing frailty in old age causes significant losses of competence, affecting the ability to perform activities of daily living (I/ADLs), and that the more vulnerable a person is the more supportive the environment should be. The concept reflects the insight that it is not the capabilities of a person or the affordances of the environment as such which determine QoL; it is rather the *relation* between capabilities and environment. Increasing frailty in old age will make persons more vulnerable to the demands of the environment, but environmental support may enable

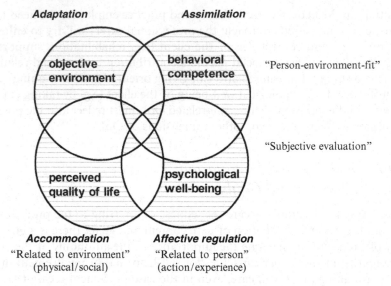

FIG. 4.1. Four sectors of good life (adapted from Lawton, 1991, p. 8).

them to "independent living". Lawton (1991) extended this basic conception further by including subjective evaluation, and describes QoL in terms of four overlapping sub-dimensions or "sectors" of the person–environment system (Fig. 4.1). The concept is explicitly multi-dimensional proposing a "four-dimensional plotting of how the person stands" (p. 12), and rejects one-dimensional concepts. He also argues for the combination of subjective and objective measures, and for a distinction of subjective and socio-political norms of evaluation, since the concept of quality implies some standard of (relative) "goodness". Lawton is not very clear about this but he seems to suggest that the subjective evaluation is applied by the person in his or her own evaluation, whereas socio-political standards are defined and used by other agencies (care systems, politicians) in a social planning context. Davies and Knapp (1981) have interpreted this framework as a *transactional model* incorporating four basic processes or functions of the person system in relation to its environment, namely, accommodation, assimilation, adaptation and affective regulation. When we combine these two approaches we get the following two dimensions of QoL, with both having two sub-dimensions:

1. *Objective "person–environment fit"*

   a. *Behavioural competence*, or the functional capabilities of the person and the potential to develop the capacities (*assimilation*);
   b. *Environment*, or the demands and opportunities of the physical and social circumstances and the potential to select and to change the environment (*adaptation*).

2. Subjective evaluation

a. *Perceived quality of life*, or the person's subjective evaluation of their past, present and future life, of their life circumstances in different life domains and the potential to adjust and to re-evaluate in new life situations (*accommodation*);
b. *Psychological well-being* or the subjective, experiential and emotional well-being, and the potential to adjust and to balance by internal dynamics both positive and negative affect (*affective regulation*).

All four sectors are components of his model of QoL, and he depicts them as overlapping and interdependent, as illustrated in Fig. 4.1. Further, Lawton discusses these sub-dimensions in three different perspectives corresponding to the three meanings of the concept of care relatedness of the Care Keys approach:

1. A general *structural model* with four sectors or sub-dimensions; the life domains combine aspects *within* each dimension depending on the study population, for example frail older people;
2. A "loose" causal model—or *production model*—with (i) the environment referring to conditions, (ii) behavioural competence and perceived QoL as the two central sectors of QoL and as mediating causal complexes and (iii) psychological well-being as "ultimate outcome";
3. A normative model, distinguishing origins of standards, namely, objective and socio-normative standards (competence, environment) and subjective and personal standards (perceived QoL, psychological well-being).

Lawton does not discuss in the context of his model the processes of communication and negotiation involved in normative evaluation; we have to return to this issue later. The causal model is admittedly "loose", and we will suggest that the four basic processes can be used to construct a more differentiated production model. For the structural model of QoL, the four sub-dimensions and their interpretation are crucial, but unfortunately, Lawton is not very clear about their theoretical status. The grouping suggested by Lawton uses two dimensions: objective versus subjective and environment related versus person related (the dimensions and the four processes we have added as a frame to Lawton's own figure). Unfortunately, Lawton makes only the first dimension (objective/subjective) explicit; a distinction of environment versus person is used explicitly only in the "person–environment fit". When Lawton (1991, pp. 8–11) describes the causal model, the four dimensions are, in fact, repeated as aspects of conditions, of intermediate factors and of psychological outcomes. For instance, psychological well-being appears itself as multi-dimensional reproducing the four structural dimensions in the perspective of the evaluating self. In later versions (Lawton, 1997) and in adoptions by other authors (e.g. Davies & Knapp, 1981; Jonker, Gerritsen, Bosboom, & Van der Stehen, 2004) an interpretation is supported which follows the structural model, and identifies its four dimensions through the causal chain, that is in the environmental potentials, in the objective QoL measures and in the subjective QoL measures. Psychological well-being, then, is conceived not as a subjective summarising evaluation (Lawton, 1991, p. 11), but as referring to emotions and moods as "major aspects of the quality of life" (Lawton, 1997, p. 95) with competence, social relations and environmental support included as further aspects. This narrower conceptualisation is introduced, interestingly enough, when Lawton applies the scheme specifically to persons with dementia, for whom a summarising subjective QoL cannot readily be obtained and observed expressions of affective responses have to take their place. This has consequences for the model of QoL, since emotions have to be integrated into the model, and subjective self-reports and evaluations have to be conceptualised in a way that they can be substituted by objective (observed) emotional expressions.

Taking up a lead from Diener (1994), the distinction of subjective versus objective should be understood as a question of *methods* (interviewed self-reports vs. observed self-expressions), and perceived QoL and psychological well-being as designating enduring features of the personality, which can be assessed by both objective and subjective methods. The inclusion of emotions is also proposed by Diener (1994), however, his discussion also shows that this may be in conflict with the concept of QoL. Emotions are typically conceived as situational, short-term psychological states, whereas psychological well-being refers to a more enduring state corresponding to the time horizon of current quality of *life*. Diener is still suggesting to integrate emotions as indicators of QoL describing "hedonic" self-expressions distinguished from cognitive self-reports, but this requires a better grounding in emotion theory than he provides. Theoretical conceptualisations of emotions have identified levels of emotional processes that can be seen as corresponding to levels of action organisation from the lowest level of behavioural operations and "hedonic" emotional responses (Diener) to a middle level of goal-oriented action with corresponding motivations and emotions, to the highest level of structured activities and emotional qualifications of experiences (see Friedlmeier & Holodynsky, 1999; Oerter, 1999). Especially on the third level, we are not only concerned with situational emotional responses (e.g. fear, comfort), or action tendencies (e.g. aggression, attraction), but with more persistent emotional dispositions which "colour" activities of the self and their relation to the physical and social environment (e.g. anxiety, joyful optimism) (Labouvie-Vief, 1999). Social theories of emotions have linked this level of emotions and the regulated triggering of lower emotional levels to social situations (Kemper, 1978) or looked at processes of social construction of emotions and their character as "transitional roles" (Averill, 1986; Harré & van Langenhove, 1999; Pieper, 1995). Thus, lower levels of emotions may be organised and regulated by higher levels, and "emotional intelligence" (Goleman) can even be interpreted as essential for a successful life (Friedlmeier & Holodynski, 1999; Oerter, 1999).

In the present context, we cannot follow these promising linkages to emotion theory, but some observations are relevant. QoL is not only subject to cognitive evaluations, but also to emotional appraisals. These appraisals should not only be seen as situational "hedonic" responses (Diener, 1994), but also as relatively persistent emotional dispositions influencing and focusing activities (Oerter, 1999). Research on emotions over the life span suggests that emotional regulation will change depending on the life history. Emotions may get more differentiated and enriched with personal growth; they may shift from an emphasis on emotions of active involvement to achieving psycho-social well-being; and they may become more selective adjusting to life situations like the loss of a partner and optimising emotional gratification under given conditions (Labouvie-Vief, 1999). Thus, QoL will reflect an "emotionality story" (Kenyon et al., 1999). The four basic processes or sectors of QoL describe relatively persistent structures of activities, for example habits of relating to oneself and the environment, and we would expect them also to regulate (the likelihood of) emotions and, in turn, be influenced by emotional dispositions. The basic processes can be interpreted as coping strategies (see later), and in the course of coping activities lower level emotional responses will vary (e.g. from fear, aggressiveness, relief to joy) depending on the initial problem and the stage of coping actions (Schmidt-Atzert, 1996), but the choice of coping strategies may reflect more general emotional dispositions related to QoL (Labouvie-Vief, 1999).

The relevance of emotion theory for QoL theory is twofold, since emotions can be integrated into the QoL model in different ways:

1. Emotions can be conceived within the context of affective regulation as one of the four basic strategies, and in this perspective achieving emotional or psychological well-being across different emotions and emotional life events constitutes an own dimension of QoL.
2. Emotions can be conceived as differentiated into four basic dimensions corresponding to action strategies such as coping, and in this perspective can be used to substitute self-reports by the analysis of self-expressions accompanying activities.

In the former perspective, following Diener, we should assess the "balance" of psychological well-being not only by subjective self-reports but also by observed emotional self-expressions. In the latter perspective, and following the lead by Lawton, we can substitute the self-reports of persons with dementia by exploiting the relationship of emotions with behavioural strategies both differentiated into "four qualities of life". One task in this perspective is to develop an instrument that relates emotional expressions to QoL of persons with intellectual disabilities. In the Care Keys project one instrument (QUALID; see Weiner, Martin-Cook, Svetlik, Saine, Foster, & Fontain, 2000) has been tested with the encouraging result that a four-dimensional model of emotions (measured by evaluation of observations over a weekly period) could be reproduced for persons with assessed mild and moderated dementia. The dimensions can be interpreted to correspond to the Lawton model, although the validity could not yet be established and awaits further analysis. The analysis (by factor analysis) identified a profile of four emotional dispositions inducing (in terms of Lawton and the WHO profile of subjective QoL):

1. emotions of aggression and irritation—interpreted as frustration of functional behaviour (physical);
2. emotions of comfort or discomfort—interpreted as responses to environmental qualities (environmental);
3. emotions of sadness and unhappiness—interpreted as feelings of psychological well-being (psychological);
4. emotions of joy with contact and interactions—interpreted as social well-being (social).

Clearly, more theoretical and empirical analysis is needed, but the conclusion can already be drawn that the description of QoL should include subjective *and* objective measurement of emotions to assess psychological well-being.

Summarising this discussion of Lawton's model, we recognise his approach as providing a valuable basis for the development of a structural model of QoL, but some clarifications have to be made. Lawton's model needs a framework that: (i) distinguishes between subjective and objective views on *all* aspects of QoL, for example including subjective evaluations of the person–environment fit; (ii) includes emotional aspects in all four dimensions and (iii) allows to apply the four dimensions to different factors in the causal chain (e.g. conditions, perceived life quality, psychological outcomes). The distinction subjective versus objective is certainly relevant, but it does not fit for the "rows" of the structural model (as described in Fig. 4.1). Furthermore, the distinction between environment related and person related has been added for the "columns" by the present authors and still needs a satisfactory interpretation. Since Lawton's approach draws on the tradition of system theory, we should check on system theory for help.

Veenhoven's Model of Four Qualities of Life

A system theoretic perspective is provided by Veenhoven (1996, 2000), who outlines a general conceptual and structural model of QoL to organise the various concepts and measures in various disciplines that are commonly associated with individual well-being or the quality of individual human lives. Veenhoven presents a fourfold taxonomy of QoL, based on two dimensions: (i) life chances and life results and (ii) outer and inner qualities (Table 4.1).

Veenhoven's framework has been applied to the QoL of older people (Vaarama, 2004; Vaarama & Kaitsaari, 2002), and it corresponds well with Lawton's approach. The life chances dimension clearly covers the two "sectors" of person–environment fit, but the life results dimension shows divergence. The "utility of life" does not find a match readily in Lawton's model, while the "appreciation of life" appears to combine both sub-dimensions of "subjective

TABLE 4.1. The "four qualities of life" by Veenhoven (2000).

	Outer qualities (related to environment)	Inner qualities (related to person)
Life chances	*Liveability of the environment*: the external conditions within which the person lives	*Life-ability of the person*: the competence of a person to cope with the problems of life or to exploit its potential
Life results	*Utility of life*: the broader value of the person's life or the meaning that a person's life has for others within the society	*Appreciation of life*: the inner outcomes of life, including subjective well-being, life satisfaction and happiness

evaluation". Reconciling the two models requires looking more closely at their theoretical basis, which has a common ground, since both models start from a view of QoL as being the quality of the person as a *living system* in an *environment*. Both are looking for dimensions of a structural model, and Veenhoven makes the two dimensions explicit, but, unfortunately, Veenhoven does not provide a theoretical derivation of the two dimensions. Veenhoven uses system theory as a heuristic scheme comparing different disciplinary models and extracting common features.

First, considering the dimension "outer" and "inner" qualities, Veenhoven provides a clear interpretation of the "columns" of the model, that is the distinction of system and environment. The problem is that the concept of environment remains ambiguous. The strength of Lawton's person–environment fit model is that it emphasises the *relation* between person and environment, for example when explaining the impact of frailty. "Outer qualities" are not conceived as being out there independently, as Veenhoven describes them, because that would imply we are not talking about the QoL *of a certain person*, but about the environment. It is only the environment in *relation* to the competences *of that person* which is relevant. Correspondingly, the "utility of life" should be related to the person in question; it is not the utility "for others" in a strict sense, as Veenhoven conceives it, that is as "externalities" others and the society get. Clearly, the relevant social context has to be identified, and it will turn out to be difficult in a pluralistic society to point out *who* is included, *which society* we are referring to and *what cultural values* are to be applied. But the decisive point is that benefits *for others* may be important in their own right, and even indirectly enhance the benefits the person receives from others, but these benefits for others are not part of the QoL of the person (see also Davies & Knapp, 1981). The utility refers, rather, to the value a person's life has *for that person* and in *relation* to the social environment *of that person*. Utility is related to the internalised social values, and to the utility attributed to its *own* social identity by the person including of one's life for others. Actually, it is this misconception that leads Veenhoven to all but dismiss this sub-dimension as "typically the playground of philosophers", and not really suitable for empirical concepts of QoL (2000, p. 14). What Veenhoven is losing here is the *social dimension* of a person, the construction and evaluation of a person's life as a social identity incorporating "external" standards. The reason is that Veenhoven operates with a "naturalistic" concept of systems which does not reflect sufficiently the nature of social systems. On the one hand, Lawton is representing this dimension more adequately in his concept of perceived QoL in different life domains, and on the other hand, Veenhoven's approach does emphasise the point that the social identity is essentially related to the social environment.

A strength of Veenhoven's model is the distinction of life chances and life results, constituting the second dimension, and forming a fourfold table when combined with the environment-related/person-related distinction. Lawton's four "circles" are overlapping to indicate interdependence, but they are not theoretically related in an explicit dimensional framework. The second distinction replaces the subjective versus objective dimension, which Veenhoven sees not as central to the model, and it solves the problems Lawton has with applying his model to the case of dementia care. For the missing theoretical foundation we can draw on social systems theory and an analysis of the "human condition" provided by Talcott Parsons (1951, 1978). On the basis of a fundamental analysis of the structure of action, he combines the dimension of external versus internal (in his terms) with the dimension of means versus ends, and develops his well-known fourfold AGIL scheme of social actions and system functions, distinguishing adaptation (efficient resource use), goal attainment (effective achievement), integration (maintenance of solidarity) and latent pattern maintenance (sustenance of values).

In the light of action theory and social system theory,

1. *Life chances* refer to the basic option of orienting towards the world in a *mode of action* and reaction (*means*), with a focus either on activities directed towards the environment, or on developing own capacities. This corresponds also to the distinction of *adaptation* versus *assimilation*.
2. *Life results* refer to the basic option to orient towards the world in a *mode of experience* and evaluation focusing either on *accommodation* to cultural patterns or on *affective regulations*, both seen as *ends* in themselves.

It is important to note that in a system theory framework, "means" and "ends" are—in this context—not considered as cause and effect in a causal chain, but as options for action (see Luhmann, 1984, for further development of this framework). Both means and ends are "valued in their own right" to use the phrase of Davies and Knapp (1981). QoL is achieved by reaching a balance between all four basic processes of assimilation, accommodation, adaptation and affective regulation. Moreover, the fourfold scheme can be applied iteratively on different levels (e.g. action, system) and to differentiate each dimension further. An example is the distinction of four kinds of emotions *within* affective regulation introduced in the previous section. The four processes should be conceived to *interact*, but also to be relatively *independent* from each other—this is Lawton's insight. High demands of the environment are not crucial, if, or as long as the person has high competences; and a person may get along even with frailty, if the environment is supportive rather than demanding (interaction). Or, one person may focus on selection of comfortable non-demanding environments; another person may develop competencies for anticipated, future situations "just to be prepared" (relative independence). The environment is always *related* to the person; many valuable or demanding features of the environment from the perspective of someone else may not be relevant for a person with a certain lifestyle.

If we look again at the distinction of environment related versus person related in this theoretical perspective, we can consider the "internalised" social environment in an analogous way. The perceived QoL in relevant life domains in Lawton's scheme refers essentially to the relations to the social environment of that person, or its *social well-being*—its roles, lifestyle, social values and cultural background constituting a social identity. Environmental relations can, thus, be distinguished according to the kind of environment involved; we have the physical-functional environment of conditions, resources and opportunities in relation to the competences and capacities of the person; and we have the social environment of lifestyles, roles, cultural meanings and values in relation to the commitments, motivations and emotions of the person. Lawton (1997, p. 95) explicitly acknowledges "social quality of life", and distinguishes these social interactions that have the "purpose in themselves" (including interactions of this quality with professional carers) from social support by services and resources (including informal care as a resource). Thus, the distinction of environment related versus person related is suitable for the interpretation of the vertical dimension in Lawton's scheme (Fig. 4.1). It refers to the basic distinction between a system (person) and the environment (of the person), which is also reflected in the way the person perceives oneself and one's life situation. Social well-being can be measured objectively by the involvement in social activities "for their own sake", and subjectively by satisfaction with the social relations or loneliness. The horizontal distinction of person–environment fit versus evaluation has received a more general interpretation of action ("means") versus experience ("ends"), reflecting whether the person looks at life as a valued state, or as having potentials for active involvement (Fig. 4.1).

The distinction of subjective versus objective is not included on the level of the two basic dimensions forming the "four qualities of life", and, actually, it dissolves into a number of quite different issues. First, the subject or person is the *reference point* for the person–environment fit, allowing the identification of person-related aspects and aspects of a selective, related (part of the) environment of that person—in distinction of objective alternative environments of *other* persons or systems. Second, subjective versus objective refers to *ways of access* to information about the person, distinguishing, for example self-reports from self-expressions or observed behaviour. Because of the privileged access a person has to his or her own experience and emotions, self-reports have a central role in the assessment of QoL justifying the special recognition of the concept of subjective QoL. But persons may also deceive themselves and others, report under the influence of biasing factors such as external environmental conditions, social expectations and internal body states (e.g. hunger, fatigue, sexual arousal) or situational emotional states (e.g. fear, discomfort), and revise their evaluation in circumstances more favourable to an "objective" self-report. Moreover, an empathetic observer (e.g. therapist), listening to connotations and reading the body language may, in fact, understand the state of the person better than that person, as they might come to agree. Therefore, even subjective QoL, that is QoL as experienced and reported by the person, should be conceptualised as accessible not only by the person. QoL and subjective QoL are not the same concept, but the latter is part of the former. Objective measures can be obtained and should be used for "improving" (Diener, 1994) or weighting (Cummins, 1997; Felce & Perry, 1997) subjective measures to gain more valid and reliable measures of QoL—and vice versa. This is also the approach taken by Lawton. QoL, in this view, is a theoretical construct referring to a persisting disposition of the person–environment system, which manifests itself in objective and subjective phenomena (see later).

Third, we have to distinguish a different meaning of objective referring to *methods* controlled for validity and reliability versus uncontrolled subjective accounts rendering information usually considered to be less reliable. Even in self-evaluations we might prefer more objective methods (e.g. psychological tests), or to communicate with "objective" others to learn about our personal states and our QoL (see later). Special scales for the assessment of subjective QoL—such as the WHOQOL (Skevington et al., 2004)—try to develop more reliable measurements of QoL through tested and controlled self-reports, containing references to both life domains and emotional dispositions, and, thus, are intended as objective scales to measure subjective evaluations. In the empirical analyses of Care Keys (see Part III), the four special dimensions of the WHOQOL scale—physical/functional, psychological, social, and environmental—could be reproduced and demonstrated to have significance in causal models. The structural model following the leads of Lawton and Veenhoven, therefore, provides a theoretical interpretation for the four dimensions of the WHO model, and the empirical evidence of the Care Keys research supports the validity of the framework.

Finally, what needs to be retained is certainly a normative sense of the client as a "subject" or a "person" to be respected even in view of physical and mental disabilities (see Kitwood, 1997). In this normative sense, a subjective report of the client is "final", and the client status as a subject has to be respected, in our care culture even "counterfactually" in case of progressing dementia. Good care has to respect the client, and the QoL of the client depends on experiencing this respect by others. In principle, the persons or clients themselves have to evaluate what aspects of their lifestyle and life situation are valuable and relevant to them, and, in fact, they have made such evaluations already by choosing a certain lifestyle, by selecting their environment and by developing a certain personality. The analysis of life histories as proposed by narrative gerontology, in fact, suggests the same four dimensions (adding the methodological dimensions of humanistic understanding and critical reflection; see Kenyon et al., 1999, p. 41). This also implies that we have not only to rely on the self-report of persons to assess their explicit and implicit evaluations but can use other methods analysing their life, too. To validate more objective assessments—for instance, observations in case of disabilities or dementia—we should also compare the individual evaluations of QoL by self-reports and self-expressions with evaluations from relevant reference groups (e.g. family members) to make sure that especially the environmental and socio-cultural "fit" is adequate. This strategy places the assessment of QoL in the normative context of the care triad (see later).

Brown's Model of Quality of Life as "Being, Belonging, Becoming"

A model of QoL proposed by Ivan Brown provides a link between QoL theory and the issue of care-related QoL referring to communication and "negotiation of order" in care relations. The model distinguishes between three main domains of life: being–belonging–becoming. It further differentiates these domains into three sub-dimensions, yielding nine (sub-) domains of life (Brown & Brown, 2003, pp. 127–128, Renwick & Brown, 1996):

Being—who a person is

1. Physical being—body and health;
2. Psychological being—thoughts and feelings;
3. Spiritual being—beliefs and values.

Belonging—the people and places in the person's life

1. Physical belonging—the places where the person lives and works;
2. Social belonging—the people in the person's life;
3. Community belonging—the resources in the person's environment.

Becoming—things the person does through life

1. Practical becoming—the practical things done in daily living;
2. Leisure becoming—the things done for fun and enjoyment;
3. Growth becoming—the things done to cope and develop.

Unfortunately, Brown does not provide a theoretical foundation for this model which would help in the interpretation of the dimensions, making it difficult to evaluate the comprehensiveness of the model and to compare it with the four-dimensional framework discussed in the previous sections. In their application of the model to persons with disabilities, Brown and Brown (2003, p. 107) choose a practice-oriented and constructivist approach considering QoL as "a concept that is a social construct...a general idea that we have created because it appears to be useful for enhancing human life". We suggest that the model can, in fact, be interpreted with reference to pragmatic philosophy and basic social theory. A structure of "Firstness" (being), "Secondness" (belonging), and "Thirdness" (becoming) is available in this theoretical background. To visualise the relationships between the three concepts we represent them in a triangle (see left side of Fig. 4.2), which is meaningful because the *relations* between the categories are also significant. The triangle can, then, be interpreted on different levels:

1. On the level of *pragmatic philosophy*, Charles S. Peirce (1931–1935, 1960; Pape, 1989) has developed the categories of "Firstness", "Secondness" and "Thirdness" as basic categories of his evolutionary metaphysics. Without taking up the philosophical discussion in the present context, we note that "Firstness" designates the idea of an immediate phenomenological experience of "Being", "Secondness" designates a relation of reaction and interaction implying a second phenomenon and (in this more general sense) "Belonging" and "Thirdness" introduces a medium of interpretation which in his metaphysics has a fundamental evolutionary character of "Becoming" (or approaching "Truth"). These three categories are applied by Peirce as a fundamental structure to all philosophical analyses. He also demonstrates—for instance, by the distinction of icon, index and symbol in the theory of signs—how the categories can be employed to further differentiate and enrich the triadic distinction to describe more complex phenomena by applying the categories iteratively. As we will see, Brown can be understood as using a quite similar strategy by applying the three dimensions again to each of the three domains. Pragmatic philosophy provides a fundamental interpretation and rationale for this strategy.
2. On the level of *communication*, the triangle helps to distinguish between expressions of signs, semantic meaning of symbols and messages and pragmatic argumentation. *Expressions* are indexical, they identify a concrete existing individual and its experience in "here" and "now". *Meaningful symbols* refer to enduring frames or languages interpreting the message; these meanings must be shared introducing the social dimension. *Arguments* place communication in the context of intentions and interaction where it can be validated (or not) as a successful performance. From the perspective of a communicating actor as conceptualised by G.H. Mead (1934), the triad represents his or her existential experience ("I") versus his or her social identity ("Me") versus his or her self-conscious reflection ("Generalised Other").
3. From the perspective of a *social triad of actors*, the triangle describes the focal role of an actor ("ego") versus the role of the communicating partner ("alter") versus the role of a "third person" validating the communication by acknowledging the authenticity of actors, confirming content of meaning and evaluating compliance with norms or values (or taking sides and enabling coalitions and "majorities") (Georg Simmel, 1950). In this perspective, the triadic structure specifies a frame of roles available to social actors which, at the same time, formulates conditions of valid communication or discourse.

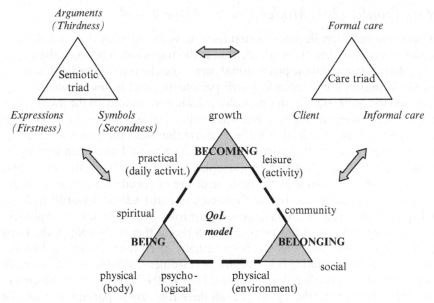

Fig. 4.2. The "being–belonging–becoming" model of quality of life (Brown & Brown, 2003), the triad of semiotics and the care triad.

Without embarking on philosophical argumentation or basic social theory in this context, we "shortcut" the argument on the relation between the semiotic triangle and Brown's QoL model by arranging his *list* of dimensions and sub-dimensions in a set of *triangles* (see centre of Fig. 4.2).

In this triadic structure, the nine sub-dimensions receive an interpretation by their affinity to the main corners or by their place on the connecting relations (e.g. practical becoming is related to being, leisure becoming is related to belonging, physical belonging (environment) is related to being, etc.). Then, we recognise that the small triangles (one for each dimension) repeat the same fundamental logic: "being" is considered as "belonging" (related) and reflected from a third perspective of "becoming" (either personal values or community culture or developmental growth). Actually, this organisation of the concepts suggests some modifications in the descriptions provided by Brown, induced also by the Lawton model and giving his model more theoretical precision. Physical belonging refers to a person's *relation* to his or her living and working environment and its resources; social belonging refers to a person's personal social relations; community refers to a person's socio-cultural context; becoming refers not only to "things done" but done *for good reasons*, making QoL an achievement in an ongoing process. This arrangement also suggests the triad as a general model or "grammar" of the existential situation of persons, of communication and of social interactions or systems, and testifies for the comprehensiveness of the framework and its applicability to the structure of QoL.

The Triadic QoL Model and the Care Triad

Taking the basic triadic model a step further, we can identify this triangle in (a general model of) the "care triad", that is the relationship between the client, the informal carer and the professional carer. The client will interpret his or her needs (being) in communication with persons relevant to his or her (belonging) and the professional carer provides guidance (reflection) in the process (see Fig. 4.2). Looking at QoL not as a static entity, but as a *process* of experience, communication and reflection make us aware that this process is a social process and that relevant other partners are necessary to find one's own identity or QoL. The sociologist and social philosopher Georg Simmel (1950) was the first to analyse the social triad as the basic structure of social relations, and—more recently—it is used for analysis in the theory of care (Adams & Gardiner, 2005; Chapters 5 and 6). Simmel distinguished the roles of "moderator", "exploiter" or "oppressor" for the third person, and in recent theory the role of the third person in conflict situations has been actually given more attention than the mediating and moderating role (Adams & Gardiner, 2005; Biggs, Phillipson, & Kingston, 1995; Corbin & Strauss, 1988; Pieper, 1997; Strauss, 1978; Strauss et al., 1963). But for the theory of QoL all three roles are important. In fact, the social triad can be interpreted as a "micro-discourse", that is as the basic triadic structure of a discourse designed to discuss a theme, to reach a consensus and to overcome conflict. When we focus on *successful* communication—in the search for understanding of QoL and for reflection on visions of the "good life", which can be validated with reference to science and/or shared social values—the moderator role is employed. However, conflicts, dependencies, power and differences of interests are also important aspects of care settings (Jochimsen, 2003; Chapter 6), and we will return to this issue.

Considering the concept of care-related QoL, we realise that "care-related" also refers to the fact that the client alone cannot really reach a sense of meaningful quality in his or her life without the communication and support of others, which assures that the personal vision can not only be experienced (Firstness), but can be *shared* with others as part of his or her social identity (Secondness), and can be *validated* as gained in an "unbiased", reflected process (Thirdness). The aspect of a shared vision refers especially to the definitions of needs and adequate ways of their satisfaction in relation to a personal lifestyle. The aspect of validation plays a prominent role in care theory and social work in establishing the reality and value base of visions of life quality. Theoretical approaches to communication like Symbolic Interactionism (except G. H. Mead), Constructivism and dialogue theories often fail to recognise that validation essentially has a triadic structure. In cases of misunderstanding in the communication and asymmetry or dependency in the interaction, we have to rely on a "third person" to mediate, either virtually by invoking shared values as binding at least in the given situation, or practically by calling upon someone for help we both can trust (for carers and managers as "third persons"; see Chapter 6). Therefore, we suggest the care triad as a *normative model* to critically analyse and practically implement processes of communication and reflection—or "discourses"—on QoL in care settings.

The theoretical fruitfulness of the basic triangle is supported by additional observations demonstrating that the social triad can be seen as a basic structure applicable to the theoretical framework of Care Keys, namely, the stakeholder perspectives in care (see Chapter 1) and the structural model of QoL based on environmental system theory, as discussed earlier.

First, the three perspectives of the triad can be related to the perspectives of main stakeholders in the context of quality of care (client/staff/informal carer; see Chapter 5) and in the context of quality management (client/staff/manager; see Chapter 6). The triad provides a basic structure for the "negotiation of order", not only for agreement, but also for conflict and change by specifying roles for stakeholders. The "negotiated order" does not just happen, it has to be achieved in a critical process recognising the legitimate interests of all parties involved. In as much as this negotiation does not occur, we have reason to doubt the validity of the communication and, in the present context, the definition of QoL in use. Thus, critical social theory enters the model of QoL when we realise that "Becoming" is not just life history unfolding and narrated. It is also about "unlived life", about "what has not been or the road not chosen" (Kenyon et al., 1999). It is about why a preferred life is not possible, and it is about authenticity, normativity and truth—the central concepts of the social philosophy of Jürgen Habermas, again mirroring the triangle.

Second, the theoretical link with the structural model might have already occurred to the reader, since inspection of Brown's model shows that the basic dimensions of QoL as distinguished in the structural model—physical, psychological, environmental, social—appear at the base of the triangle (in the terminology of the WHO concept of QoL, and as employed in the Care Keys research). The "four qualities of life" (Veenhoven) correspond to a system in balance in all four dimensions (see Fig. 4.1). The system—in view of the triangle—describes a structural model without "Becoming", disregarding growth and potentials for change and collapsing the other sub-dimensions (practical with physical/spiritual with psychological/community with physical environment/leisure activities with social relations). This we would expect in a *structural* model, and it reminds us of the alleged lack of a concept of change in social system theory (a questionable criticism often directed against Talcott Parsons). Note also that the two main dimensions of the structural model (person-environment-fit vs evalution/person vs environment) can be interpreted in view of their different relations to "Being" and "Belonging" (e.g. evaluation combines psychological and social). Without discussing the theoretical implications, we draw attention to the fact that the triangle offers two alternatives for a fourfold scheme:

1. on the axis "being–becoming" without "belonging";
2. on the axis "belonging–becoming" without "being".

The essentially "existentialistic" approach generated by the elimination of social "Belonging" collapsing the other sub-dimensions (physical environment with body/psychological with spiritual/leisure with practical activities/social change with personal growth) renders itself readily to interpretation. Correspondingly, the vision of a sociology eliminating the "Being" of concrete individuals in the concept of role and collapsing the other sub-dimensions (psychological with social/physical with social environment/practical with leisure activities/spiritual with cultural change) appears as the third option underlying, for example constructivist positions. Moreover, Lawton's approach of environmental psychology and gerontology, in this scheme, is identified as a basically "naturalistic" framework. Clearly, a comprehensive social theory and a comprehensive model of QoL have to encompass all three axes including "Becoming". Certainly, the reconstruction of theoretical approaches from the basic triadic model requires more careful analyses than these suggestions provide, but it would be interesting to follow up the relation to more differentiated system theories (e.g. Luhmann, 1984) and to "humanistic" approaches (e.g. the theory of "gerontranscendence"—see Bengtson et al., 2005; Torstam, 1996 to capture more aspects of "Becoming".

In the Care Keys approach to QoL, we chose to represent the issues in three models: (i) the structural model yields four dimensions of life quality; (ii) the production model introduces the concepts of agency, change and "final" outcomes (to be considered in more detail later) and (3) the normative model deals with problems of negotiation and openness for criticism.

Towards a Model of Care-Related Quality of Life

To summarise the reflections on three models of QoL, we note that the concept of care-related QoL is serving three functions constituting three sub-models:

1. As a descriptive or *structural model*, the concept refers to dimensions of the life of frail or care-dependent older people which have to be considered to evaluate comprehensively, and to measure adequately the quality in domains of life of this particular group.
2. As a *production model*, the concept orders the elements of QoL in relation to the impact that care and other conditions, including the role of the client, are expected to have on different elements of QoL, including effects due to the inherent dependencies in care and the production chain.
3. As a *normative model*, the concept makes aware of the process of communication and negotiation in the care triad, which generates and validates definitions and values of QoL in care settings.

A generic and comprehensive theoretical model has to assure that the structural sub-model covers all relevant dimensions of QoL and gives adequate weights (e.g. in terms of subjective relevance, utility or money equivalence); the production sub-model has to guide in the evaluation of factors as external conditions, intermediate or process factors or as "final outcomes" in a controlled process; the normative sub-model has to provide a strategy for the "negotiation of order", for example the agreement on concepts, value criteria and their measurement in practice. Moving towards a comprehensive model of care-related QoL we would like to further specify the structure and role of the three sub-models.

The Normative Model and Methodological Issues

Looking at the normative sub-model, it should be emphasised that it not only introduces normative "discourse" into the model, but also some basic guidelines for methodologies to achieve validity and reliability (in this respect reminding of the critical "logic of research" of Karl Popper). Here we want to point out that there is a systematic connection between: (i) a "critical discourse" about values unavoidably involved in the concept of quality; (ii) representing "third views" of all stakeholders and (iii) the "triangulation" of different strategies and methods to combine subjective and objective measures and to develop multi-dimensional models relying essentially on expert judgement (compare Brown & Brown, 2003). The Care Keys model of QoL includes, therefore, the additional feature of "negotiation of order" in the care triad and in quality management to give at least some conceptual basis and practical guidance to the solution of the combination and valuation problems. On the level of methods, the assessment of QoL information from different sources, especially from different perspectives in the care triad, is a prerequisite that was also addressed in the development of the Care Keys instruments (Chapter 13).

The measurement of QoL poses not only conceptual and methodological problems for the researcher, but also for the practitioner, and—most important—for the person. Evaluating one's life is not easy. The assessment has to solve implicitly or explicitly information problems (current state of self and of reference group); time problems (adequate "time window" for the assessment vs. "snap shot"); social group selection problems (previous/new/other reference group); situational problems (e.g. influences of current moods, events, other persons, environments); interaction problems between domains (e.g. health influence on social participation) and valuation problems (adequate personal aspirations, social group values). Simply to take a report by a person as "final" just means that we neglect the processes involved and do not take the person seriously. Not only in care settings, but also in "normal" social interactions we have to assume that a person seeks as much confirmation of a somewhat tentative assertion of his or her QoL as he or she is making a "final" judgement. By communicating with the older person, carers—both professional and informal—can help to clarify the state of a person: (i) in comparison with other frail older persons ("I am satisfied, since I am still better off than other people in my situation"); (ii) as influenced or not by current affects ("After a good night's sleep I will feel better"); (iii) as essentially in accordance with general life satisfaction ("The present difficulties I will overcome as I did before") and (iv) as to be expected or accepted under changing circumstances ("Now being in an institution I have to find new meaningful activities and new friends among the residents").

The assessment processes need *communication* to assure that the view on a personal QoL can be shared (even when the person itself cannot participate anymore). It needs *validation*, which means that it should be reflected in the care triad introducing a "third view", and it needs support to assure that a person does not choose inadequate coping strategies (e.g. "learned helplessness", resignation, lowering self-esteem, withdrawal). The importance of the social process of assessment implies that whenever possible a comprehensive and intensive procedure (including qualitative methods) should be preferred, and that in care settings there is a responsibility of caring persons to promote the competence and to create the context that enables reflections on the QoL and the development of adequate concepts and values of quality. After all, QoL is not only assessed in the context of care, but important decisions about further care are made. The care relationship and the dependency of the client imply an asymmetry of knowledge, power and resources, suggesting that the care triad is also employed as a conceptual and practical model in promoting reflection, empowerment and advocacy (see Chapters 5 and 6).

The care triad is essentially a normative model that should guide the development of communication and empowering practices that can solve, at least for practical purposes, the problems of combining information from objective and subjective sources and from different participants in the care triad, and problems of establishing personal and group values. The model is normative, since it does not assume that communication and discourse in care triads always function in the desired ways. It is obvious that in care settings we find also relationships of exploitation and oppression in Simmel's terms rather than of support, moderation and empowerment. The model is also a conceptual link to the model of quality of care, since it describes "good" care practices as an element of a concept of care-related QoL (see Chapter 5). The model also emphasises that the responsibility for the development of adequate values for quality judgements on life and care has to rest with the persons involved in the care process. In the literature we often find a misguiding distinction between, on the one hand, subjective evaluations of persons that just have to be taken as authentic and descriptively adequate, and, on the other hand, social policy values that have to be considered as given frame conditions and should guide the evaluation of objective indicators (e.g. Cummins, 1997; Lawton, 1991). Both are then to be combined in a comprehensive assessment of a person's QoL—but the questions are unanswered, by whom and how the combination should be made, and what procedure will guarantee the acceptance of the assessment in practice. The care triad as a normative model emphasises that these procedures have to be implemented and supported in practices of good care. There is certainly more to be said about these procedures, the refinement of methods and adequate practices of assessing and evaluating QoL. Some further considerations can be found in other chapters on the theoretical framework (Chapters 1, 5 and 6); a good and comprehensive guidance is also provided by Brown and Brown (2003) for a specific social group, that is persons with disabilities. But the normative model as sketched out is intended to provide a critical link between the issues of evaluation implied in the concept of quality, on the one hand, and the structural model and production model, on the other hand.

The Production Model and Causal Models

Looking at the production model, two causal relationships should be distinguished: (i) the causal chains linking conditions to outcomes and (ii) the internal dynamics that cope with influences of the environment and strive to realize the person's QoL. Considering the internal dynamics, the insight is important that activities in coping with the environment are, in fact, regulations of "autonomous action tendencies", that is actions on physiological and behavioural action *tendencies* triggered by the environment (see Skinner, 1999). The environment is available to the person only through its *causal involvement in a relevant environment* with which the person can cope by controlling its own (re-)actions. In this sense, the environment is already "in" the person. As we know from child psychology, the person has to learn to distinguish between itself and *its* environment. This primary causal involvement constitutes an important aspect of the "Firstness" in our relation to the environment (see earlier).

As already stated when discussing the role of emotions, we assume a hierarchy of control of cognitive *and* emotional levels, which constitute the relative autonomy of the person. The importance of a sense of control for QoL suggests integrating coping theory or resilience theory into the production model. It has been applied to older persons with frailty describing QoL as the outcome of different coping strategies (Brandstätter & Renner, 1990; Filipp & Klauer, 1991; Labouvie-Vief, 1999; Pearlin et al., 1981; Ryff, 1989; Rutter, 1995; Staudinger et al., 1999). The aim guiding this research is the identification of processes that maintain or recover a person's normal functioning level or psychological balance in response to impacts from the environment (environmental conditions, risk factors, traumatic events). The basic processes of maintaining QoL in Lawton's model already correspond to the basic options in coping theory, and can be grouped into the framework of the structural model giving an additional interpretation to the four sub-dimensions: *adaptation*—coping by adjusting the utilisation of resources and selecting environments; *assimilation*—coping by developing abilities and health; *accommodation*—coping by redefining social identity and adopting new values and *affective regulation*—coping by finding a new emotional balance (e.g. optimistic/pessimistic). A person's QoL depends on adjusting (more or less) successfully in these four dimensions to his or her life circumstances, and this achievement should be represented in a four-dimensional profile (with further differentiations of the dimensions by domains of life if meaningful for specific purposes).

The group of special interest in our context are frail or care-dependent older persons, and an important feature of their QoL is the fact that it is strongly determined by the role of care in (potentially) all dimensions and domains of their life. Care will have the function of providing an extra "buffer" supporting the resilience capacities of the client. The general model makes it possible to incorporate care into the structural model as a "frame" using the same dimensions (see Fig. 4.4), but it can also be introduced as an own factor into the production model. Considering the causal chain from conditions to outcomes, we suggest a production model that combines two *interacting chains* for care-related QoL (Fig. 4.3). Focusing on care, a chain is formed by conditions of clients and risks for disablement, care interventions, perceived care and observed well-being. Focusing on the client, a chain is formed by his or her life events and informal support, his or her resilience and his or her subjective well-being. Emotional behaviour may be further differentiated as discussed earlier to substitute self-reports (e.g. in case of dementia). The feedback effects and the relative impact of specific factors along the causal chains have to be identified by research, for example effects of institutional versus homecare settings as indicated in the literature review earlier, and investigated in the Care Keys research (Part III). It should be noted that a lot of fruitless discussions about (external) conditions versus constitutive factors of QoL can be avoided by acknowledging that this distinction depends on the research perspective. In a structural model we might like to include relevant aspects of the environment into the model of QoL, whereas in a causal production model we might distinguish conditions because of their (often only assumed) independent causal impact.

A strength of Veenhoven's model and its interpretation by social systems theory becomes apparent in the production model, that is that it specifies a *general model of quality dimensions of systems*, and opens up avenues to describe and compare different phenomena and theoretical frameworks (physical, psychological, social, political, economical, technological systems).

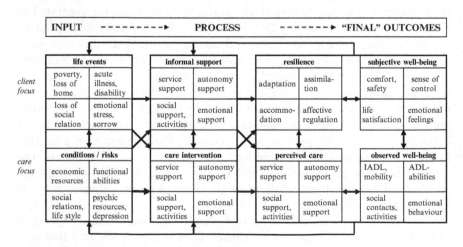

Fig. 4.3. The production model of quality of life.

The same four dimensions can, in principle, be applied to conditions, events, care interventions, coping strategies and subjective and observed outcomes including emotions (corresponding dimensions are located in the same position in the fourfold "boxes" in Fig. 4.3; characterising each dimension by an own colour—see Chapter 13—helps to identify the four dimensions along the production chain). The general model also provides bridges for the change of system reference without change of the generic quality model, for instance, in a hierarchical structure of clients, care interactions and care systems (see Fig. 4.4). The—at least heuristic—value of the four-dimensional framework across systems is the reason that the Care Keys approach prefers it on a more applied and practical level to the nine-dimensional Brown model. The advantage of this approach may be seen when comparing, for instance, the application of QoL to the level of the family by Brown and Brown (2003, p. 182). The comprehensiveness of their framework is lost, presumably, because it is too complex to handle in their practical approach, when they change to the reference system of the family. In the Care Keys project we explore the application of our quality model not only to QoL, but also to quality of care and quality of management (Chapters 5 and 6).

A Comprehensive Structural Model

The structural model can be conceptualised in a way representing all important features of the care-related QoL model (Fig. 4.4). The general four-dimensional framework makes it possible to depict an "onion model"

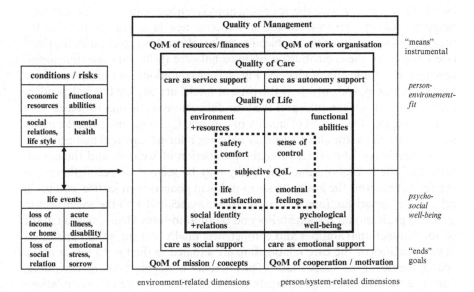

FIG. 4.4. The structural model of care-related quality of life.

of different layers involving the main stakeholders in the care setting. At the centre of the model, we find QoL as subjectively experienced in four dimensions; at the second layer QoL is represented in its behavioural involvement into the environment, and as observable by others in corresponding dimensions; on the third level we find care as a supporting frame addressing with its own four-dimensional structure the "four qualities of life" and finally, care management can be seen as the fourth layer, "setting the stage" for client-oriented care in the same dimensions based on social system theory. The model, thus, incorporates also important results of the theoretical discussion on the structure of quality of care and quality of management in the Care Keys project, which also can be conceptualised by a four-dimensional model (see Chapters 5 and 6). The model allows for easy and consistent orientation; aspects of resources and environmental support (adaptation) are always in the upper left hand sector; aspects of functional abilities, competence and autonomy (assimilation) are in the upper right hand sector; aspects of social relations, social identity and social values or value concepts (accommodation) are in the lower left hand sector; and aspects of emotions, psychological well-being, solidarity, trust and cooperation (affective regulation) are in the lower right hand sector. This "onion" with four sectors does not imply that causal chains run only within or along the same dimensions. This is clearly not the case as empirical analyses, for example in Care Keys, demonstrate. Basically, all factors can be expected to interact across layers and research has to discover the most relevant effects. The "onion" gives structure to the landscape of qualities in the care settings, and as the empirical analyses of the Care Keys project show, the four-dimensional structure can be detected also in the empirical results and even be demonstrated to have significance in explanatory modelling (see Part III). Moreover, the four-dimensional model can be employed as a heuristic strategy to introduce and to structure new layers or "frames" to the model, for instance, the QoC (subjective quality of care) as perceived by the client (see Chapter 5), the contribution of informal care (following the dimensions specified for care in the model; see Fig. 4.3) or conditions and life events from the production model, which in the present model are depicted as independent factors. Finally, we can interpret the four dimensions as themes for basic "discourses" negotiating aspects of quality of care and QoL and involving the major stakeholders, that is the client, professional carer, informal care and management, in different ways. The issues of social production of welfare, and the contribution of the household and the family may be seen as a special theme for the resource sector; the issues of socio-political goals (social justice, equity) in relation to the satisfaction of client needs are associated with the social sector; issues of professional responsibility and client autonomy clearly belong in the sector of functional abilities and competence; finally, the emotional and inter-action qualities of the care relationship are situated in the fourth sector and a special theme for the "care triad". The reference to negotiation and discourses connects the structural model again to the triadic structure of care relations involving also care management as a partner (see Chapter 6).

Summary

The concept of care-related QoL suggested three different meanings of "care relatedness". The first interpretation starts with the identification of the group receiving care, namely, frail and vulnerable older persons, and asks for a systematic concept or model of their needs. Three models of QoL by Lawton, Veenhoven and Brown were discussed and especially evaluated with respect of their comprehensiveness including dimensions covering all relevant aspects of life quality. The discussion resulted in a *structural model* of crQoL providing a framework of "four qualities of life". The essential features are that: (i) a model of subjective QoL or subjective well-being is incorporated in a more comprehensive model of QoL that allows for subjective and objective measures and (ii) the inclusion of care relations as a "frame" or "layer" of influences of care using the same general dimensions ("onion model"; see Fig. 4.4). With increasing dependency of the client (e.g. with the movement from homecare to institutional care) we expect care to become more and more an integral part of the relevant environment of the client. Thus, care relationships increasingly will be part of the QoL of the client and cannot be substituted by other relations. Additionally, the impact of socio-economic conditions and life events and risks are included as influences on the need for care, again using the same four-dimensional framework. An interpretation of the four-dimensional structure in the framework of social system theory, moreover, makes it possible to employ the dimensions as a heuristic device to add new "layers" to the "onion model", for example to introduce perceived quality of care by the client, or aspects of care management as additional influences included in the concept of care-related QoL.

The second sub-model is a *production model* with a focus on the causal relations implicit in care interventions (Fig. 4.3). This model highlights the role of the capacities of the client to cope with the conditions and events creating the need for care, and his or her capacity to make use of support from others, especially from care interventions. Care interventions in this perspective produce higher levels of coping capabilities in all four dimensions of QoL. Two interacting causal chains are focusing on the care and the client. They produce enhanced subjective QoL as experienced and communicated by the client (in self-reports or self-expressions), and observed or assessed by others with (more or less) objective methods. The distinction between subjective communications and observed QoL measures recognises the fact that especially in situations of intellectual disabilities (e.g. dementia) the capacities for communication are impaired and capacities of resilience will decrease. Thus, the carer has to rely on some form of observation and seek even support of advocacy and professional supervision. A special feature of the production model is that the same general four dimensions of the structural model are also applied to conditions, life events, care and informal support. This does not include the assumption that impacts will only arise between elements of a corresponding dimension (e.g. the life event "social loss" will have not only an impact on social aspects such as social support, accommodation, life satisfaction and social contacts, but also, for instance, on sense of control). The dimensions have the function to assure that all relevant aspects or domains are considered, even when they might not be relevant in a particular case.

The *normative model* addresses especially three issues. First, it makes aware of the fact that the views on QoL in practice are not only subjective appraisals, but also "social constructions" which arise in the interaction of the partners in the care setting, and necessarily involve normative standards of "goodness". Thus, the content of crQoL is seen essentially as generated in communication and as an element of the "negotiation of order" in care relationships. The three main partners are the client, the professional carer and the informal carer, together forming the "care triad". The three roles can be occupied by varying persons in a specific case, but the *normative* function of the model emphasises that the care setting has to satisfy certain conditions: the possibility to express authentically needs and preferences, the development and communication of shared views on QoL and the validation and evaluation of visions of QoL. The care triad provides the structure for a "minimum discourse", it allows for three persons to share the three roles implicit in critical reflection or, in this case, in the "negotiation of order" in the care setting. It combines three different stakeholder perspectives, and if each person is able to "take the role of the other", they can pursue validity, reliability and practicality concerning the descriptive content of QoL and the application of personal and social group values in the assessment of QoL.

Second, the care triad is characterised by the relative dependency of the client (otherwise he or she would not need care). This dependency raises issues of empowerment, and makes it necessary that the relationships in care can be viewed and evaluated from a "third person" perspective. This concerns all three relations in the care triad which may be subject to exploitation or oppression; also the client may be in a position to exploit, for instance, a spouse. In moving from homecare to institutional care and to intensive care we expect that the dependency increases and the "locus of control" shifts from the client to the informal carer, and then to the professional carer, and—with diminishing capacities of the client—he or she will not be able to play his or her role anymore, and an advocate has to be introduced to assure a functioning triad. The normative model of the care triad does not deny that essentially it is the person's own evaluation of his or her QoL that has to be respected, nor does it preclude the external evaluation of QoL of individuals or social groups from a comparative and social policy perspective, but it makes clear that his or her own judgements are generated on the basis of communication with others, and need support and validation in a process of critical assessment, communication and negotiation. External evaluations might fail to adequately represent the evaluation that would be produced in a "good practice" of communication and interaction of the client with the persons directly concerned and involved in the care relationships.

Finally, the common theoretical foundations of the concept of life quality and the care triad make us aware that the four-dimensional framework proposed in the crQoL model reflects a theoretical choice for a structural approach and a "naturalistic" approach in the tradition of Lawton, which will tend to neglect dimensions of change, innovation and production of welfare. The four-dimensional model was chosen because of its capacity to accommodate also aspects of quality of care and quality of management into the "onion model". However, keeping the triadic QoL model of "Being", "Belonging" and "Becoming" proposed by Brown as a more general model makes it possible to interpret the model in the light of basic social theory and pragmatic social philosophy and, thus, introduces critical discourse, growth and development into the concept of crQoL, and opens avenues to include alternative frameworks such as humanistic or constructivist theories in gerontology.

References

Abeles, R. P. (1991). Sense of control, quality of life, and frail older people. In J. Birren, J. Lubben, J. Rowe, & D. Deutchman (Eds.), *The concept of measurement of quality of life in frail elders*. San Diego, CA: Academic Press.

Adams, T., & Gardiner, P. (2005). Communication and interaction within dementia care triads. *Dementia, 4*(2), 185–205.

Atkinson, T., Cantillon, B., Marlier, E., & Nolan, B. (2002). *Social indicators. The EU and social inclusion*. Oxford: Oxford University Press.

Averill, J. R. (1986). The acquisition of emotions during adulthood. In R. Harré (Ed.), *The social construction of emotions* (pp. 98–118). Oxford: Blackwell.

Badlock, J. C., & Hadlow, J. (2002). Self-Talk versus Needs-Talk: an exploration of the priorities of housebound older people. *Quality in Ageing, 3*(1), 42–48.

Baltes, P. B., & Baltes, M. M. (1990). Psychological perspectives on successful aging: The model of selective optimization with compensation. In P. B. Baltes, & M. Baltes (Eds.), *Successful aging. Perspectives from the behavioural sciences*. Cambridge, MA: Cambridge University Press.

Baltes, P. B., & Mayer, K. M. (Eds.). (1999). *The Berlin Aging Study*. Cambridge, MA: Cambridge University Press.

Bengtson, V. L., Putney N. M., & Johnson, M. L. (2005). The problem of theory in gerontology today. In M. L. Johnson (Ed.), *The Cambridge handbook of age and ageing*. Cambridge, MA: Cambridge University Press.

Biggs, S., Philipson, S., & Kingston, P. (1995). *Elder abuse in perspective*. Buckingham: Open University Press.

Birren J., Lubben J., Rowe J., & Deutchman D. (Eds.). (1991). *The concept of measurement of quality of life in frail elders*. San Diego, CA: Academic Press.

Bowling, A., Gabriel, Z., Banister, D., & Sutton, S. (2002). Adding quality to quantity: Older people's views on their quality of life and its enhancement. Research Findings 7, Growing Older Project. <http://www.shef.ac.uk/uni/projects/gop/Bowling_F7.pdf>

Brandstätter, J., & Lerner, R. M. (Eds.). (1999). *Action and self-development. Theory and research through the life span*. Thousand Oaks, CA: Sage.

Brandstätter, J., & Renner, G. (1990). Tenacious goal pursuit and flexible goal adjustment: Explication and age-related analysis of assimilative and accommodative strategies of coping. *Psychology and Aging, 5*(1), 58–67.

Brown, I., & Brown, R. I. (2003). *Quality of life and disability. An approach for community practitioners*. New York: Kingsley.

Corbin, J. M., & Strauss, A. L. (1988). *Unending work and care: Managing chronical illness at home*. San Francisco, CA: Wiley.

Cummins, R. A. (1997). Assessing quality of life In R. I. Brown (Ed.), *Quality of life for people with disabilities. Models, research and practice*. Cheltenham: Stanley Thornes.

Davies, B., & Knapp, M. (1981). *Old people's homes and the production of welfare*. London: Routledge & Kegan Paul.

Diener, E. (1994). Assessing subjective well-being: Progress and opportunities. *Social Indicators Research, 31*, 103–157.

Faulk, L. (1988). Quality of life factors in board and care homes for the elderly: A hierarchical model. *Adult Foster Care Journal, 2*, 100–117.

Felce, D., & Perry, J. (1997). Quality of life: The scope of the term and its breadth of measurement. In Roy I. Brown (Ed.), *Quality of life for people with disabilities: Models, research and practice*. London: Stanley Thornes.

Filipp, S.-H., & Klauer, T. (1991). Subjective well-being in the face of critical life events: The case of successful copers. In F. Strck, M. Argyle, & N. Schwarz (Eds.), *Subjective well-being: An interdisciplinary perspective* (pp. 213–234). Oxford: Pergamon Press.

Freund, A. M., Li, K. Z. H., & Baltes, P. B. (1999). Successful development and aging: The role of selection, optimization, and compensation. In J. Brandstätter, & R. M. Lerner (Eds.), *Action and self-development. Theory and research through the life span* (pp. 401–434). Thousand Oaks, CA: Sage.

Friedlmeier, W., & Holodynski, M. (Eds.). (1999). *Emotionale Entwicklung. Funktion, Regulation und soziokultureller Kontext von Emotionen*. Heidelberg: Spektrum Akademischer Verlag.

Gerritsen, D., Steverink, N., Ooms, M., & Ribbe, M. (2004). Finding a useful conceptual basis for enhancing the quality of life of nursing home residents. *Quality of Life Research, 13*, 611–624.

Gubrium, J. F. (1993). *Speaking of life: Horizons of meaning for nursing home residents*. New York: Aldine de Gruyter.

Hardy, B., Young, R., & Wistow, G. (1999). Dimensions of choice on the assessment and care management process: The views of older people, carers and care managers. *Health and Social Care in the Community, 7*, 483–491.

Harré, R., & van Langenhove, L. (Eds.). (1999). *Positioning theory*. Oxford: Blackwell.

Hughes, B. (1990). Quality of life. In S. Peace (Ed.), *Researching Social Gerontology*. London: Sage.

Jochimsen, M. A. (2003). *Careful economics. Integrating caring activities and economic science*. Boston, MA: Kluwer Academic Publishers.

Jonker, C., Gerritsen, D. L., Bosboom, P. R., & Van der Stehen, J. T. (2004). A model for quality of life measures in patients with dementia: Lawton's next step. *Dementia and Geriatric Cognitive Disorders, 18*, 159–164.

Kenyon, G. M., Ruth, J.-E., & Mader, W. (1999). Elements of a narrative gerontology. In V. L. Bengtson, & K. W. Schaie (Eds.), *Handbook of theories of aging*. New York: Springer.

Kemper, T. D. (1978). *A social interactional theory of emotion*. New York: Wiley.

Kitwood, T. (1997). *Dementia reconsidered: The person comes first*. Buckingham: Open University Press.

Kitwood, T., & Bredin, K. (1992). Towards a theory of dementia care: Personhood and well-being. *Ageing and Society, 12*, 269–287.

Knapp, M. (1984). *The economics of social care. Studies in social policy.* Hong Kong: Macmillan Education.

Knapp, M. (1995). *The economic evaluation of mental health care.* PSSRU. CEMH, Aldershot.

Labouvie-Vief, G. (1999). Emotions in adulthood. In V. L. Bengtson, & K. W. Schaie (Eds.), *Handbook of theories of aging* (pp. 253–267). New York: Springer.

Lawton, M. P. (1983). Environment and other determinants of well-being in older people. *The Gerontologist, 4*, 349–357.

Lawton, M. P. (1991). A multidimensional view of quality of life in frail elders. In J. Birren, J. Lubben, J. Rowe, & D. Deutchman (Eds.), *The concept of measurement of quality of life in frail elders* (pp. 3–27). San Diego, CA: Academic Press.

Lawton, M. P. (1994). Quality of life in Alzheimer disease. *Alzheimers Disease and Associated Disorders, 8*, 138–150.

Lawton, M. P. (1997). Assessing quality of life in Alzheimer disease research. *Alzheimer Disease and Associated Disorders, 11*(6), 91–99.

Lawton, M. P., & Nahemow, L. (1973). Ecology and the aging process. In C. Eisdorfer, & M. P. Lawton (Eds.), *The psychology of adult development and aging.* Washington DC: American Journal of Psychology Association.

Luhmann, N. (1984). *Soziale Systeme. Grundriß einer allgemeinen Theorie (Social Systems).* Frankfurt: Suhrkamp.

Marshall, V. W. (1999). Analyzing social theories of aging. In V. L. Bengtson, & K. W. Schaie (Eds.), *Handbook of theories of aging.* New York: Springer.

Mead, G. H. (1934). *Mind, self and society.* Chicago: University of Chicago.

Netten, A. (2004). The social production of welfare. In M. Knapp, D. Challis, J.-L. Fernandez, & A. Netten (Eds.), *Long-term care: Matching resources and needs.* Aldershot: Ashgate Publishing.

Oerter, R. (1999). Daseinsthematische Emotionen. In W. Friedlmeier, & M. Holodynski (Eds.), *Emotionale Entwicklung. Funktion, Regulation und soziokultureller Kontext von Emotionen.* Heidelberg: Spektrum Akademischer Verlag.

Ormel, J., Lindenberg, S., Steverink, N., & Vonkorff, M. (1997). Quality of life and social production functions: A framework for understanding health effects. *Social Science and medicine, 45*, 1051–1063.

Owen, T., & NCHRDF (Eds.). (2006). *My home life – quality of life in care homes.* London: Help the Aged.

Pape, H. (1989). *Erfahrung und Wirklichkeit als Zeichenprozess.* Frankfurt: Suhrkamp.

Parsons, T. (1951). *The social system.* New York: Routledge & Kegan Paul.

Parsons, T. (1978). *Action theory and the human condition.* New York: Free Press.

Pearlin, L. I., Lieberman, M. A., Menaghan, E. G., & Mullen, J. (1981). The stress process. *Journal of Health and Social Behaviour, 22*, 337–356.

Peirce, Ch. S. (1931–1935). In Ch. Harthorne, & P. Weiss (Eds.), *Collected papers, I–VI.* Cambridge: Harvard University Press.

Peirce, Ch. S. (1960). In A. W. Burks (Ed.), *Collected papers, VII–VIII*, Cambridge: Harvard University Press.

Pieper, R. (1995). Strukturelle Emotionen, elementare Strukturbildung and strukturelle Evolution, *Protosoziologie, 7*, 181–199.

Pieper, R. (1997). Technology and the social triangle of home care: Ethical issues in the application of technology to dementia care. In S. Björneby, & A. van Berlo

(Eds.), *Ethical issues in the use of technology for dementia care*. Knegsel: Akontes Publishing.

Power, M., Quinn, K., Schmidt, S., & WHOQOL-OLD Group (2005). Development of the WHOQOL-Old module. *Quality of Life Research, 14*, 2197–2214.

Renwick, R., & Brown, I. (1996). The Centre for Health Promotions conceptual approach to quality of life: Being, belonging, and becoming. In R. Renwick, I. Brown, & M. Nagler (Eds.), *Quality of life in health promotion and rehabilitation: Conceptual approaches, issues, and applications*. Thousand Oaks, CA: Sage.

Renwick, R., Brown, I., & Nagler, M. (Eds.). (1996). *Quality of life in health promotion and rehabilitation: Conceptual approaches, issues, and applications*. Thousand Oaks, CA: Sage.

Rutter, M. (1995). Psychosocial adversity: Risk, resilience and recovery. *Southern African Journal of Child and Adolescent Psychology, 7*, 75–78.

Ryff, C. D. (1989). Happiness is everything, or is it? Explorations on the meaning of psychological well-being. *Journal of Personality and Social Psychology, 57*, 1069–1081.

Schalock, R. L., & Siperstein, G. N. (1996). *Quality of life: Conceptualisation and measurement*. Washington DC: American Association of Mental Retardation.

Schmidt-Atzert, L. (1996). *Lehrbuch der Emotionspsychologie*. Stuttgart: Kohlhammer.

Secker, J., Hill, R., Villeneau, L., & Parkman, S. (2003). Promoting independence: But promoting what and how? *Ageing and Society, 23*, 375–391.

Simmel, G. (1950) (Eds. and translated by Kurt H. Wolff). *The sociology of Georg Simmel*. Glencoe, IL: The Free Press.

Skevington, S. M., Lofty, M., & O'Connell, K. A. (2004). The World Health Organisation's WHOQOL-BREF quality of life assessment. A report from the WHOQOL group. *Quality of Life Research, 13*, 299–310.

Skinner, E. A. (1999). Action regulation, coping, and development. In J. Brandstädter, & R. M. Lerner (Eds.), *Action and self-development. Theory and research through the life span* (pp. 465–503). Thousand Oaks, CA: Sage.

Staudinger, U. M., Freund, A. M., Linden, M., & Maas, I. (1999). Self, personality, and life regulation: Facets of psychological resilience in old age. In P. B. Baltes, & K. M. Mayer (Eds.), *The Berlin Aging Study*. Cambridge, MA: Cambridge University Press.

Strauss, A. L. (1978). *Negotiations: Varieties, contexts, processes and social order*, San Francisco, CA: Jossey-Bass.

Strauss, A. L., Schatzmann, L., Bucher, R., Erlich, D., & Sabshin, M. (1963). The hospital and it's negotiated order. In E. Freidson (Ed.), *The hospital in modern society* (pp. 147–168). New York: Free Press.

Tanner, D. (2001). Sustaining the self in later life: Supporting older people in the community. *Ageing and Society, 21*, 255–278.

Tester, S., Hubbard, G., Downs, M., MacDonald, C., & Murphy, J. (2003). Exploring perceptions of quality of life of frail older people during and after their transition to institutional care. Research Findings 24, the Growing Older Project. <http://www.shef.ac.uk/uni/projects/gop/GOFindings24.pdf>

Torstam, L. (1996). Gerontrancendence – a theory about maturing in old age. *Journal of Aging and Identity, 1*, 37–50.

Vaarama, M. (2004). Ikääntyneiden toimintakyky ja hoivapalvelut. Nykytila ja vuosi 2015 (Independent living and QoL in Old Age, and the role of care. State of the Art in Finland and prospects up to the year 2015). In *Ikääntyminen voimavarana.*

Tulevaisuusselonteon liiteraportti 5 (Ageing as a resource). Valtioneuvoston kanslian julkaisusarja 33/2004. Helsinki: Edita Prima Oy. <www.vnk.fi/julkaisut>

Vaarama, M., & Hertto, P. (2003). Efficiency and equity of the care of older persons— exploring an evaluation model. Revista Española de Geriatría y Gerontología. <http://www.stakes.fi/carekeys/presentations.html>

Vaarama, M., & Kaitsaari, T. (2002). Ikääntyneiden toimintakyky ja koettu hyvinvointi. *Teoksessa* Heikkilä, M., & Kautto, M. (Toim.) *Suomalaisten hyvinvointi* (The Wellbeing of Finns). STAKES. Gummerrus Printing. Jyväskylä.

Vaarama, M., Pieper, R., & Sixsmith, A. (2007). Care-related quality of life. Conceptual and empirical exploration. In H. Mollenkopf, & A. Walker (Eds.), *Quality of Life in Old Age*. International and Multi-Disciplinary Perspectives. Dordrecht. The Netherlands: Springer, pp. 215–232.

Veenhoven R. (1996). Happy life-expectancy. A comprehensive measure of quality-of-life in nations. *Social Indicators Research, 39*, 1–58.

Veenhoven, R. (2000). The four qualities of Life. Ordering concept and measures of the good life. *Journal of Happiness Studies, 1*, 1–39.

Weiner, M. F., Martin-Cook, K., Svetlik, D. A., Saine, K., Foster, B., & Fontain, C. S. (2000). The quality of life in late-stage dementia (QUALID) scale. *Journal of the American Medical Directors Association, 1*, 114–116.

5
The Concept of Quality
of Long-Term Care

Marja Vaarama, Richard Pieper, Mona Frommelt, Seija Muurinen,
Andrew Sixsmith, Margaret Hammond and Gunnar Ljunggren

Definitions of Quality of Care

Elements of Quality of Care

To study quality of care (as well as quality of life) in a cross-national research design requires the use of some pre-defined criteria on what is or what is not good quality. This is not easy as on the one hand, quality of care has been defined in many ways, and on the other, the quality of long-term care of older people is weakly defined. Further, the definitions of quality of care from the perspectives of the clients are rare (e.g. Baldock & Hadlow, 2002; Bowling, 1997), and same regards definitions of quality from a multi-professional perspective (Nies & Berman, 2004). Regarding the quality of long-term care of older people, homecare seems to lack quality definitions (e.g. Paljärvi, Rissanen, & Sinkkonen, 2003; Thomé, Dykes, & Rahm Hallberg, 2003), more often than nursing care and institutional care (e.g. Ranz, Zwygart-Stauffacher, & Popejoy, 1999).

In health care, the definition given by Donabedian (1969, 1980) is a widely accepted framework to evaluate quality of care. According to this model, the quality of (health) care needs to be ensured in the three following aspects:

- Structure: the *stable elements* of the care system in a community that facilitate or inhibit the access to and provision of services. In health and welfare economics these factors are called inputs, meaning issues such as material resources and financial investments as well as societal goals given to the care.
- Process: the *interaction* between the client and a provider. Two dimensions are important here—the technical excellence of given care (appropriateness and skilfulness of the intervention) and interpersonal excellence (humanity and responsiveness to client preferences).
- Outcomes: *results of care* including clinical status, functional status, client satisfaction, and improved QoL of the client.

These elements are reflected in the current definitions of the quality of care and in the methods of evaluating the quality, especially regarding health care.

For example, the definition by the Medical College of Georgia (2003) implies the same characteristics: "Quality of Care is the degree to which Health Services for individuals and populations increase the likelihood of desired health outcomes and are consistent with current professional knowledge. ... Quality is achieved when accessible services are provided in an efficient, cost effective and acceptable manner that can be controlled by the ones providing it". For quality of long-term care of older persons, the multi-professional European Carmen Network (Vaarama & Pieper, 2005) suggested that a good definition of the quality of integrated care for older persons should address attributes such as

- *Structures*: well-trained multidisciplinary personnel, personnel's motivation towards constant improvement of quality, evidence-based and validated standards
- *Process*: responsiveness to needs and preferences of the client, support for autonomy and independence, respect for the client's right to dignity, client-centeredness in the planning of services, participation of the client and where appropriate their carers, empowerment, high professional quality of caring processes
- *Outcomes*: effectiveness of care, continuity of care, client satisfaction, support for QoL of a client.

The expected or desired quality of care can be defined by quality criteria and quality standards. These define the optimal or achievable level of quality, which can be used as a yardstick for evaluation of the current state. Following Donabedian (1969, 1980), quality criteria are usually connected with some desired phenomena of the structures, processes and outcomes of care. A criterion that is expressed in a measurable form to show the variation of quality is called a quality indicator. To guide care practices these indicators have to be integrated into systematic care procedures, which specify goals, define interventions and evaluate their achievements. And they have to be documented and the documentation system must be practical, that is, facilitating good care rather than absorbing time and motivation to care.

In social and health care, there are many stakeholders setting these criteria and expectations; citizens, clients, relatives, professionals, managers, taxpayers and other financiers as well as politicians. Even quality as a concept does not include any positive or negative connotations; each quality definition has a connection to the goals and values of those presenting them (Övretveit, 1998). Therefore, quality concepts have to be justified with reference to values and grounded in care theories, they have to be agreed upon by those who define and apply them, by those who finance them and those who are subjected to care.

The objective of Care Keys has not been to contribute to practices of good care on an operational level of care interventions, but rather on a more strategic level of care planning and evaluation by placing care activities in a framework of professional goal achievement. The special focus has been on the role of care documentation in the facilitation of care and on ways to improve care planning by using the information in the documentation for the evaluation of care outcomes. The guiding principle was evidence-based care, which implies that care is based on grounded theory identifying procedures and indicators of successful care and on documentation systems making evidence available when and where it is needed in practice. And as already indicated, the focus was on professional practices of long-term care in institutional and homecare settings. Care in other institutions (e.g. hospitals, rehabilitation) and non-professional care, especially informal care (e.g. by family and relatives) was not investigated. These agencies of care were included only as partners of strategies of providing a more comprehensive and integrated care.

Quality of Homecare and Institutional Care of Older People

Reviewing the literature, it is clear that quality of care has multiple definitions, and it seem that different professionals define the quality differently. Regarding homecare, there are little definitions available on the quality of homecare, and definitely there are no universal and commonly agreed definitions of the quality of homecare. This is probably because homecare is a highly contextual phenomenon, which varies over the time and location. Secondly, it has been studied within different scientific frameworks and from different paradigms, and described and evaluated from different perspectives of diverse actors, and as a part or as a dimension of the total quality of the care of older people (e.g. Paljärvi et al., 2003). During the last 10 years, there has been a growing interest also in the quality of homecare, but this has been mainly focussed on home nursing rather than on social care at home, and studies looking at both these elements of homecare are rare.

The general objectives of homecare for older people are to support their autonomy, functional capacity and personal competencies and independent living at home. Mostly, the objectives have been defined quite instrumentally as helping clients in those daily activities they need help and assistance with, but in recent years a broader objective of supporting the QoL of the clients has emerged in the definitions (e.g. Thomé et al., 2003). We can differentiate between two major elements in homecare, namely the tasks dealing with (i) housekeeping and running errands outside home, and (ii) home nursing services, which divide into specialised home nursing and basic home nursing or personal care (Weekers & Pijl, 1998). In the current definitions of quality of care, we see the dominance of the latter, while the first is weakly defined and tends to have little appreciation in professional care definitions. The limited research on quality of homecare from the perspective of the clients emphasises the importance of sufficient help in housekeeping, running errands, mobility and participation. For older clients, it is important that homecare is appropriate and responsive to their needs, but responses also emphasise the relational nature of homecare; it is not only about doing some tasks at clients' home but also about the relation between the client and the care worker, and about the socio-psycho-emotional support to the client (e.g. Bowers, Fibich, & Jacobson, 2001; Larsson & Wilde Larsson, 1998; Loewenthal, 2005; Morrow-Howell, Proctor, & Rozario, 2001; Samuelsson & Brink, 1997; Thomé and associates 2003). According to these, appropriateness and continuity of care; professional competence and skills of the care workers; the quality of interaction between the client and the care workers, the autonomy and control of the client; and safety of living at home and responsiveness of care to their needs are important elements of quality of homecare. From the perspective of personal (basic nursing) care at home, meeting certain clinical standards is an important quality factor.

Definitions of quality of care in institutional care are easier to find as nursing care theories are more developed. Still, the current approaches or models seldom cover all the characteristics of institutional care. More often just a part of the quality of care, such as nutrition, is studied. Furthermore, most of the nursing care theories are focused on acute care, missing the differentiation and specification of long-term-care. Rantz, Jensdóttir, Hjaltadóttir, Gudmundsdóttir, Sigurreig Gudjónsdóttir, Brunton, & Rook (2002) have provided a multidimensional model of good nursing home quality. The model includes the following concepts: home, environment, staff, care, communication and family involvement. According to Rantz and associates (2002), a nursing home should be as homely as possible and the environment should be clean and odour free. There should be enough staff and the turn-over of the staff should be low. The care should be individualised and the residents should be treated "as people". The communication with residents and family members should be positive and systematic, and the family should be involved in the care of the resident. Good quality in care is formed of these basic factors. Moreover, many others include the same elements as Rantz's theory, but their approach is usually narrower and describes only one part of quality of care.

Care home environment has been found to be an important factor of quality of institutional care, especially from clients' perspective (Grant, Reimer, & Bannatyre, 1996; Leppänen, Töyry, & Vehviläinen-Julkunen, 1997; Muurinen, Nuutinen, & Peiponen, 2002; Rantz et al., 2002; Tester, Hubbard, Downs, MacDonald, & Murphy, 2003). Home is described in these studies as "home likeness" of the care unit; it includes physical surroundings and equipment, pleasant milieu, cosy atmosphere and the presence of community. Tester et al. (2003) emphasise also the importance of the socio-emotional atmosphere in care homes in their study on transition from home to an institution.

Skilled and educated staff has a connection to high quality of care (Bowers, Fibich et al., 2001; Hogston, 1995; Muurinen, 2003). To assure the quality of care the staff ratio should be high enough (Bowers, Lauring, & Jacobson, 2001; Hogston, 1995; Leppänen et al., 1997). The skill-mix is also important, as the more educated carers seem to produce more rehabilitative care than the less educated carers with the same costs (Muurinen, 2003). Further, individual care and caring of the staff, which can be described also as a holistic model of care, are central to excellence in nursing care (Coulon, Mok, Krause,

& Anderson, 1996) and humane caring (Leppänen et al., 1997). Holistic care approach is defined as the "perspective that man and other organisms function as complete, integrated units rather than as aggregates of separate parts" (Coulon et al., 1996). For residents of long-stay institutions, individualised care and individuality are important factors to good QoL (Oleson, Heading, McGlynn, & Bistodeau, 1994).

Many studies emphasise communication and client–care worker interaction as a critical matter in determining of quality of care especially from the client's point of view (Bowers, Fibich et al., 2001; Caris-Verhallen, Kerkstra, & Bensing, 1997; Coulon et al., 1996: Leppänen et al., 1997). Gilloran, McGlew, McKee, Robertson, and Wight (1993) propose that the quality of care process includes among other things the following indicators: the choice offered to the clients, giving sufficient information, encouraging to independence and respecting the privacy. According to Davies, Slack, Laker, and Philp (1999), skilled staff has a potential to promote residents' personal autonomy.

It is important that care personnel support the relationship between the clients and their relatives (Muurinen et al., 2002; Rantz et al., 2002; Weman, Kihlgren, & Fagerberg, 2004). According to Lee, Lee, and Woo (2005) nursing home residents' satisfaction with social support is an important predictor of their satisfaction with care. However, clients and their relatives' participation in care do not always realise. Many relatives want to participate in the care of the clients more often than they are offered with a possibility (Laitinen, 1992).

These elements of good quality care in institutional settings are reflected also in the more recent studies of Tester and associates (2003) and Mozley et al. (2004). Tester and associates found a range of factors impacting positively or negatively on the QoL of the clients, and they can be grouped in a four-dimensional framework as follows: (i) individual resident's meaningful activities; (ii) their relationships and interactions with other residents, staff and visitors; (iii) maintaining the individual's identity and autonomy; and (iv) physical environment of the home and availability of services. Mozley and associates (2004) found that a good care home provides residents with opportunities for keeping occupied in the home; activities that are appropriate and valued; satisfaction with pleasure from things done in the home; staff working cohesively; lack of conflict; and good physical comfort.

Review of Care Theories and Models

Approaches to Care

Concepts of care and care quality have to be grounded in theory, so in addition of looking at the current understanding of the elements of the quality of care we looked also at the care theories. On the first level, we reviewed the basic paradigms of models and theories to understand their values and orientation toward care. Classifications of care theories (Marriner-Tomey, 1992; Fawcett, 1996; Meleis, 1999; Schäffer, Steppe, Moers, & Meleis, 1997) contain the following main theories

1. *Care theories of needs* (e.g. Abdellah, Hall, Henderson, Roper, Orem, Krohwinkel): These are based on need theories (e.g. Maslow, Erickson) focusing on problems, diseases, deficits and risks, and effective ways to help. The guiding question is What are care activities?
2. *Care theories of Humanistic Models* (e.g. Watson, Paterson, & Zderad): Care and receiving care are understood as an experience and expression of human existence based on existentialistic Philosophy (Kierkegaard, Heidegger, Jaspers) and humanistic psychology, and including the moral imperative, under which care, relief, welfare and support are performed in the way of human dialog. The guiding question is How is care experienced?
3. *Care theories of interaction* (e.g. Peplau, Orlando, Wiedenbach, Travelbee, Petterson/Zderad, King, Eriksson): These approaches are based on theories of interaction (G.H. Mead) or on Phenomenology (Schütz, Berger, Luckmann) and understand care as an interaction and communicative process between carer and care-needing persons establishing the social meaning of care. The guiding question is How to conduct care as relationship?
4. *Care theories of systemic conditions and outcomes* (e.g. Levine, Rogers, Roy, Johnson, Neuman): Theoretically, these are based on environmental and social system theories (Bertalanffy, Barker, Parson, Luhmann), focusing on adaptation to the environment and on outcomes of care. The guiding question is What are the contexts and effects of caring?

The theories focus in different ways on the human condition to which care is designed to make a contribution. Thus, they are in a close conceptual relationship to theories of QoL (see Chapter 4, this volume). Reviewing care theory from the point of view of clients and their expectations towards care quality, Bowers, Fibich and Jacobson (2001) distinguish three approaches: care-as-comfort, care-as-relating, and care-as-service. A closer look at this classification may justify a distinction of four approaches following the four approaches to care theory:

• Care as sustaining functional competence and autonomy
  In this perspective the rehabilitation or maintenance of capacities of the person, the competence for self-care, and autonomy are in the foreground. The important function of care has to be considered in this view of care as supporting the persons own capacities, but it includes also other supporting activities, which enhance the (relative) independence of the client, such as exercising skills, learning new ways of coping, or participation in care decisions. Looking at the care relationship, the client has to accept own responsibility in the co-production of care, whereas the carer should refrain from supporting a process of "learned helplessness" and undermining rehabilitation by over-targeting services.
• Care as supporting emotional and existential well-being
  In this perspective, usually emphasised by humanistic approaches, the need for support in the adjustment to the stress, anxieties and hopelessness generated by experiences of dependency, illness and existential threats is emphasised, and the emotional balance and integrity of the person is restored.

This aspect is especially difficult for the care relationship, because emotional support requires empathy and tends to involve the carer as a person expressing authentic own feelings. Unlike "emotional work" as part of usual services (e.g. stewardess, waitress) the emotional support in a situation of personal stress and anxiety has to have an "existential" quality in the eyes of the client and is vulnerable to perceptions of being "faked". Although much of everyday care can do without deeper emotional involvement, just like everyday in general, this quality becomes important as emotional pressures in the client increase. It requires motivations and attitudes on part of the carer, which ensue from an identification with the carer's role that "money can't buy" and must be supported by a corresponding care culture and work atmosphere. These attitudes are accomplished within education and training and conducted as well as controlled within care management tools and procedures, like proofed implementation of care models.

• Care as supporting social identity, social relations and social participation
In this perspective typically the care relationship itself is seen as an important aspect of care, since the relationship may be the only relevant social relation left to the client, for example, in case of bed-bound care in an institution. Social relation is considered here not primarily as a resource or means to other ends, but as the context in which a person finds and expresses his or her identity in a community of other relevant persons. Looking at the care relation, this social dimension seems to dissolve into giving emotional support as the client gets more and more dependent and is unable to reciprocate. However, the respect for the client on part of the carer and the client's self-esteem depend essentially on being regarded as a member of the community, even if this community is the "virtual" or "spiritual" community of a very personal, but meaningful life world or religion. As such it is not directly related to the frequency of social contacts, but to their quality.

• Care as service
In this perspective, the services and resources as well as environmental adaptations are focused. This may range from support by housekeeping activities or provision of assistive technologies (e.g. wheel chair) to adjusting to a comfortable position in bed or to feeding and giving medication. Looking at the care relationship, this concept of care goes often along with a concept of the client as a customer of care who will demand a "good service" and make choices between alternative offers. The carer, in turn, is expected to act in a professional role fulfilling a contract. Especially with increasing dependency, this customer role cannot be exercised as long as there are different options but less to not at all, if "exit" is not a viable option. While the care demand of the client increases, her dependency on the "good will" of the carer increases, too.

Again, we see care as related to the QoL of the client and, vice versa, the QoL appears as related to the quality of care, since care provides an important context for and contribution to the life of frail older persons.

Care of Older Persons with Dementia

A key issue to consider in the quality of care for older people is the care and services provided to people with dementia. Care concepts have an impact on the way a person's needs are conceptualised and the kind of care that is provided. In the "biomedical" model, dementia is characterised primarily in terms of the deterioration of the brain, which in turn results in deterioration of cognitive ability and attendant decline in the person's social and personal skills. This concept of dementia has been a powerful force that has not only shaped the way dementia is defined, conceptualised and studied, but also has had a major impact on care. If dementia is seen solely as an outcome of irreversible changes in the brain, then care becomes little more than "warehousing" (Sixsmith, Stilwell, & Copeland, 1993), providing basic support and making the person as "comfortable" as possible. The pervasive nature of the biomedical model and its underlying assumptions have been reflected in, and reinforced by, the patterns of care.

Since the late 1980s an alternative perspective on dementia has emerged (cf. Gubrium & Lynott, 1987; Kitwood, 1989; Lyman, 1989; Sixsmith et al., 1993), arguing that the biomedical model fails to account for the complexity of the experience of dementia. Kitwood and Bredin (1992) argue that, while changes in the brain determine the basic limits for cognitive functioning, other factors, such as personality and the social and therapeutic contexts, can play key roles in shaping the experience and outcome for an individual. Kitwood's work (Kitwood, 1997; Kitwood & Bredin, 1992) was also important in emphasising the subjective dimension of the experience of dementia, suggesting that many people, despite cognitive decline, are able to experience a good QoL and to "thrive". He proposed a theory of dementia based around the concept of personhood and represented by four states of being:

- A sense of personal worth, such as positive and negative views of the self and awareness of place in the world, relationships and social position
- A sense of agency or ability to exercise control over personal life, such as engaging with the physical environment and people
- A sense of confidence and hope in respect to comfort and security, relationships with people and in a spiritual sense
- A feeling of social confidence that includes an element of reciprocity with others.

These alternative perspectives have been helpful in changing approaches to the care of people with dementia with more positive, life-enhancing care interventions emerging. The idea behind this approach is that of "personhood". This is not "rehabilitation" in the sense of helping people to regain their abilities or training them to cope on their own. Rather, carers should attempt to "fill-in" the gaps in the "person" that the dementia has taken away, to make them a "whole" person again. There are several aspects to this kind of approach (Kitwood & Bredin, 1992):

- *Facilitation*: One of the frequent problems for people with dementia is that they find it difficult to communicate or carry out something that they want to do. Facilitation means helping them in what they are trying to do, to make up for the things they cannot do themselves or to make themselves understood.
- *Validation*: Caregivers acknowledge and accept and work from the person's point of view, accepting their experiences as their reality.
- *Holding*: People with dementia can experience very difficult emotional problems, such as anger, fear, anxiety and grief. It is important that the person has a safe place where they can express these emotions and where they can be worked through with a carer.

These kinds of approaches are very different from the more traditional approaches, based on the biomedical model. The emphasis is much more "person-centred", focusing on psycho-social needs of the person, their emotions and their resources, rather than on their disabilities and cognitive symptoms. Kitwood's approach can easily be reconciled with the Care Keys model of QoL based on Lawton's theory (1991) (see Chapter 4).

The special condition of dementia and the emphasis on the concept of personhood enhances the necessity to include a third-person perspective into the concept of care and care quality. Actually, it is not only in the case of dementia that frail older persons need support "to fill in the gaps", although this clearly is a most extreme case. In dementia care the concept of a "care triad" of client, informal carer and professional carer is emphasised as interacting agents of care (Adams & Gardiner, 2005; Pieper, 1997). In case of dementia, the need to define care outcomes—the QoL of clients—in more objective ways independent from subjective self-reports of clients becomes apparent and unavoidable. Subjective QoL has to be substituted by QoL as observed by "third persons", and we would require the inferred quality to be based not only on the perspective of the professional carer, but also (if possible) on the accounts of other persons who have a close relationship to the client (e.g. spouses, children, partners). In CK, we have suggested a theoretical model to include the need for "negotiation in the care triad" and an instrument (QUALID, Weiner et al., 2000) based on emotion theory to support care as described by Kitwood's approach. As discussed elsewhere (Chapter 4 and 6), the concept of the "care triad" can be generalised also beyond the case of dementia care to the situation of frail older persons and care in general.

Models of Care

Different approaches to care tend to emphasize different aspects. A "biomedical model" has a focus on health care and restoring the competencies of the person, conceiving this task mainly as a narrowly defined service, which does not necessarily include elements of social care (e.g. home help) or psycho-social support. The model of phases in patient care developed by Raatikainen (1995) combines the models of Donabedian (1969), Jantsch (1975) and van Maanen (1984).

The phases of care in the model are: Biophysical model, Personal model and Community-based model. These models represent different stages in the care path, and are cumulative. The positive characteristics of the Biophysical model are included in the Personal model, and the positive characteristics of the Personal model are included in the Community-based model. The quality of care is regarded as good when the positive characteristics of these three models are integrated. The result is that the client's physical needs are taken care of, the client is feeling emotionally and socially well, and the client and his family or community is physically, psychologically and socially rehabilitated, or can manage better by themselves. This nursing care model also comprises input, outcome and process measures like Øvretveit's model. It can be assumed that good input and process results produce good outcomes in terms of comprehensive (physical, psychological and social) well-being of the client (compare Coulon et al., 1996; Rantz et al., 2002).

These models and approaches are not mutually exclusive, but will characterise existing care provision in some kind of "mix". This implies that care has to organise a care relationship, which in important respects is not (only) an economic transaction between the provider and the client, but a social relationship between the carer and the dependent client, and in which issues of power or empowerment and of the legitimacy or ethical justification of interventions are essential aspects to address and solve.

The issue of organising a "mix" of care makes also aware of the fact that care follows not only ethical and professional standards, but also established divisions of labour. Three divisions prove to be of great influence for concepts of care and in the CK research: the division between health care and social care, professional and informal care, and institutional and home care. As Twigg (2004) for instance has shown, the medical–social boundary is closely connected to theories and discourses of the body. While medically oriented nursing focuses on "basic bed and body work", social care and social work tend to neglect "bed and body" and concentrate on psycho-social or interpersonal work. Both perspectives— including Twigg's account—fail to represent adequately household works and their substitution by—what is called—support for instrumental activities of daily living (IADL). This neglect can be understood by a reflection on the social production of welfare (Netten, 2004), which analyses the ways care services are developed out of the context of home production. Health care—and to a lesser degree—social work have made a career of professionalisation, but IADL support has still the image of unqualified, unprofessional or informal household work. Its importance is realised by now, because the lack of household support often decides on the (expensive) institutionalisation of frail older persons.

From this perspective, it seems to be about time to develop a broader understanding of the anthropology of welfare of old people (see Edgar & Russel, 1998), and based on this knowledge, a "socio-cultural care model" should be developed. This model of care would use a broad range of working methods based on gerontological knowledge to support the QoL of older clients, and make use of human, social and cultural capital the old clients still have and are happy to use.

Towards the Care Keys Model of Quality of Care

The Care Keys Quality Matrix

In the multi-perspective model of Øvretveit (1998), quality of care is divided in to three concepts: structure, process and outcome similarly to Donabedian (1969), but Øvretveit defines the model further to involve the perspectives of the clients, the professionals and the managers into quality evaluation. The client perspective in quality is defined "what clients say and want, or what is necessary in inputs, process or outcomes to give clients what they want". Professional perspective is defined as "professional's views about whether the service meets client's needs and whether staff correctly select and carry out procedures which are believed to be necessary to meet client's needs". The management perspective looks at performance at the level of the service or institution. All these perspectives should be combined for comprehensive quality evaluations (see also Currie, Harvey, West, McKenna, & Keeney, 2005; Sidani, Doran, & Mitchell, 2004). In theory, the differences between these three perspectives are clear but in practice the differentiation is often difficult. Comprehensive models of quality of care found in literature do not differentiate the concept like Øvretveit (e.g. Rantz et al., 2002). In the CK approach these three perspectives are represented as a "care triad" on the level of care management (see Chapter 6).

To clarify the framework, we introduced in Care Keys a clear distinction between the three perspectives and between subjective views and objective information or evidence. Objective indicators rely on some methods which—at least in principle—should be independent from the particular individual applying the methods. In the present case, the information provided by scales or tests and by procedures of documentation was assumed to be "objective" (although in the CK models we refer to the indicators as "documented" being aware of the biases they in fact have). What a client needs from his or her own perspective may not be the same as what he or she needs from the perspective of the care profession or management. Some desirable outcomes like non-smoking, restrictions to assure safety, or "just" sharing of scarce resources may be evaluated differently. Additionally, there is a difference between the perspective of a specific group (in the sense of their "best interest") and the subjective views of particular individuals, although both views should be recognised and evaluated for care quality. Accordingly a distinction between documented and subjective outcomes was made.

On the basis of these distinctions, and after extensive review of quality indicators in the care literature, we constructed an initial quality matrix to guide the Care Keys research (Table 5.1), which then was further developed as a care quality management tool (see Chapters 6 and 13).

In the perspective of professionals, we decided to use *documented outcome* of the care process covering the interests of the professionals. In addition, the *subjective outcome* reflected in job satisfaction is included in the final quality matrix, but it was not empirically investigated, since the design did not include interviews with the staff. The *input* includes all material and non-material prerequisites of good care, such as client-centred care concepts and ethical standards, state-of-the-art care interventions and procedures, care technologies and supportive services, and a work atmosphere sustaining motivations and team orientation. Central to the care *process* turned out to be the concept of compliance with care standards and the quality of the client–staff interaction. Outcomes, in fact, appear in the literature in three different categories: (i) the goals of client-centeredness implies that the QoL of the client is an important "final outcome", (ii) clinical outcomes reflecting

TABLE 5.1. The matrix of quality of care indicators of the Care Keys research (applied from Bowers et al., 2001; Øvretveit, 1998; Raatikainen 1995; Paljärvi et al., 2003; Vaarama & Pieper, 2005).

Evaluation perspective	Input/structure variables	Process variables	Outcome documented	Outcome subjective
Client quality	Expectations Preferences Need for compensation Resources Living conditions Psycho emotional needs	Respect Validation Control Empowerment Care support Interventions Care interaction quality	Human dignity Social identity Autonomy Competence Environmental improvements Physical safety Psychological outcomes	Well-being/quality of life outcomes Satisfaction of subjective needs and preferences
Professional quality	Concept of care Principles/ethics Professional standards	Compliance to standards Correct need assessment	Client-centred care outcomes Clinical outcomes Risk avoidance	Job satisfaction
	Evaluation procedures Work organization Information exchange Assessment tools Documentation systems	Correct interventions Good care planning Regular evaluation and updating Efficient time use	Amount of compliances	
	Care technologies Collaboration, cooperation Teamwork Informal care inclusion	Good interpersonal communication Relationship between client, care worker, and informal carer	Availability Externalities Work atmosphere	

the concerns of professionals (and their liabilities and care risks) and (iii) aspects of the work conditions that support the motivation of staff, often including the subjective view of job satisfaction. While (i) actually refers to the client perspective in the quality matrix, (ii) and (iii) describe specific dimensions of professional care quality.

There is an additional conceptual problem, because the quality of the care relation is not sufficiently reflected in the compliance to standards of good care by professionals. The Care Keys framework, therefore, included the subjective evaluation of care by the client as an intermediate outcome. This view on care quality—essentially belonging to the client perspective—served in Care Keys research as a proximate indicator for the quality of the care process, and was evaluated together with the information on staff compliance with standards (as documented in the care documentation).

Dimensions of Care

Guided by the theoretical framework and in view of the literature, we tried to systematically order the diverse features of good care, keeping the four-dimensional structure of the QoL model in mind (see Chapter 4). Good care should be *comprehensive* and make a contribution to each dimension of needs in the perspective of the client. A literature review for needs and care tasks was conducted resulting in a set of about 11 different types of care activities or care concerns. The review checked 14 different conceptualisations (including Florence Nightingale, Virginia Henderson, Nancy Roper, Monika Krohwinkel, Dorothea Orem, Martha Rogers, Imogene King) also reviewed for theoretical approaches to care (see references for care theories above). Most care theories contain a version of the ADL/IADL categories, because these are beyond dispute the main determinates of satisfaction and QoL (e.g. Baltes & Mayer, 1999), so our intention was to cover all care theories based on these parameters. We cross-walked the different ADL/IADL systems of Orem, Henderson, Roper, Juchli, Abderhalden, Krohwinkel and the Resident Assessment Inventory (RAI) system, and ended up with 13 care dimensions, specified by a large number of need/supply variables. Then the list was reduced to 44 items in 11 care dimensions (see Chapter 11), after which these dimensions were combined into four quality dimensions in correspondence to the four quality dimensions of the care-related QoL model (see Chapter 4). The dimensions correspond the QoL-dimensions of the WHOQOL-Bref (WHOQOL Group, 1998), which was selected as one of main instruments to measure QoL outcomes from the perspective of the client (see Chapter 2).

The distinction of care dimensions according to needs were

1. Physical support/care (including medical care and cure, personal care and ADL)
2. Psychological support/care (including psychological care and emotional support)

3. Social/participation support (including social support and participation needs)
4. Support services/social care (including IADL, transportation and moving outdoors).

The quality of care is regarded as good, if all parameters of needs and demands are well assessed and followed through the process of care, that is, in care diagnoses, goal definitions, care interventions and evaluations of effects and goal-achievement.

A second starting point is the satisfaction of the client with the care received. For evaluation of the quality of care from the perspective of the clients, the approach of Paljärvi and associates (2003) to quality of homecare offered a helpful taxonomy. In this approach, the following features are considered as important criteria for quality of care

• Appropriateness of care
• Continuity of care
• The professional competence and skills of the care workers
• The quality of interaction between the client and the care workers
• The autonomy and control of the client
• Safety of living at home
• Health care outcomes
• Nursing care outcomes
• Social care outcomes
• Satisfaction with care

Actually, the quality of *care* and the QoL of the client should be clearly distinguished in this list, as we suggested above. But still, *how* care is provided interacts with *what* needs are satisfied. *Respect* for the dignity of clients will support the client's self-esteem, *reliability* and *continuity* of care will enhance the autonomy, giving *adequate time* to the client will imply an increase in available services, *kindness* and *trust* in care interactions will generate emotional security. Thus, ethical standards, efficient procedures, support services, and interaction quality are *four quality dimensions of care* from the view of the client, which correspond to the QoL to the client.

A third starting point is the analysis of care as an activity, which should produce QoL as an outcome, but should also satisfy general affordances of good services. A review of the literature in this view included service quality scales providing quality dimensions, not only from the perspective of the customer (e.g. SERVQUAL scale; Picker scales), but also from the point of view of the profession (Bruhn, 2003). From this starting point, the four dimensions of quality management interrelate with care service quality (Chapter 6). Thus, the cross-walk between QoL, quality of care and quality of management revealed that the four-dimensional structure of quality—the cornerstones of the Care Keys framework—can be applied to all aspects of quality.

The relationship between the different concepts can be summarised in a model of impacts following the production of welfare approach (Fig. 5.1).

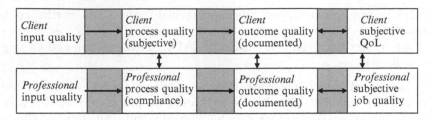

F<small>IG</small>. 5.1. Care quality concepts and their impacts.

As the arrows in the model indicate, all outcomes should be seen to interact, since the subjective evaluations are known to interact with the care outcomes as measured by more objective assessments. Similarly, the compliance of care processes to professional standards depends in a "co-production" with the client also on his or her perception of the care interaction and his or her cooperation. In Care Keys, the professional quality was measured by scales for input, process and outcome indicators using the instruments designed for extraction of data from care documentation (InDEX), and clients' subjective evaluation of care was measured by a set of measures in the client interview instrument developed in the project (CLINT). All scales were designed to cover all four dimensions of quality, and the empirical analyses gave support to this structure (see Chapter 2).

In as much as quality care is concerned with the QoL of the client as the "final outcome", professional care will strive to provide care in all four respects. From the perspective of the QoL of the client as defined by Lawton (1991), care can be interpreted as primarily addressing the dimension of environmental support and adaptations. From the perspective of the *care-related* QoL model, good care will encompass all four dimensions at least to some extent (see Chapter 4). And it is ultimately a central task of care management to facilitate good care.

Evaluation of Quality of Care from the Care Documentation

Care Documentation as Information Base for Quality Evaluation

There are many ways to evaluate the professional quality of care, and one of them is the strategy based on actual care documentation, which is quite commonly used in nursing care. There is also evidence of a connection between good care documentation and good professional outcomes. For example, Phaneuf Nursing Audit (Phaneuf, 1976), Rush Medicus Nursing Process Methodology (Jelinek, Haussman, Hegyvary, & Newman, 1974), and it's British application Senior Monitor (Goldstone & Maselino-Okai, 1986) all are examples of instruments for quality evaluation, which have been developed for evaluation of the quality of nursing care processes where all or almost all information is collected from care documentation. According to Voutilainen, Isola, and Muurinen (2004), high professional quality of care presumes also accurate documentation and up-to-date nursing care plans. In Care Keys, we wanted to investigate how well the quality evaluation based on nursing care documentation fits also to the homecare, and whether the quality of documentation has an impact on the outcomes of these two types of long-term care of older people. Additionally, Care Keys aimed to develop tools for quality management, which ultimately should lead to an improvement of the care documentation.

Usually the documenting is done in special forms, which are either electronically or manually to fill in, and the documentation of care include ideally

1. Documentation of the care needs of the client (and less often also his or her competencies)
2. Documentation of goal setting and care planning (care plan)
3. Documentation of care delivery and interventions
4. Documentation of the ways and measures for evaluation of the quality of care
5. Regular evaluation of goal-achievement and care outcomes

Already in the piloting stage of the Care Keys research we noticed that the documentation of long-term care of older people was poor and varied a lot within our five project countries (see also Chapters 7, 8, and 9). This in spite of the fact that documentation of care has legal grounding (although not always and not around Europe). For example in Finland, there are laws and statutes that determine making of care plans as a legal responsibility of care professionals, and give regulations for contents of these plans. In addition, the Finnish National Recommendation for High Quality Care and Service for Older People recommend good care planning and give instructions on how to do it (Ministry of Health and Social Affairs and Association of Local Authorities in Finland 2001; Vaarama, Luomahaara, Peiponen, & Voutilainen, 2001). Two parts of the documentation system have received special attention: the care plan and the assessment instruments—some documentation systems encompassing both.

Documentation of Care in the Care Plan

A care plan is the tool for a client centred care and service, advising in the targeting of care resources and interventions, and facilitating a goal-orientated care. The care plan ensures the continuity of care also when the care workers change, and offers an effective channel for exchange of information between the professionals and organisations as well as with the client and informal carers (e.g. Voutilainen and associates, 2002).

Ideally, a care plan is always based on the evaluation of the situation in the point when a client enters to the care system. It involves identification of the factors that cause problems to the functional (physical, psychological, social) ability of the client, including the evaluation of housing and living environments as well as clients' own resources and competencies. Based on this assessment of needs and competencies, the necessary care interventions are defined and a care plan decided. The Care Keys approach emphasises the involvement of the client in this process to empower older people in having a say in their care plans, and to facilitate the common definition of needs, setting the goals and decision on interventions. A needs-assessment is called comprehensive in Care Keys, when the clients' medical and physical, psychological/emotional/ spiritual, social, and environmental needs are evaluated. The means of collecting information for a comprehensive care plan are discussions with the client and if necessary with his or her family, the observation of the daily functional ability during the care interventions, and the use of diverse measures of functional ability and assessment systems available (see e.g. Ammerwerth, Kutscha, & Kutscha, 2001; Ehrenberg & Ehnfors, 2001; Sloane & Mathew, 1991).

To summarise, a care plan should document the goals and objectives for the care of an individual client, define the interventions and activities for achieving these goals, schedule the (gradual) goal-achievement, set strategies, schedule and give criteria for evaluation of the levels of goal-achievement. Additionally, preventive means and prophylaxes should be defined in the plan. Good care documentation

1. Concentrates on essential factors, is clear and easy to understand
2. Differentiates between the opinions or wishes of the client and relatives and the interpretations made by the care professionals
3. Defines ways and criteria of evaluation, and result of evaluations
4. Includes arguments on why the given help and interventions are undertaken
5. Assures that notes are correct and informative

The Care Keys project emphasised that care documentation should not be too burdening to professionals and should be structured to serve three purposes: (i) a set of critical indicators should be available to enable early screening for needs for purposes of prevention and eligibility for services, (ii) a more detailed documentation has to support the on-going care process, and (iii) a set of indicators should enable the regular evaluation of care achievements by the care practitioners themselves and—in an aggregated form—by quality management and by care system planners. These objectives may be combined in a comprehensive documentation system. However, at present, we have to recognise that systems are not designed to serve all functions equally well. The emphasis is typically on the functionality for the care process itself and here again, primarily for narrowly defined (and legally regulated and financed) types of care. One key task of the Care Keys research was, accordingly, to make a contribution to the definition of key dimensions and key issues of care for evaluation of the quality of long-term care of older persons.

Needs Assessment and Quality of Care

The existing services may not meet the client's needs for a number of reasons. For example, if they are based on historical factors, they may be obsolete or out of line with the client's current needs. Without re-evaluation of services, historical inequalities or errors may be perpetuated. Another possibility is that the services may be too demand-led. Here, only those who ask for the services receive them, and only the most urgent needs are met. This prevents service providers from obtaining early information about the client's physical, cognitive or social decline that may enable them to put preventative measures in place. Another problem is that needs that are obvious at a first glance may not always be the ones to cover first. Today, too little is known about many health and social services and the needs these are to cover and more research is needed. However, with a fuller picture of the client needs, preferences, QoL and quality of care, we can more easily make priorities and remodel different services to consider unmet or over-met needs. Furthermore, if the assessment is done in a comprehensive way, this gives the professionals the capability to discover risk areas that are not found if only a simple assessment is done, and prevent them (see Achterberg, van Campen, Margriet, Kerkstra, & Ribbe, 1999; Aminzadeh & Dalziel, 2002; Challis & Hughes, 2002; Hawes et al., 1997).

Evidence shows that multidisciplinary groups are preferable to single-discipline approaches in needs assessment (Fleming, Evans, Weber, & Chutka, 1995), even if they are still uncommon (Morris et al., 1997). However, the multi-dimensional approach has also been addressed as cumbersome and time-consuming (Applegate, Blass, & Williams, 1990). However, we have to look at the effects and cost of a comprehensive assessment and documentation over the whole care process, and there it can be shown that the investment of skills and time in documentation reduces time, failings and unnecessary supplies and, thus, improves quality of care (Niehörster, Garms-Homolová, & Vahrenhorst, 1998; Roth, 2001; Wierz, Schwarz, & Gervink, 2000). For professional care and care management, a comprehensive documentation enables a reliable summary description of the area or agency workload and to request and allocate resources more appropriately. The information can help to intertwine the services that are delivered by several participants in the care of the older person to achieve integrated care.

Summing up

The concept of quality of care, as it is conceptualised here, depends for its operationalisation and implementation into care practice on a good documentation system. This is often seen as interfering with the tasks of providing good care adapted to the individual needs of clients and to the conditions set by particular service organisations. In the Care Keys approach we take the position that good care should be evaluated by its outcomes, and this requires the documentation of the needs assessed, the interventions actually administered and the specification and measurement of desired outcomes. Certainly, the tasks of documentation have to be structured and organised in such a way that they are corresponding to the values and goals of care and do not reduce the client to a source of increasing needs for information in a highly bureaucratic care system. However, the reduction of information needs for good care implies that we have to look for better and more powerful indicators rather than failing to document at all. Using standardised and structured instruments and scales also facilitates and simplifies comparisons between carers, agencies, regions and nations, thus, enabling a self-critical discussion about the outcomes of interventions. In addition, this discussion about the effectiveness of care should precede any discussion about costs and savings, because the costs may be adequate when the benefits are high and the follow-up cost may be exceeding the savings. An integrated documentation system is the preferred option when several funding bodies or providers have to deliver care to an individual and therefore need to consider the benefits to optimise the resources used. This calls for discussion, negotiation and a common policy on care and care quality.

References

Achterberg, W., van Campen, C., Margriet, A., Kerkstra, A., & Ribbe, M. W. (1999). Effects of the resident assessment instrument on the care process and health outcomes in nursing homes. A review of the literature. *Scandinavian Journal of Rehabilitation Medicine, 31*(3), 131–37.

Adams, T., & Gardiner, P. (2005). Communication and interaction within dementia care triads. *Developing a theory for relationship-centered care, dementia, 4,* 185–205.

Aminzadeh, F., & Dalziel, W. B. (2002). Older adults in the emergency department: a systematic review of patterns of use, adverse outcomes, and effectiveness of interventions. *Annals of Emergency Medicine, 39*(3), 238–247.

Ammerwerth, E., Kutscha, U., & Kutscha, A. (Eds.). (2001). Nursing process documentation systems in clinical routine - prerequisites and experiences. *International Journal of Medical Informatics, 64,* 187–200.

Applegate, W., Blass, J. P., & Williams, T. F. (1990). Instruments for the functional assessment of older patients. *New England Journal of Medicine, 322*(17), 1207–1214.

Baldock, J. C., & Hadlow, J. (2002). Self-Talk versus Needs-Talk: an exploration of the priorities of housebound older people. *Quality in Ageing, 3*(1), 42–48.

Baltes, P. B., & Mayer, K. K. (Eds.). (1999). *The Berlin aging study. Aging from 70 to 100.* Cambridge: Cambridge University Press.

Bowers, B. J., Fibich, B., & Jacobson, N. (2001). Care-as-service, care-as-relating, care-as-comfort: understanding nursing home residents' definitions of quality. *Gerontologist, 41,* 539–545.

Bowers, B. J., Lauring, C., & Jacobson, N. (2001). How nurses manage time and work in long-term care. *Journal of Advanced Nursing, 33,* 484–491.

Bowling, A. (1997). Measuring health: A review of quality of life measurement scales. Buckingham: Oxford University press, 2nd edition.

Bruhn, M. (2003). *Qualitätsmanagement für Dienstleistungen (Quality management for services)*. Berlin: Springer Publisher.

Caris-Verhallen, W., Kerkstra, A., & Bensing, J. (1997). The role of communication in nursing care for elderly people: a review of the literature. *Journal of Advanced Nursing, 25*, 915–933.

Challis, D., & Hughes, J. (2002). Frail old people at the margins of care: some recent research findings. *British Journal of Psychiatry, 180*, 126–130.

Coulon, L., Mok, M., Krause, K.-L., & Anderson, M. (1996). 'The pursuit of excellence in nursing care: what does it mean?' *Journal of Advanced Nursing, 24*, 817–826.

Currie, V., Harvey, G., West, E., McKenna, H., & Keeney, S. (2005). Relationships between quality of care, staffing levels, skill mix and nurse autonomy: Literature review. *Journal of Advanced Nursing, 51*, 73–82.

Davies, S., Slack, R., Laker, S., & Philp, I. (1999). The educational preparation of staff in nursing homes: Relationship with resident autonomy. *Journal of Advanced Nursing, 29*, 208–217.

Donabedian, A. (1969). Some issues in evaluation the quality of nursing care. *American Journal of Public Health, 59*, 1833–1836.

Donabedian, A. (1980). *Explorations in quality assessment and monitoring. Volume 1. Definition of quality*. Michigan: Health Administration Press.

Edgar, I. R., & Russel, A. (Eds.). (1998). *The anthropology of welfare*. London: Routledge.

Ehrenberg, A., & Ehnfors, M. (2001). The accuracy of patient records in Swedish nursing homes: Congruence of record content and nurses' and patients' descriptions. *Scandinavian Journal of Caring Sciences, 15*, 303–310.

Fawcett, J. (1996). Pflegemodelle im Überblick. Verlag Hans Huber, Bern, Göttingen, Toronto, Seattle.

Fleming, K., Evans, J. M., Weber, D. C., & Chutka, D. S. (1995). Practical functional assessment of elderly persons: A primary-care approach. *Mayo Clinic Proceedings, 70*(9), 890–910.

Gilloran, A., McGlew, T., McKee, K., Robertson, A., & Wight, D. (1993). Measuring the quality of care in psychogeriatric wards. *Journal of Advanced Nursing, 18*, 269–275.

Goldstone, L., & Maselino-Okai, C. (1986). *Senior monitor. An index of the quality of nursing care for senior citizens on hospital wards*. Newcastle upon Tyne: Newcastle upon Tyne Polytechnic Products Ltd.

Grant, N., Reimer, M., & Bannatyre, J. (1996). Indicators of quality in long-term care facilities. *International Journal of Nursing Studies, 33*, 469–478.

Gubrium, J., & Lynott, R. (1987). Measurement and the interpretation of burden in the Alzheimer's disease experience. *Journal of Aging Studies, 1*, 265–285.

Hawes, C., Mor, V., Phillips, C. D., Fries, B. E., Morris, J. N., Steele-Friedlob, E., Greene, A. M., & Nennstiel, M. (1997). The obra-87 nursing home regulations and implementation of the resident assessment instrument: effects on process quality. *Journal of the American Geriatrics Society, 5*(8), 977–985.

Hogston, R. (1995). Quality nursing care: a qualitative enquiry. *Journal of Advanced Nursing, 21*, 116–124.

Jantsch, E. (1975). *Design for evolution. Self-organization and planning in the life of human systems*. Braziller, New York.

Jelinek, R., Haussman, D., Hegyvary, S., & Newman, J. (1974). *A methodology for monitoring quality of nursing care. Publication no. 76–25*. Bethesda, Maryland: U.S. Department of Health, Education and Welfare.

Kitwood, T. (1989). Brain, mind and dementia: With particular reference to Alzheimer's disease. *Ageing and Society, 9*, 1–15.

Kitwood, T. (1997). *Dementia reconsidered—the person comes first*. Buckingham: Open University Press.

Kitwood, T., & Bredin, K. (1992). Towards a theory of dementia care: Personhood and well-being. *Ageing and Society, 12*, 269–287.

Laitinen, P. (1992). Participation of informal caregivers in the hospital care of elderly patients and their evaluations of the care given: pilot study in three different hospitals. *Journal of Advanced Nursing, 17*, 1233–1237.

Larsson, G., & Wilde Larsson, B. (1998). Quality of care: Relationship between the perceptions of elderly home care users and their caregivers. *Scandinavian Journal of Social Welfare, 7*, 262–268.

Lawton, M. P. (1991). A multidimensional view of quality of life in frail elders. In J. Birren, J. Lubben, J. Rowe, & D. Deutchman (Eds.), *The concept of measurement of quality of life in frail elders* (pp. 3–27). San Diego, CA: Academic Press.

Lee, L., Lee, D., & Woo, J. (2005). Predictors of satisfaction among cognitively intact nursing home residents in Hong Kong. *Research in Nursing & health, 28*, 376–387.

Leppänen, T., Töyry, E., & Vehviläinen-Julkunen, K. (1997). Potilaiden käsitys ihmisläheisen hoidon keskeisestä sisällöstä. (Patients' view about the most important contents of Humane Caring Scale.) *Hoitotiede, 9*, 178–185.

Loewenthal, D. (2005). Philosophical and ethical dimensions of managing person-centred integrated care. In M. Vaarama, & R. Pieper (Eds.). *Managing integrated care for older persons. European perspectives and good practices. Stakes and the European Health Management Association (EHMA)*. Saarijärvi: Gummerus Printing.

Lyman, K. (1989). Bringing the social back in: A critique of the biomedicalization of dementia. *Gerontologist, 29*(4), 597–605.

Marriner-Tomey, A. (1992). *Pflegetheoretikerinnen und ihr Werk*. Recom Verlag, Basel.

Medical College of Georgia (2003). http://www.mcg.edu/som/fmfacdev/fd_quality.htm

Meleis, A. I. (1999). l *Pflegetheorien. Gegenstand, Entwicklung und Perspektiven des theoretischen Denkens in der Pflege*, Verlag Hans Huber, Bern, Göttingen, Toronto, Seattle.

Ministry of Health and Social Affairs and Association of Local Authorities in Finland (2001). National framework for high quality care of older persons. Helsinki.

Morris, J. N., Fries, B. E., Steel, K., Ikegami, N., Bernabei, R., Carpenter, G. I., Gilgen, R., Hirdes, J. P., & Topinkova, E. (1997). Comprehensive clinical assessment in community setting: applicability of the MDS-HC. *Journal of the American Geriatrics Society, 45*(8), 1017–1024.

Morrow-Howell, N., Proctor, E., & Rozario, P. (2001). How much is enough? Perspectives of care recipient and professionals on the sufficiency of in-home care. *The Gerontologist, 41*, 723–732.

Mozley, C., Sutcliffe, C., Bagley, H., Cordingley, L., Challis, D., Huxley, P., & Burns, A. (2004). *Towards quality care. outcomes for older people in care homes*. England: Ashgate.

Muurinen, S. (2003). Hoitotyö ja hoitohenkilöstön rakenne vanhusten lyhytaikaisessa laitoshoidossa. (Care and the staff-mix in institutional respite care for elderly) *Academic dissetation, Acta Universitatis Tamperensis 936. Tampere University Press, Tampere*.

Muurinen, S., Nuutinen, H.-L., & Peiponen, A. (2002). Omaisten mielipiteitä vanhusten hoidosta Helsingin ympärivuorokautisen hoidon yksiköissä 2002 . (Relatives perspectives in long-term care in the City of Helsinki 2002.) *Tutkimuksia 2002:2*. Helsingin kaupungin sosiaalivirasto, Helsinki.

Netten, A. (2004). The social production of welfare. In M. Knapp, D. Challis, J.-L. Fernandez, & A. Netten (Eds.), Long-term care: Matching resources and needs. Ashgate: Aldershot.

Niehörster, G., Garms-Homolová, V., & Vahrenhorst, V. (1998). *Identifizierung von Potentialen für eine selbständige Lebensführung.* Stuttgart: Kohlhammer Verlag.

Nies, H., & Berman, P. (Eds.). (2004). *Integrating services for older people: A resource book for managers.* Dublin: EHMA.

Oleson, M., Heading, C., McGlynn, K., Bistodeau, J. (1994). Quality of life in long-stay institutions in England: Nurse and resident perceptions. *Journal of Advanced Nursing, 20,* 23–32.

Øvretveit, J. (1998). *Evaluating health interventions. An introduction to evaluation of health treatments, services, policies and organizational interventions* (pp. 229–272). Buckingham: Open University Press.

Paljärvi, S., Rissanen, S., & Sinkkonen, S. (2003). Kotihoidon sisältö ja laatu vanhusasiakkaiden, omaisten ja työntekijöiden arvioimana - Seurantatutkimus Kuopion kotihoidosta. *Gerontologia, 2,* 85–97.

Phaneuf, M. (1976). *The nursing audit: Self-regulation in nursing practice.* New York: Appleton-Century-Crofts.

Pieper, R. (1997). Technology and the social triangle of home care: ethical issues in the application of technology to dementia care. In S. Björneby, A. van Berlo (Eds.), *Ethical issues in the use of technology for dementia care.* Knegsel: AKONTES Publishing.

Raatikainen, R. (1995). Hoitotyön kehitysvaiheiden luokitus. (The model of phases in patient care). *Sairaanhoitaja, 9*(95), 31–34.

Rantz, M., Jensdóttir, A., Hjaltadóttir, I., Gudmundsdóttir, H., Sigurveig Gudjónsdóttir, J., Drunton, D., & Rook, M. (2002). International field test results of the observable indicators of nursing home care quality instrument. *International Nursing Review, 49,* 234–242.

Rantz, M. J., Zwygart-Stauffacher, M., & Popejoy, L., et al. (1999). Nursing home care quality: A multidimensional theoretical model integrating the views of consumers and providers. *Journal of Nursing Care Quality, 14,* 16–37.

Roth, G. (2001). *Qualitätsmängel und Regelungsdefizite in der Qualitätssicherung in der ambulanten Pflege.* Stuttgart: Kohlhammer Verlag.

Samuelsson, G., & Brink, S. (1997). Quality attributes of home help services in Sweden and Canada—A consumer view. *Scandinavian Journal of Social Welfare, 6,* 82–90.

Schäffer, E., Steppe, H., Moers, M., Meleis, A. (Ed.). (1997). Pflegetheorien. Beispiele aus den USA, Verlag Hans Huber, Bern, Göttingen, Toronto, Seattle.

Sidani, S., Doran, D., & Mitchell, P. (2004). A theory-driven approach to evaluating quality of nursing care. *Journal of Nursing Scholarship, 36*(1), 60–65.

Sixsmith, A., Stilwell, J., & Copeland, J. (1993). 'Rementia': Challenging the limits of dementia care. *International Journal of Geriatric Psychiatry, 8,* 993–1000.

Sloane, P. D., & Mathew, L. J. (1991). An assessment and care planning strategy for nursing home residents with dementia. *The Gerontologist, 31,* 128–131.

Tester, S., Hubbard, G., Downs, M., MacDonald, C., & Murphy, J. (2003). Exploring perceptions of quality of life of frail older people during and after their transition to institutional care. Research Findings 24, Growing Older Project. http://www.shef.ac.uk/uni/projects/gop/GOFindings24.pdf

Thomé, B., Dykes, A-K., & Rahm Hallberg, I. (2003). Home care with regard to definition, care recipients, content and outcome: Systematic literature review. *Journal of Clinical Nursing, 12*(6), 860–872.

Twigg, J. (2004). The medical-social boundary and rival discourses of the body, In M. Knapp, D. Challis, J.-L. Fernandez, A. Netten (Eds.), *Long-term care: Matching resources and needs*. Ashgate: Aldershot.

van Maanen, H. (1984). Evaluation of nursing care: quality of nursing evaluated within the context health care and examined from multinational perspective. In L. Willis, & M. Lindwood (Eds.), *Measuring the quality of care* (pp. 3–42). Churchill Livingstone: Edinburg.

Vaarama, M., Luomahaara, J., Peiponen, A., & Voutilainen, P. (2001). *The whole municipality working together for older people. Perspectives on the development of elderly people's independent living, care and services*. Helsinki: Stakes.

Vaarama, M., & Pieper, R. (2005). Managing Integrated Care for Older Persons. Stakes and the European Health Management Association. Saarijärvi: Gummerus Printing.

Voutilainen, P., Isola, A., & Muurinen, S. (2004). Nursing documentation in nursing homes—state-of-the-art and implications for quality improvement. *Scandinavian Journal of Caring Sciences, 18*, 72–81.

Weekers, S., & Pijl, M. (1998). Home care and care allowances in the European Union. The Netherlands: Netherlands Institute of Care and Welfare.

Weiner, M. F., Martin-Cook, K., Svetlik, D. A., Saine, K., Foster, B., & Fontain, C. S. (2000). The quality of life in late-stage dementia (QUALID) scale. *Journal of the American Medical Directors Association, 1*, 114–116.

Weman, K., Kihlgren, M., & Fagerberg, I. (2004). Older people living in nursing homes or other community care facilities: Registered Nurses' views of their working situation and co-operation with family members. *Journal of Clinical Nursing, 13*, 617–626.

Wierz, V., Schwarz, A., & Gervink, S. (2000). Qualität in der Pflege: Beispiele aus der Praxis, Kohlhammer.

WHOQOL Group (1998). Development of the World Health Organization WHO-QOL-Bref quality of life assessment. The WHOQOL Group. *Psychological Medicine, 28*(3), 551–558.

Web Links

http:www.dh.gov.uk: The website of the UK Department of Health. For detailed information on the Single Assessment Process, go further on to Policy and Guidance, then Health and Social Care Topics, Social Care, ending up in Single Assessment Process.

http:www.nzgg.org.nz: The website of New Zealand Guidelines Group. Go further to Publications and then to Guidelines and other major publications, and there down to Gerontology, to find information on the assessment process

http:www.sheffield.ac.uk/sisa/easycare: Website of the assessment instrument EasyCARE

http:www.interrai.org: Website of the Resident Assessment Instruments, RAI.

6
Quality Management
in Long-Term Care

Richard Pieper, Mona Frommelt, Claus Heislbetz
and Marja Vaarama

Introduction

Quality management (QM) is not just a recent strategy for management tasks such as resource management, personnel management, marketing management, risk management, knowledge management or innovation management, but it has become part of a quality movement. It is currently a firm element of scientific and public discussion on quality standards and a widely accepted requirement in the provision of social and health care services. For example, Total Quality Management (TQM) has become a comprehensive management philosophy, and an approach to management encompassing all tasks within a single framework. Although the concepts and strategies of TQM are proliferating, the discussion of central concepts of quality is still proceeding without a general agreement of terms and ideas, any agreed theoretical framework or consistent body of empirical findings. The TQM approach has been developed in the manufacturing industry, transformed for use with commercial services and has in the last 10 or 15 years become pervasive within public administrations and the health care and social services (Evers, Haverinen, Leichsenring, & Wistow, 1997; Görres, 1999; Øvretveit, 1998; Peterander & Speck, 2004). The movement has generated institutions and organisations on national and international levels that define quality for different realms of production, develop systematic standards, strategies and methods for quality development and certify their successful implementation. The certification of QM procedures can also be utilised in the competition in the marketplace for consumers. Quality becomes itself a product (certification) and a sales pitch, but at the same time the independently attested quality of products and service also provides consumer protection, since the consumer often has to rely on evaluations that he or she is not in a position to make himself or herself. Clearly, not all producers compete in the marketplace with similar levels of quality; it may be only the best quality for a given low price. Therefore, it is important to keep in mind that QM does not necessarily strive for the highest quality, but for a quality standard for given costs or prices. Moreover, since quality has a price, clients may have preferences for certain levels of quality, considering the trade-off between care outcomes and other consumption alternatives (Cangialose, Cary, Hoffmann, & Ballard, 1977).

Quality only emerges as an issue when there are different alternatives and choices available. In the public sector, many of the services, such as health and social care, were traditionally provided without alternatives and at a defined standard, which was determined by administrations and politicians, particularly with a view to "minimum" or "universal" requirements within a given budget. Thus, the discussion of quality of publicly provided or financed goods and services is closely connected to the privatisation and commercialisation of public services. Five trends promote the development and implementation of QM. Firstly, public responsibility and accountability for general standards of living often imply that the quality of services has to be controlled, even when the production and distribution is delegated to a market, leading to a proliferation of agencies defining and enforcing quality standards. Secondly, cost containment policies in all European welfare regimes put pressure on services. Providers react by arguing either that quality cannot be maintained within the budgetary constraints or that cheaper alternatives or competitors provide less quality (as in the case of traditional non-profit providers arguing against new commercial competitors). In either case, quality standards are used to justify costs. Thirdly, the market for services enhances trends towards increasing professionalism and innovation, leading to an increasing influence of professions and experts (with their own interests) on the definition of quality standards. This can be observed today in the field of health care, where health care professionals defend their monopoly on defining the quantity and quality of health needs. Growing professionalism based on growing scientific knowledge and professional education is, therefore, another important trend determining the debate on quality and QM.

Fourthly, issues of QM and quality standards have been taken up by movements for consumer interests and client empowerment (Beckmann, Otto, Richter, & Schrödter, 2004; Beresford, 2004; Evers et al., 1997). TQM strategies fuel this discussion because they proclaim client orientation as being central to their approach. However, consumer power has a quite different function in the context of established markets than in the context of provision of public services and, especially, in social and health care. Empowerment in the latter context is essentially (socio-) political and concerned with the definition of rights to receive services of a certain amount and quality (an issue of "voice"), whereas in the former context, consumer influence is strengthened to allow the production of services to adapt more effectively and efficiently to changing needs and demands (an issue of "choice"). TQM approaches and professional expertise tend to form a coalition to define concepts of quality, to delegate the socio-political discussion about them to the market of demand and supply and to evade the normative and political issues raised by the empowerment movement. It thus becomes the main advocate in the negotiation of the meaning of quality and the rights to services in a more democratic or participative way, including the users or clients.

Finally, the trends of QM, professionalism, commercialisation, new markets in social and health care and consumer orientation interact and are further influenced by the cultural and technological conditions of the evolving "knowledge and information society", putting high priority on knowledge-based and technology-aided innovations. This creates a fruitful environment for QM in social and health care, but also raises concerns and arguments that the basic requirements of "good care" in social and health care services are endangered by the very impacts of these trends and the implementation of QM. Although these trends have become pervasive within the health care services and development of quality standards and QM is progressing rapidly, social care and social work services are still questioning the role of quality standards and QM, and there appears to be considerable reluctance to embark on this path. This reluctance is based on a concept of care and care quality, especially in long-term care (LTC), which is seen to be incompatible with strategies emphasising standardised information processing, quantitative measures of quality and a market orientation in care provision.

In the following sections, we will briefly sketch out first the concept of QM and of TQM as comprehensive strategy. Following the general framework of the Care Keys project, the perspective will be on QM as part of a production process and on the quality chain in different care settings. The second section will be devoted to clarifying the special affordances that care raises as an object of QM. The concept of the "care tetrahedron" and a "negotiated order" are introduced to characterise the relationship between care and QM in a management perspective. The focus is on the different actors or stakeholders in the care process and the role of management as mediating and supporting the care process. The third section, finally, takes a closer look at the dimension of quality and connects the strategy of QM to the concepts of quality of care and quality of life (QoL) in a common framework, which is then implemented in the CK quality matrix as an instrument for QM. A short conclusion will summarise the argument for QM as a necessary prerequisite and important element of "good" care services, but also for the need for a kind of QM that is sensitive to the special affordances of caring relationships.

Quality Management in LTC

Although the strategic focus, the methods and the criteria of performance will change, QM is seen as a strategy that can be applied to all levels of a care system. On the level of the *individual care process*, it is concerned with the interaction of the professional carer and the client, including informal carers whenever possible or appropriate. On the level of *care chain management*, the care process for an individual is structured, planned, monitored and evaluated along the care path, and methods such as case management are often used. On the third level of *care service management*, QM is concerned with the central care production process involving other management tasks such as personnel, resource or marketing strategies. At least on this level the distinction between large and small organisations becomes relevant, because in small organisations, QM will be the task of the care manager, whereas in large service organisations QM may be organised in some kind of special unit, and the development and implementation of strategies for integrating care services and supporting services is the task of this QM unit. In small organisations, managers typically have to be involved in "networking" in order to coordinate their services with services from *other* organisations, whereas in larger organisations coordination *within* the organisation is the predominant focus. On the fourth level of *care system management* we find great differences between welfare regimes, because the organisation and integration of services at this level may be the responsibility of a centralised care organisation, or it can be structured as a network of providers within a "mixed economy" of care operating under market conditions. Although the general principles of QM can be applied on all levels of LTC, two important conditions should be noted.

First, typically, QM assumes that it is applied *within* an organisation with a clear management structure and a hierarchy of responsibility and accountability. However, management in a *network* of more or less independent partners is very frequent in care systems, and management has to be adapted to this situation. This raises issues and problems of management of integrated care (Pieper, 2005a,b; Vaarama, 2005; Vaarama & Pieper, 2005), and also has an impact on QM in institutional care versus home care.

Second, under market conditions, management is essentially only accountable to the owners of the organisation, and management has to "keep the customer satisfied". In the social and health care services the situation is more complex, since the production of public goods and services (collective goods) implies a strong influence of the socio-political and the legal systems and ultimately of the community of citizens and tax payers. Thus, clients of services have to be considered in the role of consumers having a "choice" as well as of a citizen having a "voice". Moreover, the character of "public goods", involving principles such as human dignity and social justice, has a decisive impact on the values relevant for quality assessment, professional culture and the expectations of the clients. Clients have to be respected as vulnerable persons needing our solidarity, but also as persons with rights to autonomy and self-determination. Management has to consider the socio-political and ethical aspects of care, care organisation and care integration.

The general framework adopted in Care Keys research is the production of welfare approach. From this perspective, the quantity and quality of care are intermediate outputs in the production of welfare or QoL of the client as the "final outcome" (Chapter 1). Following a recent definition proposed for integrated care by Vaarama (2005) we may say:

Integrated quality management is a systematic method of influencing the elements (structure, process, outcomes) of a quality chain to improve and ensure the service quality, to avoid risks, and to enhance the quality of the life of the client, consumer satisfaction and system efficiency (p. 66).

The definition highlights the role of systematic methods of planning, monitoring and evaluation of quality throughout the entire production process (compare Bruhn, 2003), which is also a central focus of the Care Keys approach. However, by speaking about *influencing* rather than determining the quality chain, it also reflects the fact that management is (also) an "art" rather than (only) an applied science, and that management has to be "careful" (see later) when dealing with care.

Quite similar to the approach to QM developed in Care Keys, the strategies of TQM are characterised by an essentially four-dimensional scheme. First, TQM places great emphasis on vision and values within the organisation. As stated in the definition earlier, TQM puts the client in the centre by orienting all organisational activities, their continuous improvement and their quality evaluation, towards the satisfaction of the client (*dimension of values and quality concepts*). Second, a sound knowledge base of work organisation, procedures and risk management, systematic goal achievement, specification of quality and outcome measures, information processing and controlling and evaluation are characteristics of TQM (*dimension of professional work procedures*). Third, the strategies also contain the insight that the staff on all levels must be committed and involved in the strategy, so that issues of staff qualifications, participation and motivation are an essential part (*dimension of innovative potential*). Finally, resources, technologies and supporting services are essential (though often neglected in the discussion of "good care"), since sustainability (economic, political and ecological) provides an essential condition with social change requiring continuous innovation and a flexible "learning organisation" (Nies & Berman, 2004). This we can call as the *dimension of resource, technology and environment support*. An extensive review of the literature on innovation management of services by Reichwald and Schaller (2006) extracted quite similar dimensions indicating that high benefits for the client, systematic strategies for innovate development, adequate resources and personnel development are the important features—with client orientation being perhaps the most important feature of successful management of innovation (see also Chapter 12). Thus, TQM gives conceptual and practical support to a four-dimensional approach to QM functions. In Care Keys, these four functions were based on social systems theory, suggested by empirical research (Chapters 8 and 12) and implemented in the CK quality matrix (see later and Chapter 13). TQM will integrate QM into all structures, processes and the evaluation of outcomes involving *all* parts and levels of the organisation and phases of the production process. Vaarama also emphasises the interests and perspectives of *all* groups involved in the process, particularly a *comprehensive* client orientation, but also a staff orientation and a consideration of other relevant stakeholders.

Moreover, the chain of quality will typically cross boundaries of services and require structures and strategies of "cooperation for quality" (Pieper,

2005a,b; Vaarama, 2005). The quality chain will consist of own services, but also involve other services and informal carers and their household. Within the framework of a given service organisation, management has to determine which services it will directly offer and organise, which services it will outsource, which services it will assure by cooperation with other service providers including the household of the client, and determine those services (and corresponding needs) for which it does feel *not* responsible. Welfare regimes may differ widely in how all this is structured. Considerable differences may occur in terms of how legitimate needs are defined and who is seen as "eligible", how services are organised, how effective and efficient they are in satisfying needs, what legitimate needs are typically left unmet by the care system and what needs are considered to be outside the realm of public responsibility. Clients with more complex needs will depend on a combination or a "mix" of services from different sources, and management will not have complete control over the scope of needs and services it can effectively organise within its own realm of responsibility. This has consequences for the QoL of the client, for cooperation between partners and for the concept of quality, since the *comprehensiveness* of care—a quality criterion—will depend on the scope of available services. Arguments for *non*-responsibility have to rest on accepted professional standards, agreed divisions of labour and a "moral order" justifying neglect. A management claim that a service specialises in certain types of care (e.g. home nursing), because it can provide it "good", effective and efficient, may not be convincing for the client or the wider community with their own expectations about the comprehensiveness and the integration of care which respects the dignity of a dependent person. Accepted non-responsibilities are typically organised in a division of labour defining service types and supported by professional ethics, legal regulations and systems of financing. Management has to mediate this differentiated context of care with the affordances of client-oriented care.

Three divisions within the landscape of care are key for the conceptualisation of care and in the Care Keys research reported in this book: the division between health care and social care; professional and informal care and institutional and home care. As Twigg (2004) for instance has shown, the medical–social boundary is closely connected to theories and discourses of the body with medically oriented nursing focusing on basic "bed and body work" (p. 225), and social care and social work concentrating on psycho-social or interpersonal work (see chapter 5). Traditionally, the central role of health care is emphasised and other services are treated to some degree as auxiliary or additional. Health care, from this perspective, has a central role, because of the fundamental importance of health of the client/patient and the need of special qualifications of the personnel ("medical model"). Other services can be substituted by, for example, family care (and are therefore also in danger of being cut because of financial savings in the care system). However, this perspective becomes less and less appropriate the more LTC aims to enable frail older persons to stay at home, and it fails to represent adequately household tasks and their substitution by support for instrumental activities of daily living (IADL). In what might be called an "activation model", the focus is on the competences of clients and independence in everyday life integrating support in all activities (ADL and IADL; see also Chapter 10).

The neglect especially of IADL support can be understood by taking a closer look at the relation between professional and informal care. The social production of welfare (Netten, 2004) analyses the ways care services are developed out of the context of household production, creating a differentiation of professional and informal care. Health care and, to a lesser degree, social work have become highly professionalised, but IADL support has still the image of unqualified, unprofessional or informal household work. From this perspective, social care has a precarious role, because it is always liable to be substituted by non-professional, less qualified care. Its importance, however, is becoming increasingly apparent, because the *lack* of household support is often the deciding factor in the (expensive) institutionalisation of frail older persons. Changing household and family structures make informal support less available for an increasing number of older persons. Thus, there is no solution to the task of supporting "independent living" without the provision of household services—or the integration of informal care. And it should be emphasised that informal care has also a role in emotional support and in finding a meaningful self-identity as well a role in "negotiating order" in care. The interdependence of clients, professional social care and informal care is essential in this perspective with medical services contributing a certainly vital and indispensable basis for the QoL, the multi-dimensionality of the life situation suggesting a "Lawtonian model" (Chapter 11). Care managers in practice are well aware of these issues, but there are strong incentives to focus on a restricted health care definition of own service responsibilities and liabilities rather than taking up the challenges and risks of integrated care.

Finally, it is important to see the provision of care in terms of the distinction between home care and institutional care. Superficially, this distinction rests on the degree of dependency of the client, which eventually makes care in an institution unavoidable. But the situation is more complex, because the necessity to provide "hotel functions" depends much more on the availability of social support (e.g. the spouse caring at home) than on the degree of functional dependency. Even medical health care can, in most cases, be provided at home. In fact, in some cases of extreme dependency, where the medical profession and acute medical treatments are restricted to a supporting role, because they have no effective therapy (e.g. dementia) or are considered to be not justified anymore (e.g. hospice care), caring at home is the preferred option even from the perspective of the institutional system. Moreover, institutional care has been subjected to strong criticism that institutions tend to become "closed systems" or "total institutions", in which the narrower interests of management (in "running their business smoothly"), the particular interests of professionals (to do their job according to the "rules" and avoid risks and liabilities) and the interests of inmates (in sheer survival) evolve into a subculture of practices which totally neglect the QoL of clients (and of managers and professionals, for that matter). The only ways to control for such developments is (i) to open up the institution to external control by the community, (ii) to implement practices that empower the clients with the help of advocates (e.g. relationships with informal carer and client interest organisations) and (iii) to create a "community in care homes" as promoted by the "My Home Life" programme (Owen & NCHRDF, 2006). The essential characteristic of this approach is not that management tries to make the institution look "like a home", although that is an important feature in its own right, but that the clients participate in the "running" of the home, have partnership relations with the staff and external relations to relatives and friends. From the perspective of QM, the convergence of institutional settings becoming "home-like" and home care being extended to cover household tasks for older persons living alone implies a convergence of QM strategies in both cases. But an essential difference remains, namely, the organisational versus network structure of the cooperation between actors and the integration of care.

A Management View of the Care Relationship

Looking less from the perspective of established management strategies and more from the perspective of LTC and its characteristics, we propose to characterise the task of QM as follows:

Quality management in LTC has to provide the favourable conditions for retaining, regaining, and enhancing the quality of life of clients by supporting personal care in the "care triad" of client, professional carer and informal carer, and by mediating and negotiating the affordances of care as perceived by the "care triad" with the affordances of the service organisation, and with socio-political and socio-cultural objectives of care.

This description "encapsulates" the concept of quality of personal care into the "care triad", a concept emphasising the vital role of all three primary partners or stakeholders in the care process. Focusing on the "care triad" rather than on the individual client is useful for several reasons (see also Chapter 4). First, LTC especially in institutional settings and unlike acute health care does enter, influence and structure "normal" daily living in a long-term perspective, and in that capacity has to find ways to conceptually and practically embed care into communication and social relations of everyday life. Care is not only a bilateral issue between the professional carer and the client. Second, communication will typically happen between two partners, but from basic insights into the structure of communication and interpretation we know that the *validity* of the communication depends on a "third" perspective. G. H. Mead (1934) provided the theoretical foundation for this insight with the concept of a "generalised other" as the reference point for the evaluation of the communication between "ego" and "alter" clarifying who they are and what the meaning of their interaction is. Drawing on Georg Simmel (1950), we can extend this insight to the "social triad" as the basic unit of social interaction. It is one of the fundamental shortcomings of dialogic approaches that they underestimate or simply overlook the essential role of a "third person" in the reflection on communication. In concrete communications a third person representing the "generalised other" will not be present, but it is present in the *culturally shared* means of communication and in the *appeals to objectivity, fairness or consensus* by partners searching for agreement. Or in other words, the basic structure of a "discourse" is triadic rather than dyadic. A third communication partner will always make it more transparent to all involved that they communicate in a (more or less) shared world of meanings with others and that sharing involves agreement, negotiation and compromise.

In case of the "care triad" (see Fig. 6.1), it typically will be the informal carer (the spouse or some other friend or advocate), who will assure *both* professional carer and client that the care objectives and the care relation is in concordance with the clients views, interests and everyday life orientations, especially in case of frailty or cognitive disabilities (Adams & Gardiner, 2005; Pieper, 1997). We do not claim that the informal carer has a "right" view of a "neutral referee", but he or she will provide an "other view," which will trigger a reflection by all three persons on what is "really" meant. In this way they may mutually construct a more trustworthy and shared social reality (see Berger & Luckmann, 1966; Chapter 4).

Third, if there is an essential difference of opinion or interests, a common view and line of action or a "negotiated order" has to be created, as Anselm Strauss has so aptly described for the care relationship (Freidson, 1961; Hardy, Young, & Wistow, 1999; Maines & Charlton, 1985; Strauss, 1978; Strauss et al., 1963). Differences are to be expected, although in the descriptions of care relations there tends to dominate a view that the relations are "naturally" harmonic. Georg Simmel (1950) made an important contribution to social

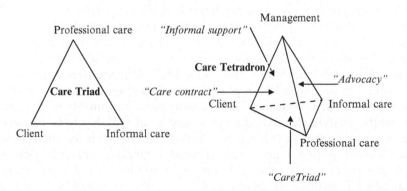

FIG. 6.1. The "Care Triad" and the "Care Tetrahedron" of quality management.

theory by analysing the role of the "third party" in the negotiation of conflict situations. If two opponents have essentially a common background of values and world views, negotiation may be cumbersome, because a lot of issues have to be clarified, but consensus is likely in the end. Where there is a fundamental difference of interests, the theory and practice of negotiation shows that the mediation by a third party is essential. Even such simple rules as the majority rule will require at least three actors. There is no guarantee that the third person may not introduce their own bias or a bias in favour of one of the partners, but still it is a good and even necessary strategy to structure practices that involve potential conflicts of interests in a way that opposing partners have access to a third party they both can trust.

"Thinking in triads" becomes especially important whenever relationships are characterised by asymmetries and dependencies, as is the case in care relationships. Following Jochimsen (2003), it is meaningful to distinguish between types of caring activities. Care may occur between persons, who could in principle help each other (e.g. between friends). Both partners, in this case, will have the capacities and resources to be in the role of the care giver, or will be able to reciprocate on another occasions. Both partners can also be conceived of as having the capacities for self-help. Although these situations have their own importance in the conceptualisation of a general theory of help and caring, the "classical cases" are the care for children, for the underprivileged, sick or impaired or for frail older persons who have some kind of *dependency* on care or help. These persons are vulnerable in the sense that *not* receiving care will bring them to some kind of precarious situation, because they cannot be expected to help themselves. Certainly, there are degrees of dependency; there may be an option to wait, to select other living conditions or to reduce the expectations on the quality or even the duration of life (for coping strategies see Chapter 4). Nonetheless, the risks for the persons are so high that they justify a moral obligation to help on part of potential carers. Not helping when being in the position to help constitutes a "moral failure", which may be accompanied by sanctions. Management has to be sensitive to this essentially moral, not only professional situation.

The conceptualisation of dependency is itself not a trivial issue—to be solved, for instance, by simply relying on biological or medical criteria of health and survival. The situation of disabled persons has taught us to recognise that functional impairments are relative to the affordances of the environment and conceptions of a "good life". A barrier-free environment can make life in a wheelchair possible and meaningful, whereas in other environments the person may be very vulnerable and unable to develop a personally satisfying lifestyle. The very concept of QoL has to be conceived in a way to incorporate this relationship of "fit" between the environment and different personal and socio-cultural evaluations of lifestyles (see Chapter 4). Thus, management has a responsibility for the living environment, which in institutional care may encompass the entire living environment of a person, whereas in home care only the apartment may be within reach of management capacities and measures of home adaptation. A central principle of care, namely, "help for self-help", can be understood as supporting a change from a situation of essential dependency to a situation of relative autonomy and "independent living". However, although this is the goal of care, it is not helpful to overlook the essential asymmetry and dependency characterising the care relationship on the road to (relative) independence. This has the implication of a responsibility of management for client empowerment as well as (supportive) professional supervision or, in other words, for making "third views" accessible.

The definition of needs or dependencies has to be made—in the first instance—within the care triad. The appropriate forms of caring or helping have to be agreed, not only derived from—say—medical assessments. This implies creating a common view of the QoL of the client, including the subjective view of the client as the main reference point, but also reflecting professional assessments and third-party views of relevant informal carers and relatives (see Chapter 4). The third party, additionally, will have the function of coping with the asymmetries and dependencies in the care relationship by being an advocate for the client and supporting care approaches that reflect the QoL of the client. This QoL will not only encompass the *care-related* QoL, but also cover domains not directly affected and involved in care (especially in home care). The position of informal carer may be rather weak and have little influence on the problems of asymmetry and dependency in the care relationship. Management, especially in institutions, will particularly influence the different aspects of the care situation, for example the work, the resources, relevant aspects of the care motivations of professional carers and the guiding care values. Considering this, it is necessary to expand the care triad into a "care tetrahedron" by introducing the relations of management to each partner in the triad (see Fig. 6.1).

Management will bring in the additional perspective of "setting the stage" and organising the care relationship (the base of the tetrahedron) as a continuing service, a set of personal relationships and a "negotiated order". The care tetrahedron has three additional triads that are important for care and each may be conceived as representing a "discourse" focusing on (but not restricted to) a specific theme. In the triad of management, professionals and clients, we expect the organisation of care to be agreed and contracted. In the triad of management, informal carer and clients, the "division of labour" involving support by relatives (or other informal support networks) and their responsibilities will be clarified; in the triad of management, professionals and informal carers, the issues of advocacy and representing the "best interest" of a client who is frail and lacking (full) autonomy have to be handled. The first of these triads is usually considered the focus of QM, and it comprises the three perspective of the CK quality matrix (see later and Chapters 1 and 13). The second triad raises the important issue of involvement of informal care, and it will be especially important in care settings (typically in home care) in which relevant care support is given by other household members rather than a professional carer. Many care systems provide a financial incentive for such household care, and this support may also be subjected to an explicit contract. It is important to realise that there is not only a division of labour at stake, but a negotiation of responsibilities and commitments. The third triad is especially relevant in cases of severe impairment and frailty such as in case of dementia. Since management and professionals are both members of the organisation, it is clear that family members or other advocates of the client play a vital role. In this situation it may be necessary, and in certain cases required by law, to introduce an advocate for the client as another independent role representing the client's interests and the interests of the community for a "fair trial". Actually, "good" QM will realise this problem and will organise adequate advocacy in the interest of the client, but also in its own interest to cope with problems of professional bias and liability towards the community and the legal system. "Thinking in triads" is, therefore, not only a heuristic guideline for stakeholder analyses in care—a typical QM method—but also a normative principle for structuring care situations (see Chapter 4). In fact, the four triads in combination—the tetrahedron—may be interpreted as a "cosmos of discourses" in QM on the four themes of care quality as identified in a system theory approach (see later, and Chapter 5) concerning care *competence* (first triad), informal care as a *resource* (second triad), client orientation as *value concept* (third triad) and the *integrative* quality of care (base triad in Fig. 6.1). The actor of the tetrahedron who is neglected in a given triad is still "virtually" present in the background and co-determining the "discourse", (i.e. management in the background of the integrative care triad and "setting the stage"; informal care in the background of the care contract triad controlling that client interests are respected; professional care in the background of the informal support triad is influencing the division of labour; client in the background of the advocacy triad acts as a reference for the "fair" representation of his or her needs—see Fig. 6.1). And, of course, the triads are "ideal types," which may be embedded in various ways in the actual roles and interactions in a given care setting.

Implications of LTC for Quality Management

The proposition on the tasks of QM introduces a distinction between management as "setting the stage" and the partners in the care triad as "doing the play". In many, especially small, organisations, managers will be engaged in care and professional carers will, conversely implement the objectives of QM in their care activities. But it is useful to maintain the distinction and to analyse the *differences* between a perspective on care and a perspective on management and to identify possible sources of conflict. The mediation of conflicts is one of the important tasks of management that is too often underestimated, because a harmonious consensus in respect to "good care" is assumed as given for all actors involved, simply because it is seen as a natural or necessary prerequisite. This point is made by Jochimsen (2003, p. 110) from the perspective of an economist, who is more apt to focus on conflicting interests:

...the task of any long-term sustainable social and economic organisation of caring situations may be described at a very general level as the task of effectively combining the motivation, work, and resource components of caring situations in such a way as to minimize asymmetry and dependency between the persons involved.

This refers to provision of the structural prerequisites of caring as the objective of management, although important characteristics of the components and the relationships involved are determined by the nature of caring. One central factor is time, as by definition LTC is required by the client over a long stretch of time, often for the rest of their life. There is, typically, no future without care, and care must provide a future or at least support the client in constructing and maintaining a sense of future and a perspective on life which is personally meaningful. A client must be able to feel confident that his or her relationship with the care service is a reliable, continuous and persistent element in his or her life. Moreover, care must be integrated into the identity of the client by reconciling it with past experiences. Being vulnerable and needing help, often after some traumatic life event, requires the person to reconstruct their own identity and find a new way of relating to other people, especially to those people on whom they are now dependent to some extent and who exert some level of control within their life (see Chapter 4). The commitment of carers to continuity in their relationship with clients has consequences for management. Strategies of "hire and fire" are not compatible, because they undermine the care culture. A good work atmosphere and participative leadership are necessary to sustain the special setting for quality care.

But "good care" is not just an issue of interaction quality; professional carers need to contribute by bringing their expertise into the care situation. The task of management is to select, qualify and organise carers who have the professional instrumental competence to cope with the problems of the client, but also the social competence to relate to the client, and the motivation to sustain this relationship over a potentially long-term period. One important element of their competence is to apply their professional knowledge to the care situation. The carer must be competent, but the carer must also be perceived, respected and trusted as competent by the client. Within the care triad, this requires that the professional carer has a competence to apply and to transform (at least part of) professional knowledge in such a way that it becomes available as a common knowledge among all the care actors. This presupposes experience with care situations and the accumulation of personal "tacit" knowledge, but it also requires what has been termed "subjectivating work" competence (Böhle, 2004). In the analysis of professional knowledge, we find that a personalised, subjectively meaningful knowledge, which (i) is adapted to dialogical communication, (ii) typically employs an associating, imaginative and experience-related way of thinking, (iii) relies on sensual perception and feeling in concrete situations and (iv) is closely related to ones own personality, is essential, especially in situations that are unplanned, new, complex and critical. The "subjectivating" competence in problem-solving is not limited to personal services, but can be found in creative problem-solving in technical professions as well (Böhle, 2004).

It is important that this competence does not simply take an everyday life perspective on the caring situation (see Pieper, 1979). Everyday life is strongly structured by habits and expectations of continuity, which may not be appropriate in the evolving situation of care. Furthermore, this view on professional competence should not be equated with what is usually understood as a "subjective" perspective in the sense that it is somewhat "irrational" and incompatible with more "objective", rational and systematic approaches to a problem. The concept of "subjectivating" competence re-introduces the professional as a subject who can relate "objective" professional knowledge to the experience of a concrete reality. The consequences of this view on professional knowledge for QM are clearly that there is no inherent incompatibility between objective evidence-based professional knowledge and procedures and subjective experiences and social competencies in professional care work. What is important is that professionals acquire the ability to combine their more formal approaches and qualifications with concrete problem-solving. This requires on part of QM that staff members are respected as *subjects* who require a certain level of autonomy in order to learn and apply their "subjectivating" competences to the caring activities. Bringing themselves as subjects into the relationship with the client makes possible the development of a shared perspective on the client's problems and the "negotiation of order" in the care triad. Moreover, the concept of "subjectivating work" competence and knowledge should not be confused with the emotional–motivational aspects of work, which are concerned with the incentives to work and important in their own right. It is more about a "style" of professional work, which can be seen as very rational and instrumental in the sense of effectively achieving aims in situations that afford the use of imagination and empathy with the client. This view on care competence emphasises that professional knowledge is a complex capacity with evidence-based scientific knowledge being an important element; that there is no inherent conflict between "objective" knowledge and client-oriented "good care" and that the development of "subjectivating" competence requires respect of management for a relatively autonomous domain of interaction in the "care triad".

The motivation of staff is crucial to "good" care, and creating motivating care situations must be a central concern of management. As Jochimsen (2003) shows, the motivation of care and especially LTC does not lend itself to a traditional economic perspective and analysis, and, thus, economic incentives alone are insufficient to motivate care givers. In reality, nursing care and social care are typically and chronically underfinanced anyway, and social care is competing with unqualified and household work within the market for care. In a time of unemployment and cheap labour arriving from less-developed new member countries to the European Union, the potential supply for rather low-paid jobs in care services may be even larger than that which socio-politicians are willing to finance. Still, care management has to be careful not to select people who are inappropriate for the job. In fact, as Jochimsen demonstrates in her analysis, there is a great danger of cheap and inappropriately motivated care personnel "crowding out" good carers. This is obvious when management looks only at the costs of care and does not select personnel according to qualifications and personal attributes, whereas it is not the overriding issue when the client is willing to pay what it takes to get qualified care (although this creates the problem of social justice for the care system; see later).

To understand the problem, it is necessary to look at care as a *relationship*, rather than at care services as a commodity. Care implies a dependency that is asymmetric. Dependency means that the care-receiving client is dependent on receiving the care, while the carer has many more options to either exploit the dependency or leave the relationship for other gainful activities. If the carer is *forced* to stay in a care relationship either by financial circumstances or by legal obligations, then this only serves to increase the danger of minimising work effort and to leave at the next available opportunity. The client has to be able to trust that the care relationship will be continuous and that the care provided meets the expectations and preferences, that is to trust in the commitment of the carer. This commitment may result from a professionalism rooted in a social valuation of the profession and a system of professional ethics (e.g. medical professions or social work). Professionalism is an important source of motivation, but in care services this professionalism has its limitations, because it implies, at least under current market conditions, that the personnel costs are high since professional education takes time, is expensive and requires substantial investment by the carer or employer. This problem is especially noticeable in long-term, socially oriented care compared with acute medical care. And expecting the professional attitude to develop in "on the job" training is just a way of restating the problem of suitable job relations.

Moreover, from the perspective of the client, professionalism as such does not totally resolve the issue, because of the importance of *personal* trust and social relationships for the client. Professionalism motivates the carer, but is not sufficient for the security and satisfaction of the client. In the care relationship, it is not only effective care that has to be produced and delivered, but also the "integrative product" (Jochimsen, 2003). This involves the additional interpretation of the caring activity as something that is socially valued and "constitutive" of the social identities of *both* the carer and the care receiver. It is not sufficient to consider care *outcomes* as "values in themselves" (Davies & Knapp, 1981), but also that the care *activity* itself contributes to the self-esteem *of the carer*. The "externality" (in economic terms) of social integration, moreover, gives the client a possibility to interpret care and help as something that he or she can readily accept without enhancing feelings of obligation, dependency and subservience. It should be emphasised that this "integrative product" is not the same as the products of the "emotional work" we have come to expect as part of a commodity (e.g. the smiles and friendliness of hostesses in airplanes). We should also distinguish it from a concept of "emotional work" focusing on the carer and the psychological stress induced by attachment, empathy and authentic display of feelings towards difficult and suffering clients that can overburden the carer to the point of "burn-out" (Wilkinson, Kerr, & Cunningham, 2005). Rather, it is about *mutual* respect, acceptance and empathy; that is the production and re-production of trust as an indispensable medium of social interaction which receives a special place in relationships that are inherently characterised by dependency, such as LTC. For QM this implies, on the one hand, the task of "setting the stage" for the creation of the "integrative product" in the care relation. On the other hand, there must be opportunities for staff to cope with the burden of emotional investments typically required by care of frail older persons. Moreover, care personnel—professionals and unqualified staff as well as volunteers—have to find themselves in a work atmosphere conducive to "good care", which implies that the motivations and values expected within the care triad will also be reflected in other practices of the service organisation and determine the concepts and approaches used within QM.

Management has to balance the needs of all involved, care givers and clients, another "sensitive point" (Jochimsen, 2003) in the care relationship. Care givers and care receivers cannot be left alone in the negotiation of needs and requirements of clients and carers. At least as far as this can be settled within the service organisation, it is in the "care tetrahedron" that a balancing of the QoL of all involved has to be achieved, that is it is a task of QM. An important prerequisite for this balance is a clear understanding of what care givers are expected to give and what clients can expect to receive, and that agreement should be reflected in a contract between the parties. Contracts do not solve the issues of the "integrative product" as described earlier, but they are an invaluable resource when it comes to misunderstandings and conflicts. Agreements below the level of formal contracts are also an important instrument for QM (not only in care, but also in general strategies of service management; see Ellis & Kauferstein, 2004). Agreements provide a structure for further negotiation and the resolution of conflicts by specifying the "arenas" and "rules" of negotiation, for example the participation in decisions by clients and staff, involvement in service development and quality circles, informal carer involvement, accountabilities and liabilities, complaint procedures, availability of advocacy and so on. Such regulations provide a "tangible" infrastructure for the empowerment of the client, for the rights of the staff as well as for the duties of management.

In all these strategies, the value orientations, the moral order and ethics play an important role suggesting even Total Value Management rather than TQM as a framework (Lachhammer, 2004). Management has to be sensitive (Jochimsen, 2003) to these characteristics and handle them with care (Jochimsen is playing on the word "care" by talking about "careful economics").

The need for sensitivity becomes even more evident, if a clear distinction is made between the moral values motivating carers and personal empathy and attachment evolving within the relationship. Management will have a responsibility for the values guiding care, since they also should reflect the values of the broader community, while the influence on personal relations will be more indirect by contributing to the work atmosphere in the service organisation. The central issue is certainly the respect of the "personhood" of all involved, not only of the client, but also of the other actors contributing to care and care services (see Chapter 5). The value of respecting the person, in a sense, includes all other values. In the care triad, basic values are mediated by the more particular cultural values and social identities of the persons involved. Religious commitments, ethnic background and personal values have to be considered in the development of the "moral order", this becoming more important as European societies develop into "multi-cultural" societies with clients, care givers and managers not always belonging to the same cultural community. The task of management is to provide guidance in the value orientation within the care triad and to specify basic value orientations in the "vision" and "mission" of the service-providing organisation. In Care Keys, these values have been incorporated into a concept of care quality that includes the following attributes or values: (i) comprehensive, need-responsive and client-oriented effectiveness; (ii) evidence-based and efficient professional standards and procedures; (iii) economic resource utilisation; (iv) integrative and innovative care practices with teamwork, collaboration and cooperation across organisational boundaries; (v) equity in the treatment of clients and among staff members; and (vi) quality concepts and strategies involving all actors in the "negotiation of order".

Perhaps the most neglected value in this list is the value of social justice or equity, since it is difficult to transform into a practical set of rules (Grand, 1991; McGuire, Henderson, & Mooney, 1988). Within a given service organisation, the exercise of social justice appears to be relatively easy, because the set of means (services and financial resources) and the needs of clients (as assessed by various methods) are quite well defined. One rule of justice would be to treat clients with equal needs equally, irrespective of their socio-economic status or other conditions for which they cannot be held responsible (for this concept of justice see Grand, 1991). Difficult issues clearly arise with the definition of "equal needs", since in many ways it can be argued that the needs of two persons can never be really equal, and that "good" care is precisely concerned with defining and providing care "tailored" to individual needs. The more pertinent questions, therefore, arise around the issue of distributing the (inevitably scarce) care resources among clients with different needs. Allocating an equal amount of resources will favour those who have few needs or already receive a lot of care. Rather than looking at distribution of resources, perhaps a more fruitful approach to equity is to look at the outcomes of care, or the benefits created by care. Here the aim would be to achieve equal benefits, or even more justifiably, to achieve equal *increases* of life quality relative to the level the client already experiences (marginal utilities in economic terms; see Davies & Knapp, 1981; Knapp, Challis, Fernandez, & Netten, 2004). But it is important to acknowledge that similar levels of "improvement" in QoL may involve quite different amounts of care and resources for different types of clients. Moreover, the definition and measurement of benefits (or utilities), especially QoL, has no generally accepted definition or solution, since clients, professionals, informal carers and local authorities all have different perspectives (Fernandez & Knapp, 2004, p. 180). In the present context, it is not possible to discuss these issues of social justice or even propose solutions, but it is important to realise that QM cannot avoid implementing, explicitly or implicitly, rules of equity. This should give additional force to the argument for fair and participative decision-making processes in the service involving clients and their advocates, and possibly the wider community. It also means that the management of equity should be included in QM, even when the specific rules implemented have to be critically evaluated and adapted to specific situations.

The Concept of Quality and the Care Keys Quality Matrix

The quality matrix, adapted from Øvretveit (1998) and expanded and interpreted within the theoretical framework of Care Keys research, is one possible approach that QM might apply to support a strategy of "continuous quality improvement", with the matrix incorporating the main aims and principles identified in the discussion earlier. The quality matrix (see Tables 12.1 and 13.1) has evolved through the conceptual developments and empirical studies carried out in Care Keys, and is still being developed. A number of central elements of the matrix require explanation in order to demonstrate how the matrix addresses the problems of QM.

Firstly, it should be noted that the quality matrix approaches the issues from the perspective of information, planning, controlling and evaluation within the service organisation. It reformulates issues in terms of "key indicators" that are needed to assess the achievement of goals in the ongoing processes of care. The collection of these indicators in a quality matrix presupposes that other strategies and methods of quality assurance are already in place to provide the information (e.g. comprehensive assessment, care plans and documentation, controlling, complaint management, quality circles, staff surveys, care outcome evaluation, etc.). Although in traditional management strategies this information often represents the "secret knowledge" of management, this need not be the case. The information may equally be used in participative practices of "negotiating order" between all participants in care (respecting data protection procedures). The matrix contains three dimensions for strategies of QM:

1. dimension 1: *production*—input/process/documented outcomes/subjective outcomes;
2. dimension 2: *stakeholders*—perspectives of client/professional staff/management;
3. dimension 3: *quality*—four sub-dimensions for quality evaluation.

Dimension 1 addresses the chain of quality in the production process. It requires QM to specify concepts of quality for each relevant phase of the care process: the provision of the structural prerequisites of care, the processes of ongoing care in a continuous pathway and the objective and subjective outcomes of care as measured by the (improvement of) QoL of the client. *Dimension 2* introduces the main stakeholders of the QM triad (see earlier), that is clients, professional carer and management. Although "good care" is primarily the task of the care triad (client, staff, informal carer—see earlier), QM has to "set the stage" for care activities. This will require concepts and indicators that will inform QM about the quality of care from the three different perspectives on care of the stakeholders, including a specification of concepts and indicators describing the achievement of management aims. Actually, informal care should be included as a fourth perspective following the "care tetrahedron"; the matrix tries to respect this by including informal care as a partner in all three perspectives, whereas other actors of the care system are included only as partners of management, but the matrix might also be extended on the basis of a more detailed stakeholder analysis. *Dimension 3* refers to the (sub-) dimensions of quality, an issue that has so far not been explicitly discussed in this chapter, and will now be addressed in order to explicate all the dimensions of the matrix and to connect the quality concept of management with the general concept of quality applied also to quality of care and QoL (Chapters 4 and 5). The quality dimension differentiates further each of the "cells" in the tabulation of dimensions 1 and 2. An additional distinction of subjective and objective outcomes leads to a total number of 48 cells (see Table 12.1 and Table 13.1).

There can be different starting points for the conceptualisation of dimensions of quality. A starting point can be the concept of QoL (see Chapter 4). Strategies of QM can be analysed according to their contribution to the QoL of clients; the dimensions of QoL will then give some order to QM strategies and activities according to their effects on QoL. Looking at the quality of care, we may also specify a conceptual scheme distinguishing dimensions of care quality, and we can again relate (the dimensions of) care activities to (dimensions of) QoL of clients (see Chapter 5) and both to QM strategies. Finally, the previous discussion has distinguished different tasks for QM. We may now ask for a conceptual scheme that provides order to the various activities and strategies included within the QM concept. For instance, the previous discussion of Jochimsen (2003) distinguishes components of motivation, work and resources in care situations and asks QM to provide a sustainable organisation for these. If we distinguish, as suggested earlier, between motivation based on "moral order" and motivation based on personal attachment (as does Jochimsen effectively in her discussion), we have four components to consider by QM: value orientations, work organisation, resource availability and personal relations in care situations.

The theoretically interesting and demanding question arising from such conceptualisations is on what grounds we can conclude that the schemes are complete covering *all* relevant dimensions. After all, a central aim of care is to provide *comprehensive* care, and an important characteristic of the quality concept is that quality encompasses "the *totality* of features and characteristics" of a given product or service which "bear on its ability to satisfy stated or implied needs" (ISO definition, emphasis added; see Chapter 4). A theoretical answer to this question is provided by system theory or, more specifically, by social system theory. A "totality" of features or functions is here described in the conceptualisation of all the (general) functions that are necessary for the survival of a system. Since the "survival" of social systems such as persons, care interactions or service organisations cannot be defined on biological grounds, we have to consider the social nature of systems. The essential difference is that social systems comprise social communications, interactions and reflections on interactions that are oriented towards valued goals and which define social "survival" criteria (Luhmann, 1984; Parsons, 1951, 1978). Maintenance of these goals, defining and re-defining them as valued or "right" orientations ("doing the right things") is one of the central functions of a social system. Additionally, goals have to be achieved (or attempted) by goal-oriented actions choosing the "right" or effective means to achieve these goals ("doing things right"). Furthermore, resources and efficient ways to utilise them from the environment are required, including the choice of favourable environments or their adaptation to needs and capacities. Finally, social systems have to function internally in a coherent and integrated way, being sufficiently free of internal conflicts and functioning as a "team".

This social system theory approach can be applied to persons or individuals, as has been demonstrated with reference to Lawton and Veenhoven for the concept of QoL (see Chapter 4). If we conceive a service organisation as a social system, it can also be applied to QM. In each case, the theoretical approach suggests that the quality (or functionality) of activities and their outcomes can be analysed with reference to exactly four (sub-) dimensions, which can then be further differentiated as necessary for the particular phenomenon. Since social system theory provides a theoretical base for most approaches to organisation, production of welfare and management, it provides a very general and powerful framework for the systematic conceptualisation of quality.

In the context of QM, an extensive review of the literature has been made by Bruhn (2003), summarising principles of QM by, for example Ishikawa, Deming, Crosby and Taguchi, and identifying the "10 Cs" of quality aspects in service organisations: consistency, congruence, coordination, communication, completeness, continuity, cost-effectiveness orientation, client orientation, consequence and competitiveness. Achieving high scores on these dimensions (describing positive features of an organisation) is seen to produce quality of services and outcomes. Authors who have discussed the management of care (see Blonski & Stausberg, 2003; Currie, Harvey, West, McKenna, & Keeney, 2005; Evers et al., 1997; Görres, 1999; Haubrock & Gohlke, 2001; Øvretveit, 1998) also emphasise interaction quality between carer and client, self-help competence of the client, inclusion of informal care and voluntary work, cooperation with other services in the community, "tailoring" of care to the individual client, their special biographical needs and the influence of life events, evidenced-based care, a comprehensive "holistic" concept of the client and socio-political values (e.g. human dignity, social inclusion, social justice). Social system theory suggests that the different factors can be organised into "4 Cs" or four dimensions of care management quality (see the management perspective in the quality matrix; Table 13.1):

1. Concepts of quality—referring to value-based orientations of TQM, especially a comprehensive, "holistic" client orientation and equity.
2. Competence and procedures—referring to rules and standards of effective, efficient, coordinated and continuous services and evidence-based goal attainment.
3. Conditions and access to resources—referring to strategies and rules of adapting to changing environments, resources and markets.
4. Cooperation and integration—referring to strategies to secure motivations and promoting integration of internal and external partners.

In practical terms, the Balanced Score Card (BSC) with its four dimensions can be interpreted in the social system theory framework. The BSC is widely used in QM, including social and health care (Friedag & Schmidt, 2004; Niven, 2003). An example is the BSC as employed in the reform of the social and health care system in the city of Helsinki (see Fig. 6.2). As has been noted by evaluations of the BSC for social services, the established interpretation of the four factors needs to be adapted. The client orientation has to take the role of "shareholder value", and financial (profit) aspects have to be re-interpreted by the concept of sustainability, whereas the factors of work organisation and staff orientation can be kept, especially, when seen in the context of TQM. Basically, the BSC approach is open to such re-interpretations, and social system theory provides a conceptual framework that is missing in the rather pragmatic approach of the BSC.

Applying this theoretical approach we get a consistent framework introducing the dimension of quality into the Care Keys quality matrix. Important "key indicators" can then be selected and organised in the management perspective, and the quality matrix can be further differentiated to include the perspective of professional care and the client perspective using the same four-dimensional quality approach. The three perspectives together will constitute the Care Keys Q-MAT instrument. As stated earlier, the quality matrix reflects also the participation of other stakeholders besides clients, professionals and management. Informal carers are introduced, at least, in the way that

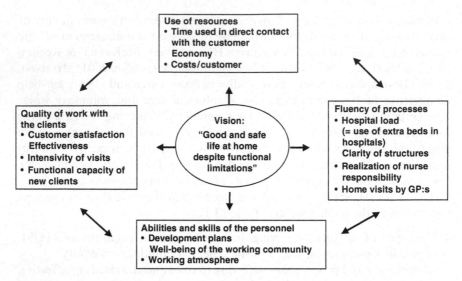

FIG. 6.2. The Helsinki Balanced Scorecard (BSC): Outcome measures of home care during the experimental period 2001–2003 (Valvanne, 2005).

their involvement and the documentation of their involvement is an indicator of quality of care (dimension of teamwork and cooperation in integrated care). Additionally, informal carers are explicitly incorporated in the case of clients with dementia (or similar impairments in their autonomy and competence) for the subjective evaluation of care. In addition, other external partners are considered and their cooperation evaluated by management. Finally, the peers of professionals can be involved by analysing and evaluating the processes of care as reflected in the care documentation. These (self-) evaluations of staff can be made the basis of quality circles and other QM strategies involving professionals, clients and management supporting the creation of a "negotiated order" and implementing the principles of the "care tetrahedron" in concrete care practices.

Quality Management in LTC: A Summary

In this chapter, QM in LTC has been analysed in three perspectives. Firstly, QM or TQM has established itself as a set of strategies which aim to facilitate a comprehensive, continuous and innovative improvement in the quality of long-term health and social care for older people (*production of welfare perspective*). QM is still not accepted without reservations, but it is part of a general trend towards professionalism and qualification within care. It is also supported by new management strategies and technologies associated with the "information society" that is at the same time an "ageing society", developing new ways of caring for an increasing number of older people in need of support. Secondly, QM will have to take up the challenge of meeting the care needs of the ageing population by developing approaches that are in keeping with the structures and affordances that are inherent within care relationships (*negotiated order perspective*). Organisations providing care cannot simply introduce QM concepts and practices from organisations in other spheres of life. Value orientations of care, the motivation to care and the acceptability of care by the client, the very concepts of "good care" and "good management" in care service organisations, cannot be adequately conceptualised within a framework of economics, or in terms of efficient standardised procedures. QM has to recognise the special nature of LTC and "set the stage" for client-centred and socially valued care practices. Strategies will also have to develop structures that will enable the participation of all parties involved, including the empowerment and support of clients by advocates, to compensate for the disadvantages of frailty and dependency in the "negotiation of order" in care. Thirdly, the demands of managing care put managers in a difficult situation. They have to find ways to reconcile economic conditions characterised by cost-saving policies of public finance, privatisation and commercialisation with a set of objectives and tasks: (i) socially defined client-oriented aims and values; (ii) the development and provision of qualified professional care; (iii) sustainable resources, technologies and care environments and (iv) the social integrative and cooperative structures and work practices which are conducive to care relationships (*four-dimensional quality perspective*).

Management will find itself in different organisational and legal contexts and has to adapt its strategies appropriately. In larger organisations, the focus will be more on improving and integrating services within the organisation, although integration with external services grows in importance; whereas in smaller services the manager will have a "networking" role in order to ensure that a comprehensive set of services is in place for frail older people with typically complex and diverse needs. The tasks and influence of management will also vary with the service setting. In home care, the services will cover only part of the life situation of the client, and cooperation with, and support by, informal care and other community services is an inherent part of home care services. In institutional care, the influence of management is stronger, but there is also an increased obligation to create a "home-like" setting and a "community of care" that respects the nature of the care triad in the provision of "good care". With increasing frailty and dependency, especially in dementia care, the role of advocacy to preserve the client "voice" is increasingly important, but so also is the obligation of management to organise care practices in such a way that the burden on carers and the dangers of emotional "burn-out" are avoided. A key focus for QM has to be to cope with the two "sensitive points" (Jochimsen, 2003) inherent in care situations: the "crowding-out" of client-oriented carer motivations by other (self-) interests and the balancing of the needs of both frail, care-dependent older people and those who provide care, both professional and informal.

References

Adams, T., & Gardiner, P. (2005). Communication and interaction within dementia care triads. Developing a theory for relationship-centred care. *Dementia, 4*, 185–205.

Beckmann, Ch., Otto, H.-U., Richter, M., & Schrödter, M. (Eds.) (2004). Qualität in der Sozialen Arbeit. Wiesbaden: Verlag für Sozialwissenschaften.

Beresford, P. (2004). Qualität sozialer Dienstleistungen. Zur zunehmenden Bedeutung von Nutzerbeteiligung. In Beckmann et al. (Eds.). (2004). Qualität in der Sozialen Arbeit. Wiesbaden: Verlag für Sozialwissenschaften.

Berger, P. L., & Luckmann, T. (1966). *The social construction of reality*. New York: Anchor Books.

Blonski, H., & Stausberg, M. (Eds.) (2003). *Prozessmanagement in Pflegeorganisationen*. Hannover: Schlüterser Verlag.

Böhle, F. (2004). Die Bewältigung des Unplanbaren als neue Herausforderung für die Arbeitswelt. Die Unplanbarkeit betrieblicher Prozesse und erfahrungsgebieteten Arbeitens. In F. Böhle, S. Pfeiffer, & N. Sevsay-Tegethoff (Eds.) (2004). Die Bewältigung des Unplanbaren. Wiesbaden: Verlag für Sozialwissenschaften, pp. 12–54.

Bruhn, M. (2003). *Qualitätsmanagement für Dienstleistungen (Quality management for services)*. Berlin: Springer Publisher.

Cangialose, C. B., Cary, S. J., Hoffmann, L. H., & Ballard, D. J. (1977). Impact of managed care on quality of health care: Theory and evidence. *American Journal of Managed Care, 3*, 1153–1170.

Currie, V., Harvey, G., West, E., McKenna, H., & Keeney, S. (2005). Relationships between quality of care, staffing levels, skill mix and nurse autonomy: Literature review. *Journal of Advanced Nursing, 51*, 73–82.

Davies, B., & Knapp, M. (1981). *Old people's homes and the production of welfare*. London: Routledge and Kegan Paul.

Ellis, A., & Kauferstein, M. (2004). Dienstleistungsmanagement. Berlin: Springer.

Evers, A., Haverinen, R., Leichsenring, K., & Wistow, G. (Eds.). (1997). *Developing quality in personal social services*. Aldershot: Ashgate.

Fernandez, J.-L., & Knapp, M. (2004). Production relations in social care. In M., Knapp, D., Challis, J. L., Fernandez, & A. Netten (Eds.). (2004). Long-term care: Matching resources and needs. Aldershot: Ashgate.

Freidson, E. (1961). Dilemmas in the doctor–patient relationship. In A. M. Rose, (Ed.), *Human behaviour and social processes. An interactional approach* (pp. 207–224). Boston: Houghton Miffling.

Friedag, H. R., & Schmidt, W. (2004). *Balanced scorecard*. Planegg bei München: Haufe.

Görres, S. T. (1999). *Qualitätssicherung in Pflege und Medizin*. Bern: Huber Publisher.

Grand, J. L. (1991). *Equity and choice*. London: Harper Collins Academic.

Hardy, B., Young, R., & Wistow, G. (1999). Dimensions of choice on the assessment and care management process: The views of older people, carers and care managers. *Health and Social Care in the Community, 7*, 483–491.

Haubrock, M., & Gohlke, S. (2001). *Benchmarking in der Pflege (Benchmarking in care. A benchmarking study of home care services)*. Bern: Huber Publisher.

Jochimsen, M. A. (2003). *Careful economics. Integrating caring activities and economic science*. Boston: Kluwer Academic Press.

Knapp, M., Challis, D., Fernandez, J. L., & Netten, A. (Eds.). (2004). *Long-term care: Matching resources and needs*. Aldershot: Ashgate.

Lachhammer, J. (2004). Total-value-management – Mittelpunkt einer Qualitätsoffensive in sozialen Einrichtungen. In Peterander, F., & Speck, O. (Eds.). (2004). Qualitäts- management in sozialen Einrichtungen. München: Reinhardt.

Luhmann, N. (1984). *Soziale Systeme. Grundriß einer allgemeinen Theorie*. Frankfurt: Suhrkamp (Social Systems).

Maines, D. R., & Charlton, J. C. (1985). The negotiated order approach to the analysis of social organisation. *Studies in Symbolic Interaction, Supplement 1*, 271–308.

McGuire, A., Henderson, J., & Mooney, G. (1988). *The economics of health care*. London: Routledge & Kegan Paul.

Mead, G. H. (1934). *Mind, self and society*, Chicago: University of Chicago Press.

Netten, A. (2004). The social production of welfare. In M. Knapp, D. Challis, J.-L. Fernandez, & A. Netten (Eds.) (2004), *Long-term care: Matching resources and needs*. Aldershot: Ashgate.

Nies, H., & Berman, P. C. (Eds.). (2004). *Integrating services for older people: A source book for managers*. Dublin: EHMA.

Niven, P. R. (2003). Balanced Scorecard – Schritt für Schritt. Weinheim: Wiley.

Øvretveit, J. (1998). *Evaluating health interventions. An introduction to evaluation of health treatments, services, policies and organizational interventions*. Buckingham, Philadelphia, PA: Open University Press.

Owen, T., & NCHRDF (Eds.). (2006). *My home life – quality of life in care homes*. London: Help the Aged.

Parsons, T. (1951). *The social system*. New York: Routledge and Kegan Paul.

Parsons, T. (1978). *Action theory and the human condition*. New York: Free Press.

Peterander, F., & Speck, O. (Eds.). (2004). Qualitätsmanagement in sozialen Einrichtungen. München: Reinhardt.

Pieper, R. (1979). Wissensformen und Rechtfertigungsstrategien. Ein Beitrag zum Vermittlungsproblem zwischen Wissenschaft, Technik und Alltag, Soziale Welt, Heft *1*, 50–69.

Pieper, R. (1997). Technology and the social triangle of home care: Ethical issues in the application of technology to dementia care. In S. Björneby & A. van Berlo (Eds.), *Ethical issues in the use of technology for dementia care*. Knegsel: AKONTES Publishing.

Pieper, R. (2005a). Integrated care: Concepts and theoretical approaches. In M. Vaar- ama & R. Pieper (Eds.) (2005). *Managing integrated care. European perspectives and good practices*. Stakes and the European Health Management Association. Saarijärvi: Gummerrus Printing Oy. pp. 26–53.

Pieper, R. (2005b). Strategies for organisational and network integration. In M. Vaar- ama & R. Pieper (Eds.) (2005). *Managing integrated care. European perspectives and good practices*. Stakes and the European Health Management Association. Saarijärvi: Gummerrus Printing Oy. pp. 113–131.

Reichwald, R., & Schaller, Ch. (2006). Innovationsmanagement von Dienstleistungen – Herausforderungen und Erfolgfaktoren in der Praxis. In H.-J. Bullinger & A.-W. Scheer (Eds.), *Service engineering*, Berlin: Springer.

Simmel, G. (edited and translated by K. H. Wolff). (1950). *The sociology of Georg Simmel*. Glencoe, IL: The Free Press.

Strauss, A. L., Schatzmann, L., Bucher, R., Erlich, D., & Sabshin, M. (1963). The hospital and its negotiated order. In E. Freidson (Ed.), *The hospital in modern society* (pp. 147–169). New York: The Free Press (pp. 147–168).

Strauss, A. L. (1978). *Negotiations: Varieties, contexts, processes and social order*. San Francisco, CA: Jossey-Bass.

Twigg, J. (2004). The medical-social boundary and rival discourses of the body. In Knapp, M., Challis, D., Fernandez, J.L., & Netten, A. (Eds.). (2004). *Long-term care: Matching resources and needs*. Aldershot: Ashgate.

Vaarama, M. (2005). Evaluating and managing quality of integrated care. In M. Vaarama & R. Pieper (Eds.) (2005), *Managing integrated care for older persons*. Saarijärvi: Gummerus Printing, Stakes and the European Health Management Association.

Vaarama, M., & Pieper, R. (Eds.). (2005). *Managing integrated care. European perspectives and good practices*. Stakes and European Health Management Association. Saarijärvi: Gummerrus Printing Oy. (pp. 64–88).

Valvanne, J. (2005). Integrating social and health care in practice – A Finnish project. In Vaarama & Pieper (Eds.) (2005). *Managing integrated care for older persons*. Stakes and the European Health Management Association. Saarijärvi: Gummerrus Printing. pp. 64–88.

Wilkinson, H., Kerr, D., & Cunningham, C. (2005). Equipping staff to support people with an intellectual disability and dementia in care home settings. *Dementia, 4(3)*, 387–400.

Part III
Empirical Results

7

Subjective Quality of Life of Care-Dependent Older People in Five European Union Countries

Kai Saks and Ene-Margit Tiit

Introduction

Ageing Europe faces a challenge of providing good care for older persons. Until recently there have been no universal standards for long-term care in the European Union (EU). Many national and European surveys indicate that health and social care for older people is primarily biomedically oriented and evaluates quality of care using health-related outcome measures (Carver, Chapman, Thomas, Stadnyk, & Rockwood, 1999; Garratt, Ruta, Abdalla, Buckingham, & Russell, 1993; Smit, 2000). Alternatively, recent research in the field of long-term care has clearly shown that quality of life (QoL) is a primary and meaningful outcome marker of care (Kane et al., 2003; Noelker & Harel, 2001). QoL can be evaluated using objective or subjective variables and indices (Lawton, 1991), but there is a growing consensus that the conceptualization and measurement of QoL in long-term care should be based primarily or exclusively on the resident's subjective assessment of his or her QoL (Kane et al., 2003). It is now recognized that QoL extends beyond a strict medical discourse into areas as psychology, environmental studies, social work and so on (Smith, 2000). For people who need help in everyday life, the quality of care can significantly influence their QoL (see Chapter 5).

Research of QoL in long-term care is usually limited to one country, one care type or even one institution, and there is lack of comparative studies in this field. The main aim of the present study was to compare QoL of older people receiving long-term care—clients of home-based or institutional care—in different regions of EU: Estonia, United Kingdom, Sweden, Finland and Germany. Estonia is a "new" EU member and other four countries are "old" members. During the study Estonia had been a member of EU less than 2 years while others more than 10 years. Estonia differed from other project countries in several socio-economic areas. The mean life expectancy in Estonia was significantly lower (Estonia 71.8, UK 84.1, Sweden 86.3, Finland 81.4, Germany 82.3 years) (List of countries by life expectancy, 2005), general life satisfaction and happiness were poorer, security and state of repair of houses were more problematic and people were less satisfied with their homes, social life and health services (InfobaseEUROPE Database Record No. 7530, 2004).

An additional aim of the study was to search, pilot and validate suitable tools for evaluating subjective QoL of older care-dependent persons. Although the need for comprehensive approach to QoL in long-term care is generally recognized there are no standardized measures available. Some QoL questionnaires, such as the World Health Organization Quality of Life Bref questionnaire (WHOQOL-Bref) (WHOQOL group, 1998) and the Philadelphia Geriatric Morale Scale (PGCMS) (Lawton, 1991) are well validated in the general older population (Skevington, Lofty, Oconnell, & The WHOQOL Group, 2004; von Heideken Wågert et al., 2005; Wong, Woo, Hui, & Ho, 2004) but in less extent with long-term care clients. Persons in long-term care probably have different needs and expectations compared with healthy older people or with patients in hospitals, rehabilitation and primary care settings.

Methods

Study Population and Research Instruments

Each partner had the aim to have a sample of 150 homecare (HC) and 150 institution-based (IC) long-term care clients from the country. Samples consisted of persons aged 65 years or more (with some exceptions) and were either random or total samples, which could be drawn from several institutions in any country. As the non-response with frail old persons especially in homecare may be quite extensive, a master sampling was used when necessary. A client in the master sample who could not be interviewed for whatever reason (e.g. sickness, death or moving to institution from homecare) was replaced with next similar *case* in the master sample.

During the preparatory stage information about practical use of QoL instruments in partner countries was gathered and analysed. Three measures were selected for piloting—WHOQOL-Bref (The WHOQOL group, 1998), PGCMS (Lawton, 1991) and Antonovsky Sense of Coherence Scale (SOC—Antonovsky, 1993). Piloting was performed in all participating countries. The results of piloting revealed that the two first measures were relatively easy to use and had also satisfactory variability rate in care-related older persons. However, a question about satisfaction with sex-life was excluded from the WHOQOL-Bref after piloting, because the response rate was very low. Five WHOQOL-Bref domains (physical health, psychological, social relationships, environment) and three PGCMS factors (agitation, attitude towards own aging—ATOA and lonely dissatisfaction—loneliness) were assessed for characterizing QoL (see Chapter 3).

The SOC scale had a number of limitations. It was too long, questions were difficult to understand, was not validated in all countries and was excluded from the final list of data collection instruments.

Data were collected using Care Keys instruments: client interview questionnaire (CLINT) and data extraction form from care documentation (InDEX). The complete version of CLINT had following parts: background information, physical environment, social relationships, hobbies and participation, functional ability and received help, quality of care, QoL (PGCMS, WHOQOL-Bref). The complete

InDEX contained information about client background and resources, social network; living environment and type of placement; functional status; functioning and personal care, health and care-related conditions, psychosocial conditions and participation; need for services and supply; care outcomes and care planning documentation.

The Mini Mental State Examination (MMSE) (Folstein, Folstein & McHugh, 1975) was used for evaluating clients' cognitive functioning if not previously documented using MMSE or some other valid method (e.g. Cognitive Performance Scale in Resident Assessment Instrument—RAI CPS) (Morris et al., 1994). A unified activities of daily living (ADL) score was calculated using data from InDEX: A mean dependency level of nine activities (toileting, dressing, eating, skin and hair care, dental and oral care, toe nails cutting, washing, moving inside, going to and getting up from bed), where 0 represents total independence and 4 extreme need for help. An instrumental activities of daily living (IADL) score was a mean dependency level of following nine activities: cooking, laundry, daily cleaning, heavy cleaning, other household chores, moving outdoors, taking care of finances, transportation and shopping and running errands (0 means no need for help and 4 means extreme need for help).

Data Collection Procedure

Each client in the master or total sample was explained the aim of the study and written permission was asked according to the ethical regulations of the country. Interviewers were researchers, staff nurses or nurse or social work students. All interviewers were given training, supplied with study protocols and supervised by an experienced researcher. Background data were collected from the care documentation using InDEX. If the cognition score was evaluated during last 6 months and it was 15 points or more by MMSE or 1–2 by CPS, client interview was started. If there were no data available about client's cognitive status, an MMSE assessment was carried out and if the score was at least 15 points an interview was commenced. Some clients with MMSE 15–18 could follow the interview, but others did not. While conducting the client interviews, interviewers were sensitive for the burden the interview could cause for the client. If the client's cognitive level turned out to be too impaired for the interview, or if the client was fatigued or anxious, and so on, the interview was paused. If the situation was such that the interview could not be continued, it was terminated. In the present study all clients whose MMSE was lower than 19 or CPS 3 or more were excluded.

The pooled database consisted of 1,527 persons (see Table 7.1) in the five countries. Because of cognitive impairment 374 persons were excluded from this study and the final database comprised 1,153 persons (15–27% of each countries), equally from HC and IC. In UK the number of HC clients was only 18, so clients of sheltered (or supported) housing (SH) were added to the sample of HC in UK. This was possible because no statistically significant (on level 0.05) differences occurred between HC and SH clients. In other countries there were no clients from sheltered housing.

TABLE 7.1. Distribution of the sample by countries and by care type.

	Frequency	Percent
Country		
Finland	418	27.4
Sweden	228	14.9
Estonia	305	20.0
UK	293	19.2
Germany	283	18.5
Care type		
Homecare	613	40.1
Sheltered housing	128	8.4
Institutional care	786	51.5
Total	1,527	100.0
Total with MMSE ≥ 19	1,153	75.5

Statistical Analyses

The complete response rate of questions concerning QoL was not very high, but in most cases only several answers were missing. In this context the EM-imputation method was used to fill in the blanks in the data (Little & Rubin, 1987). Imputation was used in cases when at least 60% of values of given instruments were present and no more than 6 values in PGCMS and 10 values in WHOQOL-Bref questionnaires were imputed.

The main analytical tool was comparison of averages. As the components of PGCMS and domains of WHOQOL-Bref were calculated as linear sums of initial variables, the assumption about normality was valid for all cases hence classical parametric methods were used.

To compare the average levels of QoL characteristics in different countries and different care-groups all characteristics were standardized to a scale 0–100, where 0 marked the lowest possible and 100—highest possible value. In all cases a significance level 0.05 was used. The following methods were used for making comparisons between countries (Toothaker, 1992)

- One-factor ANOVA for checking the influence of a country
- Contrasts and LSD (least significant difference) to compare pairs of countries
- Scheffe and Tukey multiple comparison method to build homogeneous groups

To check the differences between HC and IC in all countries the usual t-test was used. In all cases the assumption of equal variances was satisfied.

Results

Socio-Demographic and Functional Characteristics

The comparison of socio-demographic and functional characteristics of clients in different countries is presented in Table 7.2.

TABLE 7.2. Socio-demographic and functional characteristics of clients in participating countries.

Variable	Estonia	UK	Sweden	Finland	Germany	Total HC	Total IC
Male %	26.3	33.8	31.6	20.6	21.6	25.7	25.8
Age (years, mean)	75.8	84.1	86.3	82.3	82.3	81.5	81.8
Married (%)	16.9	9.1	13.2	15.5	26.3	18.1	16.9
Has a close person (%)	71.5	92.6	93.3	94.2	72.5	94.7	71.4***
ADL unified score	1.12	0.45	1.20	1.11	1.93	0.73	1.67***
IADL unified score	1.70	0.84	1.47	2.13	1.89	1.12	2.47***

***Difference between HC and IC (total sample) $P < 0.001$

The Estonian sample was younger than in other countries. Clients from UK had the best and clients from Germany the worst functional status compared with others. In Estonia and Germany fewer clients had a close person than in other countries. In the total sample, HC and IC clients did not differ in gender distribution, mean age and proportion of married persons. IC clients were significantly more dependant in ADL and IADL functions and were less likely to have someone who they considered as an informal close person.

Response Rate on PGCMS and WHOQOL-Bref

PGCMS response was complete in approximately in two third of cases and almost 90% of care-dependent persons were able to answer at least 10 of the 17 questions (see Table 7.3). The biggest number of missing answers (21.4%) were to the question 'As you get older, are things better/worse than you thought they would be?', followed by the questions, 'Are you as happy now as you were when you were younger?' (15.3%) and 'Do you feel that as you get older you are less useful?' (14.6%).

TABLE 7.3. Response rates (%) of PGCMS (total number of variables 17).

PGMS/no of responses	Finland	Sweden	Estonia	UK	Germany	Total
17	72.1	54.6	69.8	75.3	36.9	63.7
10–16	27.0	32.3	9.1	21.3	38.3	24.8
1–9	0.3	0	0.9	0	0.5	0.4
0	0.6	13.1	20.3	3.4	24.3	11.1

WHOQOL-Bref was less complete compared with the PGCMS. The questionnaire was filled in completely in a little more than half of cases. Almost 85% provided answers to at least 14 questions out of 25 (see Table 7.4). The

TABLE 7.4. Response rates (%) of WHOQOL-Bref (total number of variables 25).

WHOQOL-Bref/no of responses	Finland	Sweden	Estonia	UK	Ger	Total
25	49.1	51.5	65.1	79.2	36.9	56.5
14–24	39.0	33.3	12.5	16.6	37.4	27.9
1–13	1.8	2.0	0	0.4	1.4	1.1
0	10.1	13.1	22.4	3.8	24.3	14.5

least complete items were 'How satisfied are you with your transport?' (25.4% missing values), 'How satisfied are you with your ability to work?' (22.3%) and 'How healthy is your physical environment?' (21.3% missing answers).

These results indicate that older care-dependent people without severe cognitive impairment can and are willing to answer majority of questions of PGCMS and WHOQOL-Bref. Nevertheless, there are some questions in both questionnaires that may be inappropriate for this population.

Comparison of Estimated QoL in Different Countries

Comparison of PGCMS Scores in Homecare Clients

Mean relative values of the different PGCMS factors (agitation, attitude towards own aging and lonely dissatisfaction) for HC clients are presented on the Fig. 7.1. In all components the differences were statistically significant (by ANOVA), with the Estonian HC sample having lower QoL according to all three PGCMS factors.

Relative values of PGCMS factors in HC clients

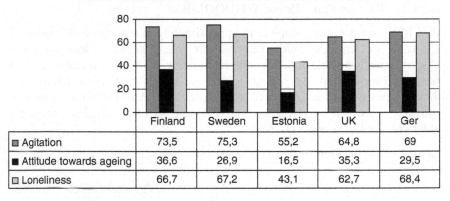

	Finland	Sweden	Estonia	UK	Ger
▨ Agitation	73,5	75,3	55,2	64,8	69
■ Attitude towards ageing	36,6	26,9	16,5	35,3	29,5
▢ Loneliness	66,7	67,2	43,1	62,7	68,4

Fɪɢ. 7.1. Average relative values of PGCMS factors (standardized to scale 0–the worst ... 100–the best) for clients of home care in different countries.

The next step was to clarify, which countries had statistically different averages and to construct homogeneous groups of countries. Method of contrasts revealed that Estonia differed from all other countries in all factors, whereas the UK differed in respect to loneliness. In addition, following significant differences were found: the agitation factor in the UK differed from Finland and Sweden; the Finnish attitude to own aging (ATOA) factor differed from Sweden and Germany and loneliness factor from Germany.

As a result of these analyses the following homogeneous groups were determined (see Table 7.5). In respect to Agitation and ATOA, two overlapping homogeneous groups formed: in the first case UK, in the second case Sweden belong to the same group as Estonia. In respect to loneliness three distinct

TABLE 7.5. Homogeneous groups formed by PGCMS scores in homecare.

Agitation		
Group 1	Estonia, UK	
Group 2		UK, Germany, Finland, Sweden
Attitude towards own ageing		
Group 1	Estonia, Sweden	
Group 2		Sweden, UK, Germany, Finland
Loneliness		
Group 1	Estonia	
Group 2		Germany, Sweden, Finland	
Group 3			UK

groups were formed. Estonia and UK differ from other three countries that form a single homogeneous group.

Comparison of PGCMS Scores in Institutional Care Clients

Mean relative values of PGCMS factors in IC homecare clients are presented in Fig. 7.2. ANOVA indicated that differences between countries in respect to ATOA and loneliness were statistically significant, but not in respect to agitation.

In institutional care the differences between countries were much less pronounced than in homecare. In respect to agitation the only significant pairwise difference was between Estonia and UK; in respect to ATOA, Estonia differed from other countries, while Sweden differed from Finland. In respect to loneliness the UK sample differed from all other countries, while Estonia and Finland differed from each other.

Relative values of PGCMS factors in IC clients

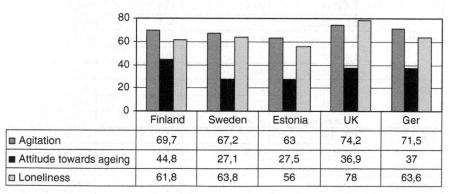

	Finland	Sweden	Estonia	UK	Ger
▣ Agitation	69,7	67,2	63	74,2	71,5
■ Attitude towards ageing	44,8	27,1	27,5	36,9	37
▢ Loneliness	61,8	63,8	56	78	63,6

FIG. 7.2. Average values of PGCMS components (standardized to scale 0–100) for clients of institutional care in different countries.

Using multiple comparisons the following homogeneous groups were formed (Table 7.6). In respect to agitation, all countries belonged to the same homogeneous group, in respect to ATOA two overlapping homogeneous groups were formed: one around Estonia and Sweden, the second around Finland, UK with Germany belonging to both. In respect to loneliness, two distinct groups appear: one contained only the UK, with all countries belonging to the second.

TABLE 7.6. Homogeneous groups formed by PGCMS scores in institutional care.

Agitation		
Group 1	Estonia, Sweden, Finland, Germany, UK	
Attitude towards own ageing		
Group 1	Sweden, Estonia, UK, Germany	
Group 2		UK, Germany, Finland
Loneliness		
Group 1	Estonia, Germany, Sweden, Finland	
Group 2		UK

Comparison of PGCMS Scores Between Homecare and Institutional Care

The next analysis was the extent to which PGCMS scores depended on care type. In Table 7.7 all PGCMS components for IC and HC clients in all countries are compared.

The differences between IC and HC clients were not large: in Finland and Estonia ATOA was much worse in HC clients; in the UK, agitation was worse in HC; and in Finland loneliness was greater in IC (Fig. 7.3).

TABLE 7.7. Comparison of PGCMS scores between institutional care and homecare.

		IC	HC	Significance
Finland	Agitation	69.7	73.5	0.260
	ATOA	44.8	36.6	0.021
	Loneliness	58.2	64.5	0.018
Sweden	Agitation	67.2	75.3	0.182
	ATOA	27.1	26.9	0.981
	Loneliness	56.2	59.3	0.590
Estonia	Agitation	63.0	55.2	0.101
	ATOA	27.5	15.5	0.001
	Loneliness	49.4	43.0	0.113
UK	Agitation	74.2	64.8	0.024
	ATOA	36.9	35.31	0.717
	Loneliness	70.3	70.68	0.895
Germany	Agitation	71.5	69.0	0.548
	ATOA	37.0	29.56	0.117
	Loneliness	55.0	56.6	0.653

Comparison of HC and IC, PGCMS

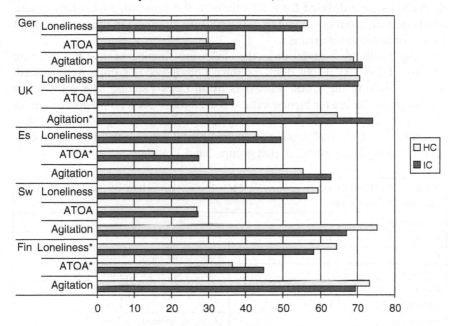

FIG. 7.3. Comparison of PGCMS components between home care and institutional care in different countries (*-significant difference).

Comparison of WHOQOL-Bref Domain Scores in Homecare Clients

Mean relative values of the WHOQOL-Bref domains (physical health, psychological, social relationships, environment) for homecare clients are presented in Fig. 7.4. ANOVA indicated that all differences between countries were strongly significant.

Relative values of WHO-QoL-Bref domains in HC clients

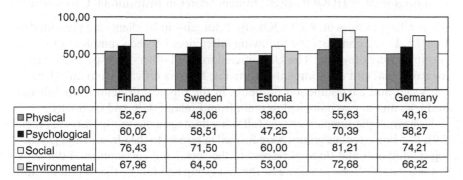

	Finland	Sweden	Estonia	UK	Germany
Physical	52,67	48,06	38,60	55,63	49,16
Psychological	60,02	58,51	47,25	70,39	58,27
Social	76,43	71,50	60,00	81,21	74,21
Environmental	67,96	64,50	53,00	72,68	66,22

FIG. 7.4. Average relative values of WHOQOL-Bref domains (standardized to scale 0–100) for clients of home care in different countries.

Finland, Sweden and Germany did not differ between each other in any domain. Estonia differed from all others in the physical, psychological and environmental domains, The UK differed from all others in the psychological and environmental domains.

Using multiple comparisons, the following homogeneous groups were formed, (Table 7.8). In all domains three homogeneous groups were formed. The first (having the lowest values) is in all cases Estonia. The core of the second group (having the highest values) is in all cases UK. A third group consists of other three countries. In the case of psychological domain all groups are distinct. In respect to the physical, social and environmental domains the third group contains Germany and Finland, so that groups 2 and 3 overlap.

TABLE 7.8. Homogeneous groups in HC formed by values of WHOQOL-Bref domains in homecare.

Physical domain			
Group 1	Estonia		
Group 2		Sweden, Germany, Finland	
Group 3			Germany, Finland, UK
Psychological domain			
Group 1	Estonia		
Group 2		Germany, Sweden, Finland	
Group 3			UK
Social domain			
Group 1	Estonia		
Group 2		Sweden, Germany, Finland	
Group 3		Germany, Finland, UK	
Environmental domain			
Group 1	Estonia		
Group 2		Sweden, Germany, Finland	
Group 3			Germany, Finland, UK

Comparison of WHOQOL-Bref Domain Scores in Institutional Care Clients

Mean relative values of WHOQOL-Bref domains in IC clients are presented in Fig. 7.5. Using contrasts the following differences between samples in the five countries were observed: The UK differed from all others in respect to psychological, social and environmental domains; Estonia differed from all others in the social and environmental domains, in the physical domain from Finland and UK, and in psychological domain from Finland, UK and Germany.

Using multiple comparisons the following homogeneous groups formed (Table 7.9). Two homogenous groups were formed in respect to the physical and psychological domains and three in respect to the social and environmental domains. Estonia was in all cases the core of the first group and UK of the second or third group. Germany, Sweden and Finland always belonged to the same homogenous group but in some cases also to overlapping groups. Three distinct groups formed in the environmental domain: Estonia, UK and all other countries.

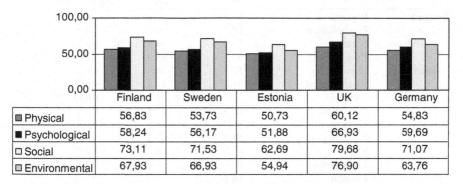

FIG. 7.5. Average relative values of WHOQOL-Bref domains (standardized to scale 0–the worst … 100–the best) for clients of institutional care in different countries.

TABLE 7.9. Homogeneous groups formed by values of WHOQOL-Bref domains in institutional care.			
Physical domain			
Group 1	Estonia, Sweden, Germany, Finland		
Group 2		Sweden, Germany, Finland, UK	
Psychological domain			
Group 1	Estonia, Sweden, Finland, Germany		
Group 2			Germany, UK
Social domain			
Group 1	Estonia, Germany		
Group 2		Germany, Sweden, Finland	
Group 3		Sweden, Finland, UK	
Environmental domain			
Group 1	Estonia		
Group 2		Sweden, Germany, Finland	
Group 3			UK

Comparison of WHOQOL-Bref Domain Scores between Homecare and Institutional Care

One further analysis examined differences in QoL between two types of care in the five countries. The results are presented in Table 7.10 and Fig. 7.6. The differences between HC and IC are not great. No significant differences were found in Finland and Sweden. In UK environmental domain was worse in HC clients. Interestingly, the physical domain of QoL was found to be better

TABLE 7.10. Comparison of WHOQOL-Bref scores between institutional and homecare.

		IC	HC	Significance
Finland	Physical	56.8	52.7	0.070
	Psychological	58.2	60.0	0.408
	Social	73.1	76.4	0.175
	Environment	67.9	68.0	0.991
Sweden	Physical	53.7	48.1	0.08
	Psychological	56.2	58.5	0.519
	Social	71.5	71.5	0.993
	Environment	66.9	64.5	0.336
Estonia	Physical	50.7	38.6	0.000
	Psychological	51.9	47.3	0.063
	Social	62.7	60.0	0.415
	Environment	54.9	53.0	0.449
UK	Physical	60.1	55.6	0.116
	Psychological	66.9	70.4	0.091
	Social	79.7	81.2	0.506
	Environment	76.9	72.7	0.011
Germany	Physical	54.8	49.2	0.021
	Psychological	59.7	58.3	0.572
	Social	71.1	74.2	0.237
	Environment	63.8	66.2	0.197

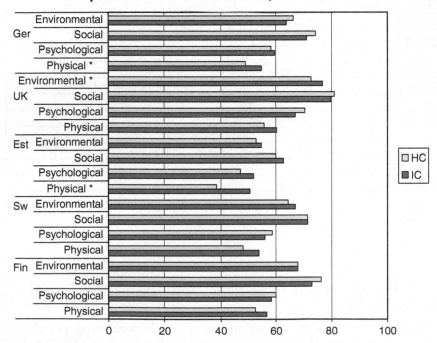

FIG. 7.6. Comparison of WHOQOL-Bref domains between home care and institutional care in different countries (*-significant difference).

among IC clients in all five countries (the difference was significant in Estonia and Germany and almost significant in the other countries).

Discussion

Two QoL assessment tools, the WHOQOL-Bref and the PGCMS, were used to evaluate the QoL of older persons in long-term care. During the pilot stage both instruments had a good response rate and were rated as appropriate tools for this sample. In the present study the general response rate was satisfactory for both instruments; more than half of persons answered all questions and the majority (more than 85%) answered more than half of questions. One question (How satisfied you are with your sexual life?) was still removed from WHO-QOL-Bref in the final data collection based on the results of piloting. Hwang et al. (Hwang, Liang, Chiu, & Lin, 2003) described similar problems with this question amongst older people in Taiwan. It can be concluded that the PGCMS and WHOQOL-Bref can be used for evaluating of QoL in long-term care. Nevertheless, some questions in both questionnaires had a rather low response rate. Further analyses should be performed to determine whether these questionnaires could be shortened for long-term care clients.

Antonovsky's SOC scale has been used widely in different studies including older community-living population, and seems to be a reliable, valid and cross-culturally applicable instrument (Eriksson & Lindström, 2005). In the Care Keys study, the SOC scale was excluded from the final list of data collection instruments after piloting, because the response rate was low and interviewers described major difficulties in using the SOC questionnaire in our target group.

In terms of the main results, a comparison of clients in long-term care in five EU countries indicated that Estonian clients were 6–11 years younger than clients in other countries. However, comparison of mean life expectancy and mean age of the national samples indicated that the remaining life expectancy of clients in all countries was rather similar.

The grouping countries by QoL scores indicated that Sweden, Finland and Germany were quite similar, but Estonia and UK differed from these others and also from each other in many QoL dimensions. In general, the QoL was the worst in Estonia and the best in UK. There may be several possible explanations of this finding.

Firstly, different national living standards in the different European regions may have an impact (InfobaseEUROPE, 2004). In particular, problems within transitional economies (Estonia) may impact on the older generation most heavily. Lower global level of QoL inevitably has an impact on the care-dependent people. On the other hand, Estonian society appears to be sensitive to a cultural paradigm that embraces a non-materialistic or spiritual dimension of life, so that existential questions and worries have become increasingly important during the past decade (Teichmann, Murdvee, & Saks, 2006). However, all the other countries were quite similar in general national QoL aspects according to infoBASE Europe. Consequently, better QoL of long-term care clients in UK cannot be explained by higher national standards of living.

Limitations in functioning have high impact on QoL of care-dependent persons (Bowling, Banister, Sutton, Evans, & Windsor, 2002). Functional dependency was highest in German clients. Nevertheless, QoL of German long-term care clients was not different from Finland and Sweden. At the same time functional status of Estonian long-term care clients was compa-rable to Finnish and Swedish samples, but QoL was significantly lower. In the survey of clients in UK, participants had fewer limitations in ADL and IADL than in other countries. Better functional status may at least partly explain better QoL among UK sample. Access to long-term care services may be easier in UK than in other countries and persons with quite low depend-ency level may be able to get formal care services and also select in which type of care institution to live. Importantly, most UK clients from HC group lived in sheltered housing where the environment was already adapted to the needs of care-dependent persons. Another possible explanation could be different approaches to care in different countries, In the UK a more social model of care may be emphasized, whereas in Finland, Sweden and Germany the care approach may be more medically oriented. Finally, differences can be explained by limitations of the national samples. One has to be careful in making any comparisons between countries based on small samples from particular localities or contexts. There was random selection of clients but not institutions in the survey and the national data may be not representative the different countries. While the national samples may not be entirely "rep-resentative" of the general population of long-term clients in each country, equally there is not reason to believe that they are untypical.

In Estonia all aspects of QoL were found to be worse (although not all differ-ences were significant) among HC clients. There may be due to problems with living conditions, or due to less developed home-care services. QoL in Estonian IC clients differed from other countries much less than those in HC. In fact, some HC clients from Estonian sample suggested that they would prefer to live in an institution setting but were unable to do so because of financial restrictions.

The most interesting finding was that QoL did not differ much between HC and IC clients (except in Estonia). On the contrary, the physical domain of QoL was found to be better in IC clients, although their objectively assessed ADL and IADL functioning was significantly worse.

The possible explanation for this could be the positive influence of an environment adapted to client needs, although there were no large dif-ferences in the environmental domain between IC and HC (except for the UK). Environments in IC facilities may support physical functioning, but the negative effect of non-homelike surroundings may offset this positive influence, so that perceived quality of environment in general is not better.

In conclusion, subjective QoL of clients is an independent outcome vari-able in long-term care that should be taken into account when monitoring effectiveness of care. Further research is needed to study how different types of care regime (medically, psychosocially or socio-culturally oriented) can influence QoL of care-dependent persons.

References

Antonovsky, A. (1993). The structure and properties of the sense of coherence scale. *Social Science and Medicine, 36*, 725–733.

Bowling, A., Banister, D., Sutton, S., Evans, O., & Windsor, J. (2002). A multidimensional model of the quality of life in older age. *Aging & Mental Health, 6*, 355–371.

Carver, D. J., Chapman, C. A., Thomas, V. S., Stadnyk, K. J., & Rockwood, K. (1999). Validity and reliability of the medical outcomes study short form-20 questionnaire as a measure of quality of life in elderly people living at home. *Age & Ageing, 28*, 169–174.

Eriksson, M., & Lindström, B. (2005). Validity of Antonovsky's sense of coherence scale: a systematic review. *Journal of Epidemiology and Community Health, 59*, 460–466.

Folstein, M. F., Folstein, S. E., & McHugh, P. R. (1975). Mini-mental state: a practical method for grading the cognitive state of patients for the clinician. *Journal of Psychiatric Research, 12*, 189–198.

Garratt, A. M., Ruta, D. A., Abdalla, J. I., Buckingham, J. K., & Russell, I. T. (1993). The SF 36 health survey questionnaire: an outcome measure suitable for routine use within the NHS? *British Medical Journal, 306*, 1440–1444.

Hwang, H. F., Liang, W. M., Chiu, Y. N., & Lin, M. R. (2003). Suitability of the WHOQOL-BFER for community-dwelling older people in Taiwan. *Age & Ageing, 32*, 593–600.

InfobaseEUROPE Database Record No. 7530 (2004). *Report on the quality of life in an enlarged European Union.* http://www.ibeurope.com/Records/7500/7530.htm.

Kane, R. A., Kling, K. C., Bershadsky, B., Kane, R. L., Giles, K., Degenholtz, H. B., Liu, J., & Cutler, L. J. (2003). Quality of life measures for nursing home residents. *Journals of Gerontology Series A-Biological Sciences & Medical Sciences, 58*, 3, 240–248.

Lawton, M. P. (1991). A multidimensional view of quality of life in frail elders. In J. E. Birren, J. E. Lubben, J. C. Rowe, & D. E. Deutchman (Eds), *The concept and measurement of quality of life in frail elders* (pp. 3–27). San Diego: Academic Press.

Little, R. J. A., & Rubin, D. (1987). *Statistical analysis with missing data.* New York: John Wiley.

Morris, J., Fries, B. E., Mehr, D. R., Hawes, C., Phillips, C. D., & Mor, V. (1994). MDS Cognitive Performance Scale. *Journal of Gerontology, 49, 3M*, 174–182.

Noelker, L. S., & Harel, Z. (2001). Humanizing long-term care: forging a link between quality of care and quality of life. In L. S. Noelker & Z. Harel (Eds), *Linking quality of long-term care and quality of life* (pp. 3–26). New York: Springer Publishing Company.

Skevington, S. M., Lotfy, M., Oconnell, K., & The WHOQOL Group (2004). The World Health Organisation's WHOQOL-Bref quality of life assessment: Psychometric properties and the results of the international field trial. A Report from the WHOQOL Group. *Quality of Life Research, 13*, 299–310.

Smith, A. E. (2000). Quality of life: a review. *Education and Ageing, 15*(3), 419–435.

Teichmann, M., Murdvee, M., Saks, K. (2006). Spiritual Needs and Quality of Life in Estonia. *Social Indicators Research, 76*(1), 147–163.

Toothaker, L. E. (1992). *Multiple comparison procedures.* Sage University paper.

von Heideken Wågert, P., Rönnmark, B., Rosendahl, E., Lundin-Olsson, L., Gustavsson, J. M. C., Nygren, B., Lundman, B., Norberg, A., & Gustafson, Y. (2005). Morale in the oldest old: Umeå 85+ study. *Age & Aging, 34*, 249–255.

WHOQOL group (1998). Development of the World Health Organization WHOQOL-BREF quality of life assessment. *Psychological Medicine, 28*, 551–558.

Wong, E., Woo, J., Hui, E., & Ho, S. C. (2004). Explanation of the Philadelphia Geriatric Morale Scale as a subjective quality-of-life measure in elderly Hong Kong Chinese. *Gerontologist, 44*, 408–417.

8
Quality of Life of Older Homecare Clients

Marja Vaarama and Ene-Margit Tiit

Introduction

The objective of enabling older people to live in their own homes as long as possible is a widely accepted guiding principle of old age policies in most western societies. "Ageing in place" is seen as a goal that accommodates the preferences of both older people themselves and society. Homecare (HC) is one of the key means to support older people who need regular external help to remain living at home. Underlying the provision of homecare, there is an implicit or explicit goal to enhance the general well-being of the clients. However, there is still little known, especially from the perspective of old people themselves, about the ways that different types of homecare and how they are organised and delivered can impact on the quality of life (QoL) of the clients.

Although patterns of homecare provision may vary considerably between European countries, reflecting different approaches to provision within "mixed economies of care", services usually range from help for housekeeping and daily activities of living to nursing care at home, as well as social, emotional and psychological support to maintain independence and autonomy. During the last two decades, most European countries have introduced policies for prioritising or targeting client needs in order to allocate the available scarce resources to those in most need (e.g. Evers & Svetlik, 1993; Pacolet, Bouten, Lanoye, & Versieck, 1998). For example, in Finland, a shift from a publicly provided social model of home help towards a more medically orientated care at home is apparent, as well as a shift from public provision towards a more mixed economy, involving providers from both the public and private sectors (Vaarama & Noro, 2006). For "better targeting of care", eligibility for formal homecare is increasingly targeted on those people with highest needs in respect to personal daily activities (PADL—help with personal hygiene, going to the toilet, etc.), whereas those persons needing help in housekeeping and other instrumental daily activities (IADL) are increasingly likely to be cared for by families or to buy the services privately. Importantly, services that support the psycho-social and environmental and housing needs of clients tend to be ignored.

These changes have been rationalised by efficiency objectives, but whether this type of homecare is efficient in the provision of well-being for older clients and in meeting their needs is an area that has received little attention by researchers. Moreover, given the high priority and expectations placed on homecare within government policies for older people, it is very striking as to how little research has been carried out that examines homecare from the client's perspective (Baldock & Hadlow, 2002; Bowling, 2004; Hellström & Hallberg, 2001).

As discussed earlier in this book, the entire concept of homecare is cultural relative, and lacks a clear definition, whereas there are also no commonly accepted criteria for quality of homecare (Paljärvi, Rissanen, & Sinkkonen, 2003; Thomé, Dykes, & Rahm Hallberg, 2003). Furthermore, even care theories assume a connection between good care documentation and good care outcomes (e.g. Goldstone & Maselino-Okai, 1986); such standards of documentation are lacking within homecare. As a consequence of poor documentation, homecare tends to remain invisible behind walls and closed doors, often hiding problems of poor service quality and unmet needs.

Given the rapid ageing of European populations and the expected increase of care needs, current underdeveloped structures and processes in homecare need to be replaced with knowledge-based interventions, accompanied with valid instruments to measure the outcomes of care. This knowledge should also be based on the views of older people themselves, as only they can evaluate their own well-being and the role of care in their QoL. More information is required about how older people perceive why homecare is needed, what types of care they prefer and about their experiences of how care can have positive impacts on their QoL. Moreover, although it is evident that the meaning of the concept of homecare is culturally dependent, it still may be worthwhile to try to develop some more "universal" definitions and quality criteria for it, especially as homecare is as a cornerstone of the future care systems for older people.

Objectives and Theoretical Base

The aim of the research presented in this chapter was to investigate: (i) the determinants of subjective QoL among old homecare clients and the role of homecare in the production of their QoL; (ii) the determinants of homecare quality that have most impact on the QoL of the clients; (iii) the management inputs that provide best care outcomes and (iv) the key variables for evaluation of care outcomes from the perspectives of the clients, professionals and management.

Current general understanding of QoL emphasises multi-dimensionality (e.g. Skevington, Lofty, & O'Connell, 2004; WHOQOL Group, 1998). However, current theories on QoL have been criticised for failing to fully take into account the role of the conditions of QoL of frail older people (Bowling, 2004; Hughes, 1990). Where research has been carried out, the results suggest that the dimensions of QoL in old age are the same as those in the younger population, but factors such as mobility, being able to manage homecare and personal care, personal optimism and morale, barrier-free living environment, access to leisure activities and outings, loneliness, recent positive or traumatic life events and receiving enough care are all important determinants of QoL in frail old people living at home (e.g. Birren & Dieckmann, 1991; Cummins, 1997; Hughes, 1990; Löwenstein & Ogg, 2003; Vaarama, Pieper, & Sixsmith, 2007; Chapter 4).

The Care Keys research has a multi-dimensional approach to life quality and, following Lawton (1991), a model of care-related QoL has been developed to highlight the special conditions and needs of care-dependent old people. This model was used as a reference model in the research presented in this chapter, more specifically, a "production of welfare model" was used, where subjective QoL was considered as the "final outcome" and the driving objective of homecare, whereas the quality of care (QoC) as reflected in the care documentation (docQoC) and care management (QoM) were seen as the means (intermediate outcomes) to realise this goal (see Davies, Bebbington, & Charnley, 1990; Chapter 1). The evaluation was client centred and the intermediate outcomes were evaluated against their effectiveness in having a positive impact on QoL of old clients (Fig. 1.3).

Although it is difficult to evaluate the role of care in the production of QoL without a longitudinal design, it is still worth examining variation in QoL to identify the role that care plays in shaping QoL. The aim is also to try to bridge the differences and boundaries between care systems by searching for key determinants of homecare quality that the Care Keys data might suggest as being "universal" or common among the different project countries representing different care systems.

The focus is on the identification of key indicators, therefore, the investigation of the four-dimensional structure of care and management quality (Chapters 5 and 6) was not a priority, although the results provide some evidence supporting the general four-dimensional model and identifying key indicators in all dimensions.

Data and Methods

The data were collected in the five Care Keys countries in late 2004 to early 2005, using the data collection instruments described earlier in this book: client interview instrument CLINT-HC, documentation extraction form InDEX-HC and management survey instrument ManDEX (see Chapter 2). The homecare data consist of the complete database of five countries (Estonia, Finland, Germany, Sweden, UK), where only clients with reasonable cognitive function (MMSE $\geq$ 15) were included. Almost all data were EM imputed, and besides the original data, several calculated variables (e.g. calculated I/ADL scores, problems with house and environment) were used. The sample size was 513 complete cases (clients): female 77%, mean age 81 years, married

18%, widowed 52%, primary education 40%, post-secondary and higher education 20%, IADL score mean 11.5 (range 0–36), ADL score mean 7.5 (range 0–36), MMSE mean 24.6 (range 15–30). The response rates of the instruments were satisfactory, but for InDEX (care documentation) it was only 45.2% (see Chapter 3). This may be attributed to the poor level of documentation of homecare in the project countries.

The following six measures were used as dependent variables characterising subjective QoL of the clients (all but WHOQOL Global scaled 0–100, higher values indicating better QoL):

1. WHOQOL-Bref domains: physical, psychological, social (slightly modified as the question of sexuality was replaced with loneliness), environmental.
2. WHOQOL Global: GobalQoL (single item question: How would you rate your QoL? Scaled 1–5, where 5 indicates the best QoL).
3. WHOQOL-Bref General: GQoL (calculated as weighted sum of the four dimensions of WHOQOL-Bref). This variable was created because it was noted that a linear combination of all WHOQOL-Bref variables provides better models than the single-variable Global QoL that includes more random variability.

As potential arguments the following variables were used:
A. Client-specific circumstances

1. Client background variables (BG), mostly treated as binary variables, total number 18: Country, gender, age, marital status, living alone, cohabitation (with whom the client cohabits).
2. Client's physical functional ability: IADL score and ADL score calculated as indexes (sums of values of need variables from InDEX or from CLINT with higher values showing more problems), health status (currently ill or not).
3. Client's psychological well-being: Factor 2 of the Philadelphia Geriatric Centre Morale Scale (PGCMS, Lawton, 1975): Attitude towards own ageing (ATOA), including five initially measured variables; cognition score, depression score.
4. Client's social well-being: Variables characterising the social networks and participation (S), total number 22: Existence of close persons, frequency of contacts, participation in leisure activities, hobbies at home and outside.
5. Client's physical environment: (E), total number 15: House or flat ownership, problems with heating, dump, missing lift, difficult stairs, barriers to indoor and outdoor mobility, distance to transport and local amenities.
6. Life events: Variables connected with traumatic life experiences of clients during the last 2 years (LE), total number 9: Death of spouse, serious illness of client or his or her close relation, financial problems.

B. Care and client preferences

1. Subjective quality of care (sQoC), total number of variables 23: Continuity of care, QoC relationship, client autonomy and control, satisfaction with care, appropriateness of care (sufficient amount and access to care).
2. Documented professional characteristics of care (docQoC) including a long list of different actions as presented in individual care plans (CP) and documents, total number 64: Pain management, different prophylactic means, degree of goal orientation in care, QoC plans, organisation of cooperation between different care actors and informal care, clinical care outcomes (pressure ulcers, falls, loss of weight, usage of sleeping pills, suffering pain).
3. Sources of other help, total number 13: Help from spouse, children, friends, paid nurse, church, also need and supply of volunteers' help (H).

C. Management of Homecare

1. Variables describing the management of homecare, total number 43: Management strategy, structures and processes for quality, cooperation and collaboration, self-efficacy of the management. These variables were not used in the final models, as they were only measured for about half of the sample and could not be imputed as dropout was not random.

As many previous research, also the model of care-related QoL developed in Care Keys emphasises the role of psychological well-being for subjective QoL (see Chapter 4) or "successful aging" (Baltes & Baltes, 1990). We explored with a factor analysis on WHOQOL-Bref and PGCMS instruments whether these two instruments measure subjective QoL similarly. In the analysis, the loneliness factor of the PGCMS loaded together with WHOQOL-Bref domains, suggesting that they measure QoL "outcomes", and other PGCMS factors loaded on different factors. Therefore, we included the factor ATOA from the PGCMS in the present analyses as an independent variable indicating psychological resources for subjective QoL. According to Lawton (1975), the measure addresses the individual's perception of changes taking place in his or her life and his or her evaluation of those changes. Single items of the PGCMS have been used also in previous research, for example in BASE (Baltes & Mayer, 1999) and in norLAG (Solem, 2003). As expected, the loneliness measure alone had a statistically very significant negative correlation with GlobalQoL ($r = -0.37^{***}$). However, in the present study, loneliness was not included as a separate variable but it participates in the WHOQOL-Bref social dimension and in the general QoL measure. This is because the Care Keys study replaced the question on "sexual activity" of the social dimension of WHOQOL-Bref instrument with the question "How alone do you feel in your life". The reason for this was that the sexual activity question had a very low response rate in our pilot research, and similar low response rates have been reported also by other researchers (see Chapter 2). The question is also not included in WHOQOL-OLD (Power, Quinn, Schmidt, &WHOQOL Group, 2005).

To analyse the quality and management of homecare, we used factor analysis with Varimax rotation, along with linear regression analysis for modelling, where stepwise selection (combination of forward and backward selection rules) of arguments and significance level 0.05 were used. The quality of factors is described by Cronbach's alpha (if possible) and quality of the models is assessed by the determination coefficient R^2. Only statistically significant models with all significant terms are discussed. The list of potential explanatory variables contains 293 variables. In general, the correlations between explanatory variables are quite weak, so the multicollinearity is not a serious problem in the case of smaller models, but may arise in comprehensive models. As dependent variables (WHOQOL domains) are normally distributed in the data (this fact has been tested using skewness and kurtosis), the linear regression models give the best results. In some cases, logistic regression analysis was also used. Taking the special focus of this study into account, analyses began by examining the connections between intermediate and final outcomes, and then considered the impact of care management and client's life circumstances.

Results

QoC and Its Impact on QoL in Homecare Clients

The central questions were which features of homecare did the client find to be of high quality and which were most influential on their QoL. We differentiated between the subjective care evaluations of the clients (sQoC) and the professional homecare quality as reflected in the documentation of homecare (docQoC) (see Chapter 1).

Key Dimensions of Subjective Quality of Homecare

A four-dimensional model of sQoC was suggested by a four-factor solution with three first factors having a good internal consistency (Table 8.1). The first factor describes the quality of interaction between the client and the care worker, and the professional skills and trustworthiness of the care workers, highlighting the importance of a good care relationship for client satisfaction with care. The second factor describes the importance of homecare in being responsive to client expectations of comfort and cleanliness, and the third reliability and continuity of care. The fourth factor describes self-determination in terms of clients' control over his or her day, including enjoyable meals. The general description rate of analysis (51.2%) is satisfactory. The Cronbach's α-coefficients show that, in general, the variables are quite well distributed among factors, but too many correlated variables appear to have been measured, given that half of all variables belong to the first factor.

TABLE 8.1. A four-factor solution of subjective quality of care (sQoC).

	1. F	2. F	3. F	4. F
The first factor, description rate 22.1%, Cronbach α = 0.89				
Care workers' kindness	0.76	0.049	−0.126	0.137
Care workers' honesty and trustworthiness	0.705	−0.018	−0.131	−0.021
Care workers treat client with dignity and respect	0.705	0.097	0.078	0.086
Care workers are good at what they do	0.656	0.261	0.35	0.146
Care workers have a good understanding of client and client's needs	0.653	0.294	0.307	0.077
Client would recommend this service	0.633	0.166	0.276	0.146
Care workers do the things that client wants to be done	0.59	0.321	0.377	0.046
Satisfaction with care	0.58	0.346	0.197	0.034
Care workers deliver the services as promised	0.564	0.313	0.413	0.063
If client raises concerns, does he or she feel that care worker listens	0.556	0.111	0.346	0.066
Care workers give you enough information about care	0.511	0.105	0.495	0.12
The second factor, description rate 11.3%, Cronbach α = 0.71				
Client able to keep as clean as he or she would like	0.204	0.756	−0.141	0.172
Client able to keep as well dressed as he or she would like	0.187	0.732	−0.076	0.077
Client's home as clean and tidy as he or she would like	0.144	0.707	0.143	0.058
The third factor, description rate 11.3%, Cronbach α = 0.68				
Client mainly sees the same care workers	0.067	−0.186	0.703	−0.037
Care workers keep their appointments as promised	0.238	0.141	0.606	0.074
Care workers have enough time for client	0.312	0.371	0.541	0.118
Client has person in charge of care	−0.037	−0.185	0.388	−0.165
The fourth factor, description rate 7.4%, Cronbach α = 0.48				
Client gets the right amounts to eat	−0.016	−0.178	0.049	0.722
Client gets to eat at the times that suit for him or her	0.11	0.174	0.144	0.68
Client able to get up and go to bed at times that suits him or her	0.259	0.106	−0.169	0.52
Client enjoys meals	0.03	0.265	−0.04	0.509

Variables of Subjective Quality of Homecare with Most Impact on Subjective QoL of the Clients

The analyses demonstrated a strong relation between subjective quality of homecare and QoL. The description rate of QoL domains by QoC variables varied between 21% and 29%. For all domains, the most important variable was "Client able to keep as clean as he or she would like", and the gain to the description rate (ΔR^2) of this variable varied between 14% and 19%. The description rate of this single variable was lowest in social and psychological domains and highest in the physical domain. Other variables had much less descriptive power. However, variables "being able to be as well-dressed as one likes", "clean home", "enjoyable meals" and having care workers who "understand and listen", who "treat the clients with dignity" and "keep promises in terms of appointments" were connected with satisfaction with care, and they were important within the different dimensions of the QoL of the clients.

For global QoL, "being as clean as one likes", "control over own bed-times", having an "honest and trustworthy care worker" and being satisfied with care were important, but these variables explained only 17% of the variation. The model for GQoL explained 35% of the variation, and contained only six explanatory variables from three care quality factors. Again, the most important explanatory variable was "Client able to keep as clean as he or she would like" ($\Delta R^2 = 0.24$), but all explanatory variables belonged to the set of most important variables in previous models for QoL domains.

Further modelling revealed that only ten initially measured variables added to the description of QoL domains by more than 1%. In terms of descriptive power, the best variables belonged to the second factor (client clean and well dressed, home clean). In the second place was the first factor (QoC relationship and skilfulness of the care workers); and in the third place was the fourth factor (self-determination). The remaining third factor had a rather marginal descriptive power (Table 8.2).

Further modelling indicated that the QoC variables given in Table 8.3 were the most influential for clients' QoL.

Documented Professional Quality of Homecare and Client Outcomes

The Care Keys Concept of Professional Quality of Homecare

In Care Keys, professional quality of homecare was measured through the examination of care documentation (docQoC) checking whether there was a reference to certain elements of care quality, care risk or outcomes in the documentation. A five-factor solution suggested that the use of external resources from the wider community and especially the involvement of the informal carers were important dimensions of docQoC (first factor), but so were also the quality of individual care plans and the degree of goal orientation in care (second factor) as well as the processes of evaluation of the quality of homecare (third factor). The fourth factor appears to combine involvement of physician and teamwork, connected with two clinical outcomes: pressure ulcers and falls. The fifth factor describes active prevention strategies and monitoring of changes in clients' conditions. None of the factors have a good internal consistence, although the first three are close to it (Table 8.4).

Again the factor analysis distributes the analysed items quite evenly among the factors, but the three clinical outcome factors (usage of sleeping pills, loss of weight and pain) do not load on any factor. These five factors give a 44% description rate (49%, if not counting the last three variables). With the exception of the clinical outcome measures, the factor solution supports to some extent our theoretical concept of professional quality of homecare (see Chapter 5). The absence of the three clinical outcome measures may be due to the poor care documentation in current homecare practices, which we assume to be associated with low response rate in InDEX-HC.

TABLE 8.2. Descriptive power (ΔR^2) of subjective quality of care (sQoC) variables by dimensions of WHOQOL model.

	Global	Physical	Psychological	Social	Environmental	GQoL	Sum	Factors
Client able to keep as clean as he or she would like	0.131	0.188	0.144	0.144	0.039	0.245	0.890	Second F 1.147
Client able to keep as well dressed as he or she would like		0.016	0.011		0.148	0.013	0.188	
Client's home as clean and tidy as he or she would like		0.033		0.008	0.009	0.018	0.069	
Satisfaction with care	0.024	0.013	0.008		0.017	0.026	0.088	First F 0.177
If client raises concerns, does he or she feel that care worker listens		0.011			0.008	0.009	0.028	
Client would recommend this service				0.011			0.011	
Care workers do the things that client wants to be done				0.023			0.023	
Care workers have a good understanding of client and client's needs					0.011		0.011	
Care workers' honesty and trustworthiness	0.007						0.007	
Care workers treat client with dignity and respect				0.008			0.008	Fourth F 0.136
Client enjoys meals	0.011	0.023	0.036	0.011	0.013	0.035	0.117	
Client able to get up and go to bed at times that suits to him or her		0.009					0.019	
Client mainly sees the same care workers			0.007			0.007	0.007	Third F 0.016
Care workers keep their appointments as promised				0.009		0.009	0.009	
Sum	0.172	0.292	0.205	0.214	0.246	0.346	1.1477	

TABLE 8.3. The key variables of subjective quality of homecare with most impact on QoL.

Variables	Sum ΔR^2	Factor
Client able to keep as clean as he or she would like	0.890	F2
Client able to keep as well dressed as he or she would like	0.188	F2
Client enjoys meals	0.117	F4
Satisfaction with care	0.088	F1
Client's home as clean and tidy as he or she would like	0.069	F2
If client raises concerns, does he or she feel that care worker listens	0.028	F1
Care workers do the things that the client wants to be done	0.023	F1
Client able to get up and go to bed at times that suits him or her	0.019	F4
Client would recommend this service	0.011	F1
Care workers have a good understanding of client and client's needs	0.011	F1

Documented Quality of Homecare and Subjective Care Outcomes

The connections between documented quality of care (docQoC) and sQoC and QoL were generally weak, although also some significant connections were found. Overall, docQoC explained only a little of the variation in QoC perceived by the clients (top-ten variables) as the models had R^2 values in the range 1–10%. On average, the models contained 2–3 explanatory variables, none of which were predominant. The most influential docQoC variables were "teamworking" and "co-operating physician nominated in the documentation"; after these came use of prophylaxes and needs assessment, but these had a very weak impact. Similarly, the linear models built for each care factor (see Table 8.1) by docQoC variables were weak, having R^2 values in the range 3–7%. Logistic analyses failed to give any different results. In addition, models of QoL by docQoC variables were quite weak, having a description rate of less than 10%, but nine variables had statistically significant explanation power on QoL. Most influential docQoC variable was "Does the client suffer from pain", which described on average 2.7% of the variation of the various WHOQOL measures. Second was "Does the care plan record change in client condition and needs", with 1% average description rate (Table 8.5).

In this analysis, suffering pain was the best predictor of QoL. As pain did not appear in our previous analyses of the most important dimensions of documented quality of homecare, we may conclude that pain is an important determinant of QoL for old homecare clients, but current homecare documentation practices seem to fail to account for it properly. From this we may conclude further that pain management may be currently inadequate in homecare. Further, the quality of individual care plans and respect of client preferences impacted on both QoC and QoL. From this it can be concluded that careful care planning that involves the evaluation of the client preferences can lead to positive care outcomes, as assumed in the care theories discussed in Chapter 5.

TABLE 8.4. The factor analysis of professional homecare characteristics by documentation (docQoC).

Variables	1	2	3	4	5
The first factor, description rate 10.7%, Cronbach α = 0.697					
Does CP make reference to use of external resources?	0.775	0.08	0.056	−0.099	−0.094
Does CP make reference to need for external services?	0.738	0.056	0.049	−0.127	−0.095
Does documentation show involvement of informal care?	0.532	0.252	0.047	0.088	0.103
Does the regular evaluation consider the adequacy of involvement of informal carer?	0.523	−0.044	0.443	−0.176	0.106
Does CP include informal carers?	0.446	0.07	0.315	0.075	−0.266
The second factor, description rate 10.2%, Cronbach α = 0.689					
Does CP record interventions?	0.16	0.684	0.131	0.036	0.022
Does CP make reference to prophylaxis?	0.09	0.61	−0.006	0.152	0.224
Does CP separate the activities client can do independently and those in which he or she needs help?	0.093	0.608	0.021	−0.172	−0.129
Does CP include needs assessment?	−0.122	0.542	0.543	−0.04	−0.04
Does CP include documentation of methods of care (interventions)?	−0.297	0.524	0.041	0.01	−0.102
Does CP include strategies and methods for teamworking?	0.235	0.5	−0.05	0.259	0.185
Does CP explicitly consider all four goals?	0.376	0.4	0.247	−0.049	0.046
The third factor, description rate 9.4%, Cronbach α = 0.622					
Do regular evaluations take place?	0.122	0.021	0.772	0.088	0.046
Has CP been reviewed and updated?	0.133	0.017	0.714	0.313	0.024
Does evaluation consider client's preferences?	−0.036	0.087	0.581	−0.31	−0.023
Does CP demonstrate regular evaluation of prophylaxis?	−0.046	0.311	0.349	0.334	0.247
Does CP evaluate attainment of four goals?	0.307	0.191	0.345	0.092	0.218
The fourth factor, description rate 7.1%, Cronbach α = 0.364 (without the variable has the client fallen, having opposite scale)					
Does CP identify a cooperating physician?	−0.095	−0.075	−0.022	0.583	−0.383
Does documentation show teamwork?	0.026	0.178	0.212	0.573	0.25
Has a pressure ulcer occurred?	0.02	0.266	0.09	0.551	−0.017
Has the client fallen?	0.032	0.128	0.026	−0.49	0.128
The fifth factor, description rate 6.1%, Cronbach α = 0.341					
Is everything done to avoid loss of weight?	0.109	−0.064	−0.073	0.013	0.624
Is everything done to avoid sleeping pills?	−0.069	0.063	0.074	0.044	0.503
Does CP record changes?	−0.156	0.056	0.103	−0.057	0.5
Variables not included to factors					
Usage of sleeping pills	−0.335	0.092	0.082	−0.176	−0.042
Loss of weight	0.054	−0.008	−0.013	−0.173	0.294
Does the client suffer from pain?	−0.143	0.004	0.114	−0.17	0.031

Management of Homecare and the QoC Outcomes

The Care Keys Concept of Management of Homecare

The full list of the management variables (QoM) taken from the ManDEX instrument contained more than 100 variables measured on the level of providers. It was possible to combine the QoM data with data on 245 clients, but in almost all cases, a series of variables were missing. Due to their special character (nonrandom pattern of missing data) it was not possible to use EM imputation. Still, it was possible to find a set of 43 variables having

TABLE 8.5. The description rates (ΔR^2) of docQoC variables by subjective (WHO)QoL domains.

Variables	Global	Physical	Psycho-logical	Social	Environ-mental	GQoL	Sum
Does the client suffer from pain?	0.02	0.065	0.012	0.015	0.013	0.036	0.161
Does CP record changes?		0.014			0.026	0.016	0.056
Does CP include needs assessment?	0.007		0.011				0.018
Does CP include strategies?					0.014		0.014
Does documentation show teamwork?	0.014						0.014
Does evaluation consider client's preferences?			0.013				0.013
What are client's and helper's activities?	0.013						0.013
Does CP include informal carers?				0.012			0.012
Does CP make reference to prophylaxis?			0.008				0.008
Sum	0.054	0.078	0.044	0.027	0.053	0.052	0.308

listwise sample size of 100 cases. This set was used in analyses of the connection between care management and care outcomes. Factor analysis produced a three-factor solution with a description rate of about 65%, which is very high. This is seemingly for the reason that the cases were not independent, but grouped by providers. When interpreting the results, it is important to remember that in all the models containing QoM variables only a (nonrandom) sub-sample (100 cases) is used instead of the total sample (513 cases) (Table 8.6).

The factor solution is difficult to interpret as the factors are quite mixed, suggesting a need to clarify the management concept used within Care Keys, but the results correspond to some extent the four management dimensions defined in Care Keys (see Chapters 6 and 12). The first factor seem to describe effective quality management with reference to quality standards (dimension I), the second factor to deal with management structures and resources (dimension III) and the third with administrative practices, formal procedures and management outcomes (dimension II). Interestingly, dimension IV (cooperation or teamworking or informal care inclusion) does not form an own factor but is spread across the first and second factors. Another interesting result is that many of the items in the first factor correspond with the results of clients' perception of quality of care (sQoC), that is the factor reflects a client orientation in accordance with the dimension I of management quality. The Cronbach's α-coefficients are not calculated, as the variables belonging to the same factor have both positive and negative correlations (and also factor loadings).

Subjective QoC and Management of Care

According to the analyses, management variables explained 6–35% of the variation of sQoC. The selected statistically most powerful predictors are presented in Table 8.7.

TABLE 8.6. Factor analysis of selected care management variables.

Variables	1	2	3
The first factor			
Fall-prophylaxis	−0.876	−0.043	0.162
Client-centred care—setting of goals	0.857	0.211	0.181
No client received services he or she did not need	−0.85	−0.019	0.189
Thrombosis prophylaxis	−0.829	0.068	0.175
Evaluation of material resources	0.828	0.196	0.414
Work process—setting of goals	0.824	0.334	0.364
QMS includes hospitals	0.806	0.141	−0.035
QMS can be produced on request	0.775	0.275	0.447
Having a primary carer	−0.768	−0.057	−0.172
Multidisciplinary team in care planning	0.673	0.644	−0.124
Informal carers' participation in care planning	0.67	0.636	−0.057
Good quality of services, adequate time for them	0.66	0.072	0.581
Pneumonia prophylaxis	−0.626	−0.011	0.26
QMS includes institutional care, day care, etc.	−0.62	0.397	0.044
Meetings with informal carers	0.604	−0.187	0.167
Cooperation was satisfactory	−0.584	0.057	−0.388
Client's participation in care planning	0.534	−0.298	0.037
The second factor			
Total number of personnel converted into full-time employees	−0.268	−0.905	0.088
The resources were adequate	0.208	−0.894	−0.005
Number of care personnel converted into FTE	0.175	−0.883	0.242
Services support autonomy	0.247	0.879	0.059
Concept of care performance	0.206	0.863	0.341
Explicit goals, regular evaluation	0.159	0.788	0.442
Care-oriented case conferences (last 6 months)	0.338	−0.729	−0.132
Living conditions reviewed, adaptations implemented	−0.618	0.718	−0.011
Access to e-mail communication provided by organisation	0.069	−0.7	0.418
Pain management	−0.01	−0.67	0.62
Problems with cooperation—informal carer or family	−0.602	0.658	−0.101
Use of external resources from the wider community	0.046	0.635	0.406
Problems with cooperation—institutional care	−0.48	0.536	−0.468
QMS includes informal carer	0.069	0.59	0.341
All clients needing a service received it	−0.184	−0.461	0.033
The third factor			
No possibility to improve services without worsening them for others	0.303	0.002	0.777
Identification by administrative service groups	−0.365	0.339	−0.747
Services correspond to needs	0.428	0.008	0.647
Formal appraisal talks with employees	0.377	−0.334	0.641
Identification by special client groups	−0.5	0.19	−0.619
Pressure ulcers prophylaxis	−0.271	−0.476	0.59
QMS includes GPs	0.177	−0.154	−0.518
Induction of new employees	−0.082	0.216	0.388
External counselling staff	0.082	−0.216	−0.388
Includes procedures for complaint management	−0.058	−0.009	0.32
Services within agreed time	0.032	−0.172	−0.216

TABLE 8.7. Most powerful QoM predictors for subjective quality of care (sQoC) variables, linear models (sub-sample data, $N = 100$).

	B	ΔR^2
Dependent: Client able to keep as clean as he or she would like, $R^2 = 0.151$		
Constant	2.572	
Identification by administrative service groups	−0.239	0.151
Dependent: Client able to keep as well dressed as he or she would like, $R^2 = 0.275$		
Constant	3.288	
Services support autonomy	−1.231	0.172
Work process—setting of goals	0.948	0.103
Dependent: Client's home as clean and tidy as he or she would like, $R^2 = 0.146$		
Constant	3.189	
Use of external resources from the wider community	−0.427	0.146
Dependent: Client would recommend this service, $R^2 = 0.108$		
Constant	3.885	
Services support autonomy	−0.488	0.108
Dependent: Care workers have a good understanding of client and client's needs, $R^2 = 0.142$		
Number of care personnel converted into FTE	0.019	0.142
Dependent: Client mainly sees the same care workers, $R^2 = 0.256$		
Constant	−1.556	
Pain management	−0.473	0.154
QMS can be produced on request	1.057	0.102

Client groupings may refer to, for example the charging policy (administrative groups), or may classify clients in a way that allows care workers to better differentiate the individual needs of different clients (special client groups). Support of clients' autonomy refers to the care concept or care standard in use. Goal-oriented working processes, pain management and a written quality management strategy (QMS) describe the standards of care quality implemented. Regarding resources, both sufficient amount of care personnel and use of external resources from the wider community seem to be important facilitators of a good-quality homecare.

QoL of the Clients and Management of Homecare

In general, QoM variables had quite a modest influence (on average 14%) on the dimensions of QoL. The most influential variable was the standard "services support autonomy". This was followed (in general, three times less influential) by the standard "work process—setting of goals". General QoL depended on the two most influential ManDEX variables: "services support autonomy" and "work process—setting of goals", with a relatively good description rate of 20%. The QoL domain that depended most on management was the environmental domain (Table 8.8).

When this list is compared with Table 8.7, it is apparent that many items are the same, but Table 8.8 also includes three new variables: "Formal appraisal talks with the employees" (leadership), "Client's participation in care planning" (empowerment) and "Informal carer's participation in care planning" (collaboration). For homecare to have a positive impact on clients' QoL,

TABLE 8.8. Linear models of QoL variables by QoM variables (sub-sample data, $N = 100$).

Dependent variable: Global QoL (variable)	B	ΔR^2
Constant	4.237	
Access to e-mail communication provided by organisation	−0.288	0.07
Evaluation of material resources	−0.143	0.025
$R^2 = 0.095$		
Dependent variable: Physical domain		
Constant	31.47	
Services support autonomy	9.188	0.082
$R^2 = 0.082$		
Dependent variable: Psychological Domain		
Constant	46.49	
Use of external resources from the wider community	7.625	0.062
Formal appraisal talks with employees	−5.497	0.023
$R^2 = 0.085$		
Dependent variable: Social Domain		
Constant	58.68	
Services support autonomy	14.39	0.071
Work process—setting of goals	−11.5	0.039
$R^2 = 0.110$		
Dependent variable: Environmental Domain		
Constant	53.21	
Services support autonomy	12.8	0.19
Work process—setting of goals	−12.1	0.072
Client's participation in care planning	−6.219	0.023
Informal carers' participation in care planning	5.194	0.029
$R^2 = 0.314$		
Dependent variable: General QoL (GQOL)		
Constant	45.76	
Services support autonomy	13.94	0.135
Work process—setting of goals	−10.69	0.065
$R^2 = 0.200$		

it seems to be important that care managers communicate with their care workers, that the clients are empowered to participate in their own care planning and that the informal carers are also involved in this process. Pain management as well as client's and informal carer's involvement in the care planning also seem to be important for all stakeholders, the clients, the professionals and the care management, and it seems to be important that the management strategy includes both goals and processes for realisation of these goals in practice.

An interesting result is that management variables had stronger impact on the QoL of the clients than the documented care quality, but it is not possible to draw too many conclusions on this due to the low response rate in care documentation and due to the small sample size used in management analyses (see also Chapter 12). However, that such a small sample generated many important connections between management and care outcomes is a remarkable result, which allows us to conclude that good homecare management is important for the achievement of good care outcomes.

Dimensions of QoL in Old Homecare Clients

Before moving on to the comprehensive analysis, the impact of two background variables, physical living environment and source of help for QoL were analysed separately in order to pick up the most important aspects for the summary models.

Influence of Background Variables on QoL

The analysed background variables had a rather weak influence on the different domains of QoL in homecare clients. The description rates varied between 9% and 17%, and their ΔR^2 values were very small, with the exception of the influence of the country of residence. Being resident in Estonia had a negative impact on QoL, whereas old age had a generally positive impact on QoL. Living alone or with spouse had a positive impact, although living with children or others had a negative impact on subjective QoL. Men had somewhat higher QoL than women. It seems that in general in this data, living with children was not a good situation for older homecare clients. The poorer QoL scores for people in Estonia appear to reflect the particular situation of a country that is experiencing political, social and economic transition. The financial situation of clients was analysed as a being part of traumatic life events, where having financial problems decreased the QoL of the clients.

Influence of Environmental Variables on QoL

Information on physical living environment was obtained both from clients and from the care documentation. In linear models, the description rate of environmental variables on global QoL was 15% and on GQoL 24%, which is rather high and emphasises how important the circumstances associated with physical environment are for the QoL in care-dependent old people. Further analyses demonstrated that the variables "How easy is it to get to local services and amenities", documented "Problems with kitchen" and "Inadequate heating or cooling" experienced by the client had most impact on QoL. A logistic regression analysis confirmed further that in all domains of QoL, and both for persons over and under 80 years of age, the barriers for indoor mobility had a strong negative impact on their subjective QoL. The same result was seen for difficulties in access to local amenities, but this appeared to decrease the QoL in the younger age group (under 80 years of age) more than that in the oldest group.

Influence of Subjective Adequacy and Source of Help on QoL

The previous analyses suggested sQoC and the involvement of informal carer to have a strong influence on the subjective QoL of the clients. A further logistic regression analysis confirmed that all domains of QoL depend strongly on clients' satisfaction with the help they receive. Getting enough help increased the clients' probability of positive QoL compared with those getting inadequate help. In persons over 80 years of age, getting help from close relatives increased significantly the probability of a good QoL compared with those getting help from some other sources.

Comprehensive QoL Models

To build up comprehensive care-related crQoL models, the most significant variables suggested by the previous analyses were chosen for each of the boxes (physical, psychological, social, environment) defined in the theoretical reference model (see Fig. 1.3). Daily functional ability was included as sum indexes of IADL and ADL problems. Need and supply of care variables were not explicitly included, but were part of the "satisfaction with care" and "would recommend the home care" variables. As has already been seen, these were closely connected with clients getting what they wished. As described earlier, loneliness participates in the WHOQOL-Bref measures, and ATOA is used to describe the psychological well-being of the client. Management variables were not included as they were measured only in a sub-sample. Altogether 41 independent variables were used, firstly to analyse the dependence structure within the set of potential independent variables and, secondly, stepwise linear modelling was used to build up comprehensive QoL models. This was done both with and without the subjective health variable in order to ascertain how this impacted on the results. This generated three models of Global QoL, having description rate between 30% and 36%, and three models for General QoL with a description rate of 55–63%. The General QoL results are presented in Table 8.9, but the variables explaining Global QoL were very similar to those explaining general QoL.

When subjective health was not included, positive ATOA was the best predictor of a good QoL. Advanced age, participation in clubs and activities outside home, individual hobbies at home, having siblings as well as satisfaction with homecare (to the extent that the client was prepared to recommend the service to others) all had additionally a positive influence. Problems with housing (bathroom, inadequate heating or cooling, high doorsteps), difficulties in access to local amenities, financial problems and lack of close relatives all had a negative effect.

When subjective health was added, the description rates of the models were improved. The predictive power of ATOA decreased in model 2 by 22% and of age by 4.1%; siblings and inadequate heating or cooling dropped out. Three new variables appeared in model 3: lack of telephone decreased QoL, and documented quality of professional care was represented by two variables. Where the care plan recorded changes in a client's condition, this was negatively connected to QoL. This may reflect documentation practice, where changes were documented only for clients with significant problems. In this situation, the explanation comes from the fact

TABLE 8.9. Determinants of QoL in older homecare clients (general QoL).

Model 1 Total R² = 0.548	M1	ΔR²
Constant	34.53	
Attitude towards own ageing (higher values better)	3.401	0.338
Age	0.228	0.053
How easy is it to get to local services and amenities (1—easy, 3—difficult)	−1.353	0.041
Satisfaction with care (1—very satisfied, 5—very dissatisfied)	−1.072	0.027
Participated in clubs or social activities (1—yes, 2—no)	−3.46	0.022
Problems in bathroom and WC (0—no such problem, 1—problem exists)	−3.528	0.018
Life experience had financial problems (1—yes, 2—no)	3.083	0.013
Client would recommend this service (1—yes, definitely, 5—no, definitely)	−1.37	0.008
Inadequate heating or cooling (0—no such problem, 1—problem exists)	−0.421	0.007
The client has someone feel close to care worker (0—no, 1—yes)	−0.3	0.006
The client has someone feel close to sibling (0—no, 1—yes)	0.372	0.005
High doorstep (0—no such problem, 1—problem exists)	−0.653	0.005
Undertaken individual hobbies at home in past 2 weeks (1—yes, 2—no)	−1.51	0.004
Model 2 Total R² = 0.611	**B**	**ΔR²**
Constant	30.22	
Satisfaction with health (higher values better)	3.288	0.382
Attitude towards own ageing (higher values better)	2.52	0.118
Life experience had financial problems (1—yes, 2—no)	3.399	0.03
Satisfaction with care (1—very satisfied, 5—very dissatisfied)	−1.151	0.018
Problems in bathroom and WC (0—no such problem, 1—problem exists)	−3.514	0.015
Participated in clubs or social activities in past 2 weeks (1—yes, 2—no)	−2.463	0.013
Age	0.136	0.009
Undertaken individual hobbies at home in past 2 weeks (1—yes, 2—no)	−1.645	0.007
The client has someone to feel close to care worker (0—no, 1—yes)	−0.267	0.007
High doorstep (0—no such problem, 1—problem exists)	−0.586	0.006
How easy is it to get to local services and amenities (1—easy, 3—difficult)	−0.892	0.004
Client would recommend this service (1—yes, definitely, 5—no, definitely)	−0.898	0.003
Model 3 Total R² = 0.630	**B**	**ΔR²**
Constant	26.48	
Satisfaction with health (higher values better)	3.2	0.382
Attitude towards own ageing (higher values better)	2.409	0.118
Life experience had financial problems (1—yes, 2—no)	3.272	0.03
Satisfaction with care (1—very satisfied, 5—very dissatisfied)	−1.073	0.018
Problems in bathroom and WC (0—no such problem, 1—problem exists)	−2.898	0.015
Participated in clubs or social activities in past 2 weeks (1—yes, 2—no)	−2.12	0.013
Age	0.145	0.009
Undertaken individual hobbies at home in past 2 weeks (1—yes, 2—no)	−1.377	0.007
The client has someone to feel close to care worker (0—no, 1—yes)	−0.32	0.007
High doorstep (0—no such problem, 1—problem exists)	−0.55	0.006
Does CP record changes? (0—no, 1—yes)	−5.736	0.004
Does documentation show teamwork? (0—no, 1—yes)	3.737	0.003
Telephone (including GMS) (0—no, 1—yes)	2.708	0.004
The client has someone to feel close to siblings (0—no, 1—yes)	0.342	0.004
Client would recommend this service (1—yes, definitely, 5—no, definitely)	−1.045	0.004
How easy is it to get to local services and amenities (1—easy, 3—difficult)	−0.866	0.003
Inadequate heating or cooling (0—no such problem, 1—problem exists)	−0.307	0.003

TABLE 8.10. Model for attitude towards own ageing (ATOA) by subjective quality of care (sQoC) variables.

	B	ΔR^2
Constant	2.812	
Client able to keep as clean as he or she would like	−0.246	0.084
Client enjoys meals	−0.328	0.046
Care workers do the things that client wants to be done	−0.287	0.019
Care workers keep their appointments as promised	0.196	0.01
Client's home as clean and tidy as he or she would like	−0.135	0.007
$R^2 = 0.166$		

that the client's problematic condition decreases his or her QoL. Documented teamwork in homecare was associated with an increase in the QoL of the client, as seen in previous analyses. The result also demonstrates that subjective health is one, but not the only, important condition for QoL among homecare clients.

ATOA was found to be very important for QoL. An explorative analysis was carried out to determine whether the quality of homecare had an impact on ATOA, and it found positive connections between five variables of the top-ten QoC variables and ATOA (Table 8.10). Following on from this, good subjective quality of homecare is connected with positive ATOA, but the direction of this relation cannot be confirmed without further research.

Key Variables for Effective Homecare

A major aim of the research was to find key variables describing the QoL of older homecare clients and the key features, structures and processes of homecare that have most impact on their QoL. A preliminary set of 53 variables common for both homecare and institutional care had been defined by statistical testing (Chapters 3 and 9). To take the specific conditions of frail old people living at home into account, this list was combined with the results of the theoretical modelling in the present study. As a result, a total of 76 items were identified as relevant for care-related QoL in homecare. Most were single variables, but some were part of a set of variables (such as need and supply for care, QoL scales). From these variables, 47 were drawn from the client interview questions, that are their subjective evaluations of the issues; 14 items resulted from the analyses of care documentation, and the list was added with five clinical outcome measures as, even our data quality did not allow us to confirm their importance, they are regarded as important in care theories (Chapter 5); 10 management quality variables were results of the management analyses of the present study. With these items it is possible to study the QoL in homecare clients, and the quality of homecare from the perspectives of the clients, professional care and care management (Tables 8.11 and 8.12).

TABLE 8.11. The key variables of care-related quality of life (QoL) (information source: client).

Background variables
 1. Country (in cross-national research)
 2. Age
 3. Gender
 4. Cohabitation (alone or with spouse, children, siblings, other)

Physical functional ability and subjective need for care
 5. Subjective IADL functionality
 6. Subjective ADL functionality
 7. Subjective need for homecare
 8. Subjective need for rehabilitation (mobility, socio-psychological)

Psychological resources (ATOA)
 9. Things getting worse as person got older (PGCMS2)
10. As much energy as last year (PGCMS2)
11. When getting older getting less useful (PGCMS2)
12. When getting older, things get better or worse than one thought (PGCMS2)
13. As happy now as were when person was young (PGCMS2)

Social networks and participation
14. Activities and hobbies undertaken at home in past 2 weeks
15. Participation in clubs and other activities outside home
16. Having a close person (relative, friend, care worker)
17. Being visited by someone close in past 2 weeks
18. Access to informal help (spouse, church, volunteers)

Living environment
19. Problems with housing (kitchen, bathroom, WC, high doorstep or stairs, heating or cooling, no lift)
20. How easy is it to get to local services and amenities
21. Need for safety alarm
22. Access to telephone

Life events
23. Life experience—become seriously ill
24. Life experience—had financial problems

Care and client preferences—client satisfaction with care
25. Client able to keep as clean as he or she would like
26. Client able to keep as well dressed as he or she would like
27. Client enjoys meals
28. Satisfaction with homecare
29. Clients home as clean and tidy as he or she would like
30. If client raises concerns, does he or she feel that care workers listens
31. Care workers do the things that client wants to be done
32. Client able to get up and go to bed at times that suits to him or her
33. Client would recommend the homecare to others
34. Care workers have a good understanding of client and client's needs

Subjective QoL
35. How would you rate your QoL? (WHOQOL-Bref)
36. Does the client suffer from pain? (WHOQOL-Bref)
37. Is the client currently ill? (WHOQOL-Bref)
38. Perceived health (WHOQOL-Bref)
39. Amount of medical treatment to function in daily life (WHOQOL-Bref)

(continued)

TABLE 8.11. (continued)

40. Enjoying life (WHOQOL-Bref)
41. Feeling alone (WHOQOL)
42. Enough energy for everyday life (WHOQOL-Bref)
43. Able to accept bodily appearance (WHOQOL-Bref)
44. Satisfaction with the support getting from friends (WHOQOL-Bref)
45. Satisfaction with access to leisure activities (WHOQOL-Bref)
46. Satisfaction with access to transportation (WHOQOL-Bref)
47. Satisfaction with access to health services (WHOQOL-Bref)

TABLE 8.12. The key variables of professional quality of care (QoC) and care management QoM.

Care planning and documentation (information source: care documentation)

Assessed care needs
1. IADL score
2. ADL score
3. Cognition score
4. Depression score
5. Assessed need for homecare by dimensions (including need for rehabilitation)

Documented QoC
6. Does CP record clinical care outcomes, including pain and pain management?
7. Does CP record changes?
8. Does CP include needs assessment?
9. Does CP include setting of goals for care and teamwork?
10. Does documentation show teamwork?
11. Is CP evaluated regularly, including client's preferences?
12. Are client's and helper's activities separated in CP?
13. Does CP include informal carers?
14. Does CP make reference to prophylaxis?
15. Has a pressure ulcer occurred during the last year?
16. Has the client fallen during the last 3 months?
17. Is the client using sleeping pills?
18. Unintended loss of weight during the last 6 months?
19. Does the client suffer from serious pain (making daily activities difficult)?

Homecare management (information source: care managers)
20. Clients are identified in different needs or administrative groups
21. Services support autonomy of the clients
22. Goal-orientated interventions and work processes
23. Services delivered within an agreed time frame
24. Use of resources of wider community
25. Number of care personnel (FTE)
26. Formal appraisal talks with the employees
27. Pain management
28. Clients and informal carers participate in care planning
29. Use of prophylaxes (especially falls)

Our results suggest many of the dimensions of the QoL of clients of home-care to be similar to those of older adults in general, but the particular situation of being care dependent is clearly visible: daily functional ability, acute illness, pain, need of medication, need of homecare services, together with psychological and social factors and physical living environment are the special conditions impacting on the QoL of care-dependent older people.

With respect to care documentation, the key variables point to the necessity for comprehensive needs assessment and careful planning of care, in which both clients and informal carers are involved. Prophylaxes, and especially actions to prevent falls, are important as is the recording of pain and pain management (Table 8.12).

It was possible to analyse the impact of management on outcomes of home-care only in a sub-sample of 100 cases from 5 countries, so especially these results must be seen as exploratory. The results suggest that the care concept (services support autonomy), goal-oriented working processes and sufficient resources were important structural factors in good-quality homecare. Further, it appears to be important that there are structures and processes in place that involve the clients and informal carers in care planning, and ensure effective pain management, but additional research is required for more detailed conclusions.

Summary of Results

The aim of this study was to investigate the determinants of subjective QoL among older clients of homecare services, to examine the role of homecare in production of their welfare and to find out the features of good-quality care that have the most positive impact on the QoL of the clients. The approach to evaluating the QoC particularly emphasised the perspective of the older clients.

The results demonstrated that the dimensions explaining QoL of home-care clients (such as functional ability, psychological resources, social relationships and subjective economic situation) were broadly similar to those of adult population in general, suggesting that a general model is applicable and that frail older people living at home should not be seen as too "different" to the rest of the adult population (Chapter 4). However, the results highlight a number of factors that are important when one is frail and care dependent. Acute illnesses, problems with daily functional ability, problems with housing and living environment, restricted possibilities to participate in social life, a passive lifestyle (no hobbies or exercises at home or outside) and a lack of close relatives all had a negative influence on the QoL of care-dependent old people. Positive attitude towards one's own ageing and satisfaction with home-care both had a strong positive impact on the QoL of the clients. These results are in line with previous research in the field (Baldock & Hadlow, 2002; Birren & Dieckmann, 1991; Cummins, 1997; Hughes, 1990;Vaarama et al., 2007), with the basic model of QoL outlined by Lawton (1991) and support the model of care-related QoL developed in the Care Keys research (Chapter 4).

Regarding the role of homecare in production of QoL, the results indicate that client satisfaction with homecare was highest when services were responsive to their expectations. Subjective QoL of older homecare clients was positively connected with adaptation to ageing (or accommodation, see Chapter 4), but more research is needed on how and to which direction this connection works. In general, our results suggest that a more client-oriented approach to care and psycho-social support are effective ways of improving care outcomes.

One of the remarkable results in the study was the strong relationship between subjective quality of homecare and the QoL of the clients. Whether this is a one-way causal relationship we do not know, but the result at least confirms the assumption that care has a very important role in production of welfare in old homecare clients. Homecare had a positive impact on QoL when the client was as clean as he or she would like, his or her home was as clean as he or she would like, he or she dressed as he or she would like, he or she went to bed and got up as he or she would like and he or she felt that the care workers listened to and understood what he or she would like. Fundamentally, this is not just a matter of being clean and tidy and well dressed, but rather it is about having a responsive care that reflects the personal preferences of the client. From the client perspective, responsive care, good care relationships and continuity of care appear to be important determinants of care quality, and realisation of these can have a positive impact on their QoL. At the present time, these items are seldom included in regular evaluations of the quality and effectiveness of care, and we strongly suggest that these quality measures should be used in addition to the usual clinical outcome measures.

It was possible to define 47 key variables which, from the perspective of the clients, had an impact on their QoL; 37 of these describe client-specific conditions and perceived QoL, and 10 evaluate the quality of homecare as experienced by the clients. Practical experience within the Care Keys project suggests that the developed instruments are easy to administer with frail older people and within care routines. Regular use of these client quality measures, together with measures of clinical and other professional care outcomes, would give a more multifaceted picture of quality and effectiveness of homecare, and give clients a stronger voice and role within the management of their own care and the development of homecare in general.

The results indicate that the involvement of informal carers in care planning and evaluation was considered to be important for the quality of homecare by all stakeholders: the clients, the professionals and the managers. This suggests that homecare should develop a family orientation, as also suggested by Hellström and Hallberg (2001). The research instruments used with clients in Care Keys could also be used for collecting information from informal carers or other key informants.

The low response rate and missing values in the care documentation instrument (InDEX-HC) was due to the generally poor standards of documentation in homecare. This was especially the case in Estonia, but was also evident in other countries. Even so, the results highlighted some positive connections between documented professional care quality and subjective care outcomes. Although the connections were weak they were significant and pointed to a positive effect when individual care plans included needs assessment; separated between the activities client can perform independently and activities in which he or she needs help; included references to use of prophylaxes (especially falls); included strategies and methods for teamworking and showed evidence of teamwork; involved informal carers; recorded pain and pain management and involved evaluation and recording the preferences of the clients. As in the case of institutional care (Chapter 9), these results are among the first to show a positive connection between homecare documentation and homecare outcomes, but taking the low response rate in InDEX into account, the results need to be seen as exploratory. Before the relationship between care documentation and care outcomes can be analysed in more depth, it would seem unavoidable that the documentation needs to be improved. For example, although clinical outcome measures, such as usage of sleeping pills and loss of weight, did not appear in the list of key variables, it is not possible to conclude that these are unimportant, as the result may be a consequence of poor care documentation. Still, the research highlighted 14 key items for the documentation of homecare, and we kept the 5 clinical outcome measures included for further investigations of importance. All in all, the results correspond with care theories and it is possible to conclude that careful planning and documentation of individual care interventions and the regular evaluation of achievements that involve both the client and informal carers are important facets of good-quality, professional homecare. Furthermore, pain management proved to be a very important factor in the QoL of older clients, but pain was inadequately documented and perhaps also inadequately managed.

Management of homecare was connected with both quality of homecare and subjective QoL of the clients. Most frequently, quality standards such as "services support autonomy" (care concept or regime), "setting the goals for care" (degree of goal orientation in care) and "services within agreed time" (continuity) and "number of care personnel converted into FTE" and "sufficient material resources" as evaluated by the manager emerged as important features. In addition, structures and processes for pain management and for participation by clients and informal carers in care planning, written quality management procedures and contact between management and employees were connected with good homecare outcomes. These results show that management plays an important role in providing the right context for the realisation of good homecare outcomes. The impact of management was stronger on QoL than the impact of documented care quality, but it is not possible to determine how much this was due to weaknesses in the data, notably the low response rate in care documentation. There were ten key variables to document and evaluate the quality of management of homecare, and the results correspond adequately with the management concept used in Care Keys. Even though the results should be seen as tentative, they still point to directions for development of homecare management.

The similarities in the nature of QoL between care-dependent people and the adult population in general has implications also for the instrumentation of QoL research. For instance, general measures of QoL, such as the WHOQOL-Bref (WHOQOL Group, 1998), were broadly applicable to the target population in the Care Keys research. However, the additional determinants of QoL that were highlighted in the present research should be included in the instrumentation when dealing with care-dependent older people. Our results demonstrate gaps in current instrumentation, including the newly developed WHOQOL-OLD measure (Power et al., 2005), and we provided a client interview instrument with 47 items to help filling in these gaps. Regarding subjective quality of homecare, perceived QoC measures such as SERVQUAL and Pickert (see Chapter 2) are available, but the Care Keys research is, besides Netten, Francis, Jones, and Bebbington (2004), among the first ones to specify measures for quality and performance of homecare as experienced by clients. Gerontological research on QoL is currently very active, so it can be expected that QoL instrumentation develops continuously, and we hope the models and measures presented in this chapter can contribute to this development.

The experience gained from the Care Keys research suggests that the model of crQoL was a very valuable conceptual framework for research on QoL in the study population. The set of potential variables was very rich and the large number of potential arguments means that the number of possible models was huge. Because of this, the models selected and presented in this chapter represent a larger set of models that may differ slightly from the given model, including different explanatory variables. But in general, the stability of the models was confirmed, as the variables belonged to the same groups and more or less measured the same features. This also confirms the usability and flexibility of the conceptual framework and the model of crQoL in research on the QoL of old, care-dependent people. A key challenge will be to test it in longitudinal design to determine whether the measures and instrumentation are sufficiently sensitive to capture the nuances of care, its quality and its outcomes.

Conclusions

The results suggest that homecare has a great potential to support and enhance the QoL of older clients, but in order to do this, care has to be responsive to client needs and expectations. To this end, it is important that ageing and old age should not be seen purely as a biomedical process but also as a complex psychological and social process, which takes place within different social and cultural contexts. High-quality homecare that is responsive to the complex needs of the people it serves has to take this issue seriously. A care philosophy based on a socio-cultural, rather than on a medical model of ageing would allow a more holistic understanding of the needs and competencies of older clients and involve clients, families and society in more preventative care strategies. This implies giving more priority to the clients' own expertise, authority and preferences in order to empower them to get the kind of care and support that assists them to live according to their own wishes and expectations, rather than to provide task-oriented, superficial care. Sufficient information to the clients about alternatives and choices about care are important elements of the socio-cultural model of care, as well as rehabilitative interventions to prevent premature decline of physical, psychological, cognitive and social functional abilities. Working methods to achieve this include also non-medical interventions with cultural gerontological work, of which there are promising examples (e.g. Edgar & Russel, 1998; Pitkälä, Routasalo, Kautiainen, Savikko, & Tilvis, 2005). A change of care philosophy is also necessary within medical care as this is crucial in supporting older people with chronic illnesses who live at home, and where good collaboration with homecare is important. For example, Kane and Kane (2001) suggest a change in the philosophy of long-term medical care from an acute care model towards chronic care that supports both compensatory and therapeutic interventions.

As an important step in this direction, we would strongly argue that homecare should have the explicit goal of enhancing the QoL of the older clients, and the degree of achievement of this goal should be included in the criteria for measuring the effectiveness of homecare (see also Thomé et al., 2003). In the evaluation of care outcomes, besides clinical and other professional care outcome measurements, client feedback on effectiveness and QoC should also be regularly measured. Giving an effective "voice" to clients should be a cornerstone of the socio-cultural model of care, together with the multi-actorial evaluation of structures, processes and outcomes of care. The Care Keys models and instruments provide useful tools in this respect. The research presented here supports the Care Keys theoretical model of crQoL as a useful conceptual framework for the research of QoL among care-dependent people living at home.

References

Baldock, J. C., & Hadlow, J. (2002). Self-talk versus needs-talk: An exploration of the priorities of housebound older people. *Quality in Ageing, 3*(1), 42–48.

Baltes, P. B., & Baltes, M. M. (1990). Psychological perspectives on successful aging: The model of selective optimization with compensation. In P. B. Baltes, & M. Baltes (Eds.), *Successful aging. Perspectives from the behavioural sciences.* Cambridge: Cambridge University Press.

Baltes, P. B., & Mayer, K. K. (Eds.). (1999). *The Berlin aging study. Aging from 70 to 100.* Cambridge: Cambridge University Press.

Birren, J. E., & Dieckmann, L. (1991). Concepts and contents of QoL in later years: An overview. In J. E. Birren, J. E. Lubben, J. Cichowlas Rowe, & D. E. Deutchmann

(Eds.), *The concept and measurement of QoL in the frail elderly*. San Diego, CA: Academic Press Inc.

Bowling, A. (2004). *Measuring health: A review of QoL measurement scales* (3rd ed.). Buckingham: Open University Press.

Cummins, R. A. (1997). Assessing QoL. In R. I. Brown (Ed.), *QoL for people with disabilities. Models, research and practice*. Cheltenham: Stanley Thornes.

Davies, B., Bebbington, A., & Charnley, H. in collaboration with Baines, B., Ferlie, E. Hughes, M. & Twigg, J. (1990). *Resources, needs and outcomes in community-based care. A comparative study of the production of welfare for elderly people in ten local authorities in England and Wales*. PSSRU, University of Kent at Canterbury. Avebury: Aldershot.

Edgar, I. R., & Russel, A. (Eds.). (1998). *The anthropology of welfare*. London: Routledge.

Evers, A., & Svetlik, I. (Eds.). (1993). *Balancing pluralism. New welfare mixes in care for the elderly*. Vienna, Avebury: European Centre.

Goldstone, L., & Maselino-Okai, C. (1986). *Senior monitor. An index of the quality of nursing care for senior citizens on hospital wards*. Newcastle upon Tyne: Newcastle upon Tyne Polytechnic Products Ltd.

Hellström, Y., & Hallberg, I. R. (2001). Perspectives of elderly people receiving home help on health, care and QoL. *Health and Social Care in the Community, 9*(2), 61–71.

Hughes, B. (1990). QoL. In S. M. Peace (Ed.), *Researching social gerontology: Concepts, methods and issues* (pp. 46–58). London: SAGE.

Kane, R., & Kane, R. (2001). Emerging issues in chronic care. In: R. Binstock, & L. George (Eds.), *Handbook of aging and the social sciences*. USA: Academic Press.

Lawton, M. P. (1975). The Philadelphia Geriatric Centre Morale Scale: A revision. *Journal of Gerontology, 30*, 85–89.

Lawton, M. P. (1991). A multidimensional view of QoL in frail elders. In J. E. Birren, J. E. Lubben, J. C. Rowe, & D. E. Deutchman (Eds.), *The concept and measurement of QoL in frail elders* (pp. 3–27). San Diego, CA: Academic Press.

Löwenstein, A., & Ogg, J. (Eds.). (2003). OASIS. Old age and autonomy: The role of service systems and intergenerational family solidarity. Final report. Haifa: University of Haifa. <www.dza.de/forschung/oasis_report.pdf>

Netten, A., Francis, J., Jones, K., & Bebbington, A. (2004). Performance and quality: User experiences of home care services. Final report. PSSRU Discussion Paper 2104/3. April 2004. <www.PSSRU.ac.uk>

Pacolet, J., Bouten, R., Lanoye, H., & Versieck, K. (1998). *The state of the debate on social protection for dependency in old age in the 15 EU member states and Norway*. Leuven: Hoger Instituut voor de arbeid.

Paljärvi, S., Rissanen, S., & Sinkkonen, S. (2003). Kotihoidon sisältö ja laatu vanhusasiakkaiden, omaisten ja työntekijöiden arvioimana—Seurantatutkimus Kuopion kotihoidosta (The contents and quality of home care as evaluated by the older clients, their relatives and the care professionals. A follow-up study of home care in the city of kuopio, Finland). *Gerontologia, 2*, 85–97.

Pitkälä, K., Routasalo, P., Kautiainen, H., Savikko, N., & Tilvis, R. (2005). *Ikääntyneiden yksinäisyys. Psykososiaalisen ryhmäkuntoutuksen vaikuttavuus*. (*Loneliness in old age. The effectiveness of psycho-social rehabilitation*). Vanhustyön keskusliitto. Geriatrisen kuntoutuksen tutkimus- ja kehittämishanke. Tutkimusraportti 11. Vaajakoski: Gummerus.

Power, M., Quinn, K., Schmidt, S., & The WHOQOL Group (2005). *Development of the WHOQOL-OLD module. QoL Research 14*, 2197–2214.

Skevington, S. M., Lofty, M., & O'Connell, K. A. (2004). The World Health Organisation's WHOQOL-BREF QoL assessment. A report from the WHOQOL group. *QoL Research, 13*, 299–310.

Solem, P. E. (2003). *Forskningsinstrumentene I norLAG. (Research instruments in nor-LAG). Den norske studien av livslöp, aldring og generasjon.* Oslo: NOVA.

Thomé, B., Dykes, A-K., & Rahm Hallberg, I. (2003). Home care with regard to definition, care recipients, content and outcome: Systematic literature review. *Journal of Clinical Nursing, 12*(6), 860–872.

Vaarama, M., & Noro, A. (2006). Care of older persons. In S. Koskinen, A. Aromaa, J. Huttunen, & J. Teperi (Eds.), *Health in Finland.* Helsinki: KTL, Stakes and Ministry of Social Affairs and Health.

Vaarama, M., Pieper, R., & Sixsmith, A. (2007). Care-related QoL in old age. Conceptual and empirical exploration. In H. Mollenkopf, & A. Walker (Eds.), *Quality of life in Old Age.* International and Multi-Disciplinary Perspectives. Dordrecht, The Netherlands: Springer. pp. 215–232.

WHOQOL Group (1998). Development of the World Health Organization WHOQOL-BREF quality of life assessment. *Psychological Medicine, 28*, 551–558.

9
Quality of Life in Institutional Care

Kai Saks, Ene-Margit Tiit, Seija Muurinen, Susanna Mukkila,
Mona Frommelt and Margaret Hammond

Introduction and: Theoretical Basis

It is generally accepted that most old people prefer to live independently in
their own homes. However, institutional care in nursing or residential homes
is often the only option available for frail and dependent people, who require
higher levels of support. Moreover, social and demographic changes throughout Europe show a weakening of family and community networks, resulting
in a reduction in informal support from family and friends to allow frail old
people to remain at home.

Care institutions provide adapted and safe environments and provide a
range of care, such as support in everyday activities and medical procedures.
In addition to these instrumental issues, increasing attention has also been
paid to the general quality of life (QoL) of clients through facilitating social
participation, leisure activities and, supporting clients' lifestyles, while trying
to preserve individuals' autonomy and control. At the same time however,
the individual has to conform to the social roles and rules prevalent in the
institution. Among older people, this process can lead to "induced dependency" whereby the person undergoes psychological changes, loss of personal
competence and even physical deterioration.

Residents of care institutions commonly have serious limitations in their
abilities to take care of themselves because of the illnesses or frailties of
advanced age. These conditions and associated functional decline inevitably
have an impact on QoL. As well as physical functioning, other factors such
as psychological, social and emotional changes can have an impact on well-
being and satisfaction with life.

The World Health Organization's general definition (1995) of QoL
emphasizes the individual's own perception of their position in life and their
goals, expectations, standards and concerns. This definition also includes
the culture and value systems in which an individual lives. QoL in the context of institutional care differs from general QoL and from health-related
QoL. Multidimensional QoL models for older persons include a broad

variety of factors, both objective and subjective, which influence the QoL (Faulk, 1988; Hughes, 1990; Lawton, 1975, 1991; Veenhoven, 2000). Care can influence only part of these factors (see Chapter 2) in care planning and management. An individual approach can ensure optimum outcome for the client. Nevertheless, such an individual approach should rely on evidence regarding how different care-related factors impact on QoL of frail older care-dependent persons.

The assessment of how care impacts on a person's well-being and QoL is not straightforward. In Donabedian's (1969) model of quality of care (QoC), input and process factors produce certain care outcomes and Øvretveit (1998) has used this same theoretical basis in his QoC model. According to these models QoC indicators may be used as professional measures for characterizing clients' QoL. Although there is no commonly agreed definition of QoC, there are many characteristics of QoC in different models (Currie, Harvey, West, McKenna, & Keeney, 2005). These characteristics can be easily monitored if care documentation corresponds to recommended standards.

Recent research indicates that the client perspective should be prioritized when monitoring QoL in long-term care (Kane et al., 2003). This means that in addition to professional (objective) QoC, perceived (subjective) QoC and subjective QoL should be included when evaluating the outcome of care. However, there has been no specific valid instrument for monitoring QoL in institutionalized clients, although recent work in this area has been carried out in several research centers (Kane et al., 2005). The research presented in this chapter has the following aims:

1. To determine which care-related factors influence the QoL of cognitively well persons in institutional care (IC)
2. To define key variables for QoL (KVQL) and QoC in IC settings

Methods

Database

Data for the study were collected using Care Keys data collection instrumentation CLINT-IC and InDEX-IC, following data collection guidelines (see Chapters 2 and 3). Modeling was performed several times using different databases: during the piloting stage a pooled database from three countries was used (Estonia, Sweden and UK) along with national Care Keys databases. For the final modeling, the complete Care Keys database of five countries (Estonia, Finland, Germany, Sweden and UK) was used, although only clients with reasonable cognitive function (MMSE $\geq$ 15) were included. The sample size was 435 complete cases (see Chapter 3).

Modeling of QoL and QoC in IC Clients

Final modeling was performed by two research teams—in Helsinki (Finland) and Tartu (Estonia). In Helsinki, factor and correlation analyses were used to find key variables for subjective and professional QoC. The framework for modeling was the Production of Welfare model together with the Combined Nursing Model based on Øvretveit's Three-Dimensional Quality of Care Model and the Model of Phases in Patient Care (Muurinen, Valvanne, & Mukkila, 2004; Øvretveit, 1998). Logistic regression analysis with backward (Wald) option was used. In modeling of QoL the following dependent variables were used:

• Philadelphia Morale Scale (PGCMS; Lawton, 1975): sum of 17 variables
• Single variable: How would you rate your QoL?
• Single variable: How satisfied are you with your health?
• Single variable: How much do you enjoy life?
• Single variable: In general, how satisfied are you with this care home?
• Horizontal target efficiency (TEFF H; characterizing the proportion of met needs among all needs) (see Chapter II)
• Mean of four dimensions of needs (medical, daily activities, psycho-social, environmental) (see Chapter II)
• Clinical outcomes: usage of sleeping pills, suffering from pain, pressure ulcers, falls

The Tartu team used the data to build models for nine dependent variables of QoL: four from the World Health Organization Quality of Life brief questionnaire (WHOQOL-Bref; WHOQOL group, 1998), three from the PGCMS, and two single variables defined in WHOQOL-Bref, but not included in the domains. All dependent variables were scaled to interval 0–100, where bigger values correspond to better client QoL.

• WHOQOL-Bref domains: physical, psychological, social, environmental
• PGCMS factors: agitation, attitude toward own ageing, loneliness
• Single variable: How would you rate your QoL?
• Single variable: How satisfied are you with your health?

The following variables were used in the Tartu analysis:

Background variables of clients (BG): country, gender, age, marital status, mother-language (common for given country or not). Most were treated as binary variables, total number = 9.
Variables connected with traumatic life experiences of clients (LE): divorce, death of spouse, illness of client or his or her close relatives, financial problems, injustice, and so on, total number = 9.
Variables characterizing the physical environment of the client (E): living in single or shared room, having own WC and bathroom, ease of getting outdoors and so on, total number = 12.
Correct allocation of services (if client has need then this need is met, etc.) in different areas (dimensions) (NS): medical, care in ADL, care in IADL,

safety, legal, social psychological and emotional counseling, free time activities, social events and so on, total number = 49.

TEFF values in the same dimensions (T), total number = 11.

Subjective satisfaction with different aspects of care that were selected during the Care Keys piloting stage (QC): Personal characteristics of care workers (kind, honest, treats with dignity, etc), quality of their work (clean and tidy environment, clients clean dressed, enough time to eat, enough time for clients, etc.), clients would recommend their care, total number = 36.

Professional characteristics of care including a long list of different actions and organizational steps (PC): Pain management, different prophylactic means, QoC planning and care documentation, organization of cooperation between specialists inside and outside of institutions and so on, total number = 55.

Variables characterizing the communication and social activities of client (C): Existence of people to whom the client feels close, frequency of visits, getting along with other residents and care persons, also leisure activities and so on, total number = 23.

Linear regression analysis was used as the modeling methodology (using SPSS), using step-wise selection (combination of forward and backward selection rules) of arguments and significance level 0.05. The dependent variables' distribution was estimated and satisfactory closeness to normal distribution, especially in the case of WHOQOL domains was observed. The quality of models was assessed by the determination coefficient R^2. Only statistically significant models with all significant terms were considered. The list of potential explanatory variables contained more than 200 variables.

The reason for using different modeling schemes by the two research teams was to create a range of different models for selecting the most important key variables that is those that were present in several different models. The Tartu team was primarily responsible for QoL modeling and the Helsinki team for QoC modeling.

Defining the Key Variables

Forty-three variables described QoL and the number of conceptually meaningful domains (linear combinations of initial variables) was between 4 and 7 (by different theoretical approaches). Using the linear models and defining the descriptive power of all initial variables for all other variables, the most useful 10 initial variables were selected (ensuring, that all domains/dimensions were covered). The overall description rate was about 70–75%.

All other variables (explanatory variables) were divided into groups (using correlation and factor analyses), where each group consisted of variables measuring the same or similar features. Using the traditional step-wise selection process and the original concept of descriptive power, the most informative subsets from all exploratory variables of each group were selected to forecast (i) the initial domains of QoL and (ii) the predicted key-variables domains of QoL.

Results

QoL Models

The best models containing only statistically significant terms had, in most cases, a description rate of about 40–50% (average for WHOQOL domains 47%, and for PGCMS 41%) and contained between 16 and 26 explanatory variables (average for WHOQOL-Bref—21, for PGCMS—20 variables). In Table 9.1 the most important characteristics of models have been given for all QoL components.

Although the number of variables measuring professional QoC was the highest (28), the usability rate (the rate of variables presented in models compared with all potential variables) was the lowest (45%). The usability rate for different groups was 45—200%. These results indicate that the list of theoretically selected important variables can be reduced in most categories of variables.

Background Variables

Surprisingly, background variables had a rather weak influence on QoL. The only exception was "being currently ill" determining 16% of the Physical domain and 8% of Attitude toward own ageing. Other variables from this

TABLE 9.1. The most important characteristics of QOL components in IC.

QoL indicators	R^2	Number of explanatory variables from groups								
		BG	LE	E	NS	T	QC	PC	C	Total
WHOQOL-Bref Physical	0.450	3	2	2	2	2	4	2	0	17
WHOQOL-Bref Psychological	0.448	0	4	4	5	1	6	4	2	26
WHOQOL-Bref Social	0.440	0	3	4	6	3	2	5	2	25
WHOQOL-Bref Environmental	0.538	0	3	1	1	0	4	4	3	16
PGCMS Agitation	0.323	1	2	1	5	0	4	2	3	18
PGCMS Attitude toward ageing	0.437	1	3	3	4	1	3	4	1	20
PGCMS Loneliness	0.465	0	1	2	8	1	5	4	1	22
Total		5	18	17	31	8	28	25	12	144

BG, background variables; LE, variables connected with traumatic life experiences; E, variables characterizing the physical environment; NS, correct allocation of services; T, TEFF values; QC, subjective satisfaction with care; PC, professional characteristics of care; C, variables characterizing the communication and social activities.

group were not included in the top-five explanatory variables in any model. Language was included in one model, indicating that people speaking the native language of a country have higher QoL. However, the country of residence did not appear in any model. From this it can be concluded that national differences are not simply country-specific, but due to different care conditions, or possibly due to the different historical and cultural backgrounds of clients.

Life Experiences

Life experiences may have a long-term influence on peoples' QoL. Illness of a family member, financial problems and bereavement (other than spouse) were the most influential variables, determining the 3–4% of QoL. Illness of family members, serious illness of self, and becoming widowed were also important, appearing in 5 of the 7 models.

Physical Environment

While there were only a few variables describing the physical environment, some of these had an important role. Living alone or sharing a room determined about 4% of QoL being in the top two variables in several models. Almost as important was "Easy to get outdoors," being in the top-two several times and determining 4% of QoL. Well-lit, spacious, clean and tidy rooms, and good indoor air had a positive relationship with the QoL of clients.

Correct Allocation of Services (Fitting of Need and Supply)

Variables measuring the correspondence between need and supply appeared in all models, but not as the most influential ones. Only two of these variables were in the top-five: safety alarm and cleaning. Medication, legal and psychological counseling, were influential, along with cardiovascular and respiratory care and different ADL and IADL services. Need and supply variables were recorded according to care documentation, and poor quality of the documentation may have influenced these results. There may also have been different opinions between professionals and clients about their needs and supply of care.

TEFF Variables

The TEFF variable was modified in order to use in the various models while not losing information. If originally TEFF variables, defined by ratio, exist only in cases when the denominator differs from zero, then in modified TEFF variables the missing values are substituted by highest value 1. TEFF variables were not particularly influential, being represented in QoL models through the emotional dimension, delirium, memory and IADL and having only the eighth highest position in the models. As TEFF values can only be determined using good care documentation the generally poor quality of documentation may have influenced results.

Subjective Quality of Care

Variables from this group were the most influential on client QoL. In all models, the first explanatory variable, describing 6–26% of QoL, was from this group: satisfaction with care (18% and 13%), recommendation of the institution (26% and 13%) and good understanding by care-workers (10% and 6%) each appeared twice as the most influential variables. The last of these belonged in the top-five influential variables in a total of five models. Also being dressed as one preferred, enjoying meals, keeping clean, and the possibility to plan one's own day were amongst the top-five influential variables, with day-planning describing 17% in one model.

Professional Care

Only a few professional care variables were influential: "Do regular evaluations take place" is in second place in one model, describing 5% of QoL, and in 5th place in another. Additionally, "Does regular evaluation consider the adequacy of involvement of the informal carer?" and "Does the care plan record interventions aimed at supporting and increasing the client's own resources?" were also within the top five variables. It would seem that the influence of variables from this group acts indirectly through the subjective QoC variables.

Communication

From this group only a few variables were influential: having close relationship with care-workers, having enough things to do (in two models) and getting along with residents.

Small Models for QoL Dimensions

In this section, the "best-5" explanatory model for each QoL variable is provided. All dependent variables (QoL dimensions) are scaled 0–100. Two characteristics of the models are shown in the results tables: the regression coefficient B and the increase R^2.

PGCMS Factor: Agitation

The model (Table 9.2) describes 21.1% of the total variation of Agitation, with the first explanatory variable, "care worker's good understanding," has a description rate of almost 10%. In the most favorable case the prognosis of Agitation is 88.6.

PGCMS Factor: Attitude Toward Own Ageing

According to this model (Table 9.3) in the most favorable case, the estimated score for Attitude toward own ageing equals 79.3. Illness decreases the score by 15 points and problems in household chores by 18.5 points.

TABLE 9.2. Model for PGCMS factor: Agitation.

Explanatory variables	Scale	B	Increase R^2
(Constant)		99.5	
Care workers have a good understanding of client and client's needs	1-yes, always…5-never	−7.7	9.8
Satisfied with living alone/share a room	1-yes, 2-I cannot say, 3-no	−9.9	14.1
Life experience – serious illness of close family member	0-no, 1-yes	−13.2	17.1
Client able to keep as well dressed as he or she would like	1-yes, always…5-never	−4.5	19.1
Nursing hospital—supply	0-no, 1-yes	11.2	21.1

TABLE 9.3. Model for PGCMS factor: Attitude toward own ageing.

Explanatory variables	Scale	B	Increase R^2
(Constant)		40.0	
Currently ill	1-yes, 2-no	15.4	7.7
Care workers have enough time for client	1-yes, always…5-never	−5.0	11.8
Other household chores—correct allocation	0-no, 1-yes	18.5	15.8
Quality management strategy includes hospitals as partners	0-no, 1-partly, 2-yes	−11.00	19.3
Client able to get up and go to bed at times that suits to him or her	1-yes, always…5-never	−4.5	21.7

TABLE 9.4. Model for PGCMS factor: Loneliness.

Explanatory variables	Scale	B	Increase R^2
(Constant)		112	
Satisfaction with care	1-very satisfied…5-very dissatisfied	−8.4	18.2
Care workers have enough time for client	1-yes, always…5-never	−5.7	23.6
Satisfied with living alone/share a room	1-yes, 2-I cannot say, 3-no	−8.5	27.4
Enough things to do	1-yes, always…5-never	−3.5	29.7

PGCMS factor: Loneliness

In this case (Table 9.4), a 4 variable explanatory model has been given due to its high description rate. The first explanatory variable "Satisfaction with care" determines the value of the Loneliness score by more than 18%. The most favorable case is when all variables have a value of 1, then the score value of Loneliness is 86.0.

WHOQOL-Bref: Physical Domain

In the most favorable case the estimated score of the Physical Domain equals 71.6. The most influential variable is illness with a description rate of 16.5%. (Table 9.5) and decreases the score by 11 points. Changes of 1 point in all other variables only decreases the score by about 2 points.

WHOQOL-Bref: Psychological Domain

In the most favorable case the estimated score for the Psychological Domain equals 83.6. The first explanatory variable, "satisfaction with care," describes 13%, and the 5-argument model 26%, of total variance of the Psychological Domain (Table 9.6).

WHOQOL-Bref: Social Domain

The first explanatory variable, "client would recommend this service," describes 12.5%, and the 5-argument model 26%, of total variance of Social Domain (Table 9.7). In the most favorable case the estimated score of Social Domain equals 89.3.

TABLE 9.5. Model for WHOQOL-Bref: Physical domain.

Explanatory variables	Scale	B	Increase R^2
(Constant)		59.3	
Currently ill	1-yes, 2-no	11.0	16.5
Client can plan his or her day	1-yes, always...5-never	−2.7	25.0
Client enjoys meals	1-yes, always...5-never	−2.4	28.4
Easy to get outdoors	1-yes, definitely...5-no	−1.9	31.2
Care workers have a good understanding of client and client's needs	1-yes, always...5-never	−2.6	32.9

TABLE 9.6. Model for WHOQOL-Bref: Psychological domain.

Explanatory variables	Scale	B	Increase R^2
(Constant)		77.1	
Satisfaction with care	1-very satisfied...5-very dissatisfied	−3.4	12.7
Client able to keep as clean as she/he would like	1-yes, always...5-never	−3.1	18.5
Easy to get outdoors	1-yes, definitely...5-no	−2.0	22.2
Does the regular evaluation consider the adequacy of involvement of informal carer?	0-no, 1-yes	8.4	25.0
If client raises concerns, does he or she feel that care worker/s listens?	1-yes, always...5-never	−3.2	23.9
Does the care plan record interventions aimed at supporting and increasing the client's own resources?	0-no, 1-yes	6.5	26.2

TABLE 9.7. Model for WHOQOL-Bref: Social Domain.

Explanatory variables	Scale	B	Increase R²
(Constant)		72.4	
Client would recommend this service	1-yes, definitely...5-no	−4.1	12.5
Do regular evaluations take place?	0-no, 1-yes	10.1	17.3
Client has someone that he or she feels close to	0-no, 1-yes	7.5	21.0
If client raises concerns, does he or she feel that care worker/s listens	1-yes, always...5-never	−3.2	23.9
Does the care plan record interventions aimed at supporting and increasing the client's own resources?	0-no, 1-yes	6.5	26.2

TABLE 9.8. Model for WHOQOL-Bref: Environmental Domain.

Explanatory variables	Scale	B	Increase R²
(Constant)		87.4	
Client would recommend this service	1-yes, definitely...5-no	−4.2	26.3
Care workers have a good understanding of client and client's needs	1-yes, always...5-never	−4.9	34.2
Life experience - had financial problems	0-no, 1-yes	−8.9	38.4
Getting along with other residents	1-very well... 5-very poorly	−2.5	40.8
Do regular evaluations take place?	0-no, 1-yes	6.3	42.8

WHOQOL-Bref: Environmental Domain

In the most favorable case the estimated score of the Environmental Domain equals 72.9. The first explanatory variable, "client would recommend this service," describes 26.3%, and the 5-argument model 42.8%, of total variance of Environmental Domain (Table 9.8). This model is the best of all the 5-argument models based on its description rate.

Models of QoC and QoL

The results of modeling of QoC and QoL by the Helsinki team, with sum variables, are presented in Table 9.9 and with single variables in Table 9.10. Client-centered action had a positive relationship on all QoL and QoC variables. Atmosphere and social environment influenced subjective QoL in two models. Quality of the documentation had an impact in one QoL and three QoC models. A number of single variables had a significant impact on QoL, specifically "ease of getting outdoors" and "perceiving that care worker had enough time for the client." Surprisingly, the quality of the care documentation had a direct influence on QoL.

TABLE 9.9. Results of modeling QoC and QoL with sum variables.

Predictors			
Input variables	Process variables	Outcome variables	Nagelkerke R^2
Social environment Atmosphere	Quality of documentation Client-centered action	PGCMS17*	0.332
Atmosphere Social environment	Quality of care in ADL Client-centered action	Subjective QOL*	0.395
Atmosphere	Client-centered action	Satisfaction with care**	0.424
Physical comfort (-)	Client-centered action Quality of documentation	TEFF—H*	0.134
Physical comfort (-)	Client-centered action Quality of documentation	No sleeping pills***	0.141
	Quality of documentation	No pressure ulcers***	0.047
Physical comfort	Client-centered action	No falls***	0.142
–	–	No pain***	0

TABLE 9.10. Summary of models with single variables.

Predictors			
Input variables	Process variables	Outcome variables	Nagelkerke R^2
Getting along with care workers	Enough time	PGCMS17*	0.382
Easy to get outdoors Enough things to do Client can plan his or her day	Quality of documentation		
Getting along with other residents	Enough time	Subjective QOL*	0.504
Good quality of indoor air	Care workers do things that client wants to be done		
Easy to get outdoors	Quality of care in ADL		

Correlations Between Documentation Quality, QoL, Clients' Satisfaction and Care Planning Quality

The modeling revealed a number of correlations between QoL and QoC. This finding deserved further analysis, as some of the documented QoC items not only highlighted the quality of documentation but were also indicators of the QoC planning. To determine whether the quality of documentation per se was correlated with clients' QoL, satisfaction with care and QoC planning, correlation analysis was carried out to examine the impact of missing values in InDEX-IC. InDEX-IC includes a comprehensive set of data that are considered necessary for facilitating good care in long-term care settings, according to previous research and care theories.

Four of the seven dimensions of QoL had significant correlations with missing values in care documentation: attitude toward own ageing, physical domain, psychological domain and environmental domain (Table 9.11).

TABLE 9.11. Correlations between the completeness of InDEX-IC and QoL dimensions.

QoL factor or domain	Correlation coefficient (r)	Significance (P)
Agitation (PGCMS)	0.018	0.742
Attitude toward own ageing (PGCMS)	0.140	0.009
Loneliness (PGCMS)	0.092	0.088
Physical (WHOQOL-Bref)	0.145	0.009
Psychological (WHOQOL-Bref)	0.129	0.021
Social (WHOQOL-Bref)	0.079	0.157
Environmental (WHOQOL-Bref)	0.243	0.000

TABLE 9.12. Correlations between the completeness of InDEX-IC and clients' satisfaction with the environment.

Environmental variable	Correlation coefficient (r)	Significance (P)	Scale
Satisfied with living alone/share a room	−0.114	0.022	1-yes...3-no
Pleasant physical environment	−0.126	0.011	1-yes, definitely...5-no, definitely not
Clean and tidy physical environment	−0.156	0.002	1-yes, definitely...5-no, definitely not
Good quality of indoor air	−0.092	0.066	1-yes, definitely...5-no, definitely not
Too noisy in care home	0.100	0.046	1-yes, always...5 - never
Easy to get outdoors	−0.153	0.002	1-yes, definitely...5-no, definitely not
Visiting hours suit to you and your visitors	−0.183	0.000	1-yes, definitely...5-no, definitely not
Client can plan his or her day	−0.068	0.173	1-yes, definitely...5-no, definitely not

The correlations between documentation quality and specific environmental items were mostly significant (Table 9.12).

In addition, significant correlations between clients' satisfaction with care and documentation quality were found (Table 9.13). Clients' satisfaction with care workers' personal qualities such as dignity, honesty and respect did not depend on the quality of documentation. At the same time an association was found between the quality of documentation and clients' satisfaction with care and meals.

Looking at correlations between overall documentation quality and QoC planning, all results were significant and expected: the more complete the documentation, the higher the standards of good care planning ($r = 0.117$–0.268; $P = 0.019$–0.000). In addition, correlations were observed between general documentation quality and variables relating to clients' clinical outcome: pressure ulcers ($r = -0.099$; $P = 0.047$), and suffering from pain ($r = -0.160$; $P = 0.001$). Frequency of usage of sleeping pills had no correlation with the quality of documentation.

TABLE 9.13. Correlations between the completeness of InDEX-IC and clients' satisfaction with care.

Variable (scale:1-yes, always...5-never)	Correlation coefficient (r)	Significance (P)
Care workers are good at what they do	−0.115	0.021
Care workers' honesty and trustworthiness	−0.080	0.108
Care workers treat client with dignity and respect	−0.019	0.700
Care workers have a good understanding of client	0.000	0.993
Care workers do the things that client wants to be done	−0.103	0.039
If client raises concerns, does he or she feel that care worker/s listens	−0.039	0.438
Satisfaction with care	−0.114	0.022
Client would recommend this service	−0.121	0.015
Client gets to eat at the times that suit for him or her	0.185	0.001
Client gets the right amounts to eat	−0.116	0.031
Enough time to eat	0.096	0.075
Client enjoys meals	−0.157	0.004
Client able to keep as clean as he or she would like	−0.074	0.169
Client able to keep as well dressed as he or she would like	−0.126	0.020
Client able to get up and go to bed at times that suits to him or her	−0.106	0.050
Privacy respected	−0.076	0.163

The results of the analysis showed not only the expected correlations between quality of documentation and QoC but also many significant correlations between general quality of documentation and clients' QoL, satisfaction with care and care environment.

KVQL and QoC in Long-Term Care Institutions

As a result of the statistical analysis it was possible to reduce the initial list of variables by about 10 times, yet still preserve 75% of useful information. The final list of key variables addresses the results of modeling QoL drawing on the Care Keys final pooled database, national databases of Finland, Estonia and UK and also an analysis of client satisfaction using final pooled database by the UK team.

KVQL represent all the domains of WHOQOL-Bref and the PGCMS factors and all meaningful variables found in the factor analysis of the initial dataset. There were no high correlations between KVQL variables. The list of key variables of QoL in institutional care is presented in Table 9.14. The list includes 3 variables from PGCMS and 7 variables from WHOQOL-Bref. The description rate of QoL key variables in IC was 48–83% (Table 9.15).

TABLE 9.14. List of QoL key variables for clients in long-term care institutions.

No.	Variables source (instrument and question number)	Variable description
1.	PGCMS 3	Feeling lonely
2.	PGCMS10	Being as happy when person was younger
3.	PGCMS17	Getting upset easily
4.	WHOQOL-Bref g4	Satisfaction with health
5.	WHOQOL-Bref f2_1	Enough energy for everyday life
6.	WHOQOL-Bref f4_1	Enjoying life
7.	WHOQOL-Bref f7_1	Able to accept bodily appearance
8.	WHOQOL-Bref f11_3	Amount of medical treatment
9.	WHOQOL-Bref f14_4	Satisfaction with support of friends
10.	WHOQOL-Bref f19_3	Satisfaction with access to health services

TABLE 9.15. Original factors/domains of QoL and the description rates using statistically significant linear models by KVQL variables (on level 0.05).

Factor/domain/variable	Description rate by R^2
Agitation (PGCMS)	0.59
Attitude toward own ageing (PGCMS)	0.49
Loneliness (PGCMS)	0.62
Physical Domain (WHOQOL-Bref)	0.72
Psychological Domain (WHOQOL-Bref)	0.83
Social Domain (WHOQOL-Bref)	0.69
Environmental Domain (WHOQOL-Bref)	0.61
QOL variable g1—How would you rate your quality of life? (WHOQOL-Bref)	0.48

Combining the results of the different analyses (Tartu group, Helsinki group, piloting data, analyses on national databases) and using the theoretical framework of crQoL, the list of key variables for the assessment of QoL and QoC in institutional care was compiled (Table 9.16). Some variables that were deemed essential from a theoretical point of view and on the basis of previous studies, but were not included in the potential variables in the present study, were also inserted in the list (marked with *). These key variables constituted the basis for data collection instruments for assessment of QoL and QoC in institutional care—CLINT-IC and InDEX-IC (see Chapters 2 and 13).

Discussion

QoL is a multivariate concept and its dimensions depend on many different factors; some of which can be measured and characterized using a range of different instruments. Generally, it is assumed that good care inputs and process will result in good outcomes, in terms of the comprehensive (physical, psychological and social) well-being of the client (Øvretveit, 1998; Rantz et al., 2002).

TABLE 9.16. KVQL and quality of care assessment in care institutions.

Input	Process	Outcome
Client perspective	Getting along with other residents	WHOQOL-Bref:
Language of communication	Able to keep well dressed	Satisfaction with health
Serious illness	Able to keep clean	Enough energy for everyday life
Serious illness of a family member	Can plan his or her day	Enjoying life
Financial problems	Enjoys meals	Able to accept bodily appearance
ADL	Satisfied with care	Amount of medical treatment
IADL	Satisfied with help in moving inside	Support of friends
Cognition	Satisfied with help in moving outside	Access to health services
Depression		PGCMS:
BMI*		Feeling lonely
Date of admission*		Being as happy as in younger age
		Getting upset easily
Professional perspective	*Adequate need-supply*	*Clinical outcomes*
Suitable living room (single, twin etc.)	*(TEFFI):*	Usage of sleeping pills
Own WC, shower	Dressing and undressing	Falls
Clean environment	Dental and oral care	Suffering from pain
Good quality of indoor air	Skin and hair care	Pressure ulcers
Easy to get outdoors	Cutting toe nails	Nosocomial infections
Visiting hours suitable	Moving inside	*TEFF-dimensional*
Enough things to do	Moving outside	
	Medication	
	Respiration procedures	
	Cardiovascular procedures	
	Pain management	
	Falls prophylaxis	
	Depression	
	Emotional support	
	Spiritual, religious support	

Leisure activities

Contact with other people

Documentation:

Distinguish activities which
client does himself or
herself and where help is needed

Care plan record interventions aimed at
supporting and increasing
the client's own resources

Regular evaluations take place, care
person in charge and client are involved

Evaluation consider client's
preferences and lifestyle

Documentation show
involvement of informal care

Documentation show
evidence of team work

Care plan make references to prophylaxis

Client centered action :

Care workers have enough time

Care workers have a
good understanding
of client and client's needs

Care workers do the things
that client wants to be done

Care worker listens

The aim of the research presented in this study was to identify the most important factors influencing the QoL of clients in institutional care. The set of potential variables was very extensive, but fortunately the explanatory variables were not highly correlated and multicollinearity was not a major problem. The large number of potential arguments meant that the quantity of all possible models is also very extensive (e.g. more than 2.6 billion 5-term models can be created from 200 variables!). This means that each model presented represents a large set of models, all of which only slightly differ from the given model. This includes some different explanatory variables, but, in general, these come from the same group and measure almost the same features. The description rate of the constructed models of QoL was quite high − 40–50%.

The most important explanatory variables for QoL in IC clients related to subjective QoC. "Care workers' good understanding of the client," "doing things that client wants to be done", "listening if client raises concerns" and "having enough time" were the most important factors on the provider side. Many studies emphasize communication and client–care worker interaction as a critical matter in determining QoC, especially from the client's own point of view (Bowers, Lauring, & Jacobson, 2001; Caris-Verhallen, Kerkstra, & Bensing, 1997). However, in some studies, the client-centered approach has still not been shown to have a significant effect on resident well-being and satisfaction (Boumans, Berkhout, & Landeweerd, 2005).

Satisfaction with personal hygiene and dressing had fundamental influence on clients' QoL. For ADL-dependent persons the most important variables in this area were: "satisfaction with help in moving indoors," "dressing and undressing," "dental and oral care," "skin and hair care" and "cutting toe nails." The other interesting finding was that the person's ADL score itself was not amongst the top variables influencing QoL. Nagatomo, Kita, Takigawa, Nomaguchi, and Sameshima (1997) have published similar results, indicating that QoL of older long-term care residents was influenced by subjective symptoms, but not by the ADL score. However, it should be noted that the present study has limitations regarding the analysis of the influence of ADL score on QoL, as routine care documentation was used, where the ADL score was missing or was measured by different instruments.

From the medical perspective, the major influences were helping with medication, cardiovascular and respiratory care. These results may be explained by the high prevalence of these medical needs in the sample. Medical needs are of course individual and supply should correspond to assessed needs. Moreover, a client's satisfaction with received help also had impact on their QoL and should be assessed in addition to professional assessment of the adequacy of care.

Satisfaction with help in participating in leisure activities had a direct influence on QoL. This is of great relevance for care practice, as it indicates that even among care-dependent persons some aspects of their life could serve as 'strengths' that compensate for losses in other areas and which could be used for optimizing their QoL. An international study of social engagement among nursing home residents described essential differences in the level of social engagement between countries (Schroll, Jonsson, Mor, Berg, & Sherwood, 1997). This indicates that different care models are used in different countries, which have different perspectives and emphases in respect to QoL of clients.

Our study revealed a strong influence of enjoyment of meals on QoL. Eating and the dining experience are an integral part of the resident's life in a nursing facility. This is more than a matter of nutrition; allowing residents to select their food, dining times, dining partners and other preferences may also improve the QoL (DePorter, 2005).

Importantly, professional QoC was found to have a direct influence on clients' QoL both on the level of the quality of documentation and clinical outcomes. In the survey, needs assessment, interventions aimed to support a client's own resources, regular evaluations of care that include the client, considering the preferences of the client and information about informal carers were all found to have a direct influence on QoL. Moreover, the general quality of documentation per se had a direct correlation with the clients' QoL and satisfaction with care. From this it is possible to conclude that good documentation is not only an outcome variable for QoC as shown by other researchers (Voutilainen, Isola, & Muurinen, 2004), but is also an important determinant of clients' QoL. Although this has been presumed within various theoretical models, the research carried out within the Care Keys project is probably among the first, which has shown this clear connection between good documentation, good QoC and good QoL. Good documentation is an indicator of good care; a client-centered approach is not only documented but also used in everyday practice.

Control and autonomy have long been identified as important contributors to psychological well-being. Gilloran, McGlew, McKee, Robertson, and Wight (1993) proposed that QoC process includes, among other things, the following indicators: choice is offered to patients, giving information, encouraging independence. The results presented in this chapter corresponded well with these suggestions and indicate that these factors have an impact on persons' well-being. It is important that care process supports the maintenance of relationships of clients and their relatives (Muurinen, Nuutinen, & Peiponen, 2002; Rantz et al., 2002; Weman, Kihlgren, & Fagerberg, 2004). Clients and their relatives' participation in care do not often realize. It is noteworthy that in Finland many relatives of clients in long-term care wanted to participate more frequently in the care of their relative, but had little opportunity to do so (Voutilainen et al., 2004). The present research shows that involving informal carers in the care process may have a positive impact on the QoL of clients in institutional care.

The research has demonstrated a relationship between subjective well-being and some widely recognized clinical outcome indicators in long-term care: usage of sleeping pills, falls and pain. All these are generally accepted outcome indicators of care and influence QoL through subjective symptoms.

Among the variables related to living environment, "easy to get outdoors" was one of the most important factors influencing QoL. Several models showed that good indoor air also had a relatively large impact on QoL. In addition, satisfaction with personal living arrangements (living alone or sharing room, having own WC and shower) had a direct influence on clients' QoL. Home and environment are important factors of QoC from clients' perspective (Muurinen et al., 2001; Rantz et al., 2002). Home is described in these studies as homeliness of the care unit and includes the physical surroundings and equipment, pleasant milieu, cosy atmosphere and the presence of community. However, our research found that ease of access to outdoors influenced the QoL of clients in care institutions at least as much as having a pleasant atmosphere inside.

Among input variables associated with the person, "being currently ill" had the most important impact on QoL. Age, gender and country did not have any significant influence. A number of studies of health-related QoL have shown that subjective feeling of being ill is one of the most important factors influencing a person's QoL. For example, Subasi and Hayran (2005) were unable to find any influence of common socio-demographic characteristics (such as gender, socio-economic status) on life satisfaction of elderly people living in nursing homes. At the same time, negative events in the recent past (illness of a family member, financial problems, other bereavements) described the QoL of IC clients by 3–4% in our study; these same problems may also have been the reason for the client's admission into institutional care.

Conclusions

The QoL of clients living in institutional care settings, such as nursing homes, depends on many factors. The best possible models presented in this chapter describe 30–60% of the different domains of the QoL. Subjective QoC has a major role in this, explaining about 75% of the variability of the models. At the same time, care documentation quality was shown to be an independent factor influencing clients' well-being and satisfaction with care. Involvement in care by relatives plays an important positive role and should be given greater consideration as a resource in care planning. In order to evaluate the effect of care, both the client's subjective view and professional quality need to be measured. A short questionnaire for clients (CLINT) and data extraction instrument from routine care documentation (InDEX) allow the evaluation of all significant dimensions of QoL and QoC. These instruments are not a substitute for comprehensive instruments for assessing the client's needs. However, they allow care managers to extract data from available care documentation and client assessments and to collect data about clients' satisfaction with care and QoL, which can then be used to analyze the impact of the care provided. The evaluation of care outcomes in long-term care facilities should also bear in mind the concept of care-related QoL rather than health-related QoL. The results of empirical modeling of QoL presented in this chapter correspond well with the Care Keys theoretical framework. The research shows that QoL of persons living in long-term care institutions is dependent on a diverse set of factors that go beyond medical and health-related factors.

References

Boumans, N., Berkhou, A., & Landeweerd, A. (2005). Effects of resident-oriented care on quality of care, well-being and satisfaction with care. *Scandinavian Journal of Caring Sciences, 19,* 240–250.

Bowers, B. J., Lauring, C., & Jacobson, N. (2001). How nurses manage time and work in long-term care. *Journal of Advanced Nursing, 33,* 484–491.

Caris-Verhallen, W., Kerkstra, A., & Bensing, J. (1997). The role of communication in nursing care for elderly people: a review of the literature. *Journal of Advanced Nursing, 25,* 915–933.

Currie, V., Harvey, G., West, E., McKenna, H., & Keeney, S. (2005). Relationships between quality of care, staffing levels, skill mix and nurse autonomy: literature review. *Journal of Advanced Nursing, 51,* 73–82.

DePorter, C. H. (2005). Regulating food service in North Carolina's long-term care facilities. *North Carolina Medical Journal, 66, 4,* 300–303.

Donabedian, A. (1969). Some issues in evaluation the quality of nursing care. *American Journal of Public Health, 59,* 1833–36.

Faulk, L. E. (1988). Quality of life factors in board and care homes for the elderly: A hierarchical model. *Adult Foster Care Journal, 2,* 100–117.

Gilloran, A., McGlew, T., McKee, K., Robertson, A., & Wight, D. (1993). Measuring the quality of care in psychogeriatric wards. *Journal of Advanced Nursing, 18,* 269–275.

Hughes, B. (1990). Quality of life. In S. M. Peace (Ed.), *Researching social gerontology: concepts, methods and Issues* (pp. 46–58). London: SAGE.

Kane, R. A., Kling, K. C., Bershadsky, B., Kane, R. L., Giles, K., Degenholtz, H. B., Liu, J., & Cutler, L. J. (2003). Quality of life measures for nursing home residents. *Journals of Gerontology Series A-Biological Sciences & Medical Sciences, 58, 3,* 240–248.

Kane, R. L., Rockwood, T., Hyer, K., Desjardins, K., Brassard, A., Gessert, C., & Kane, R. (2005). Rating the importance of nursing home residents' quality of life. *Journal of American Geriatric Society, 53,* 2076–2082.

Lawton, M. P. (1975). The Philadelphia Geriatric Centre Morale Scale: a revision. *Journal of Gerontology, 30,* 85–89.

Lawton, M. P. (1991). A multidimensional view of quality of life in frail elders. In J. E. Birren, J. E. Lubben, J. C. Rowe, & D. E. Deutchman (Eds.), *The concept and measurement of quality of life in frail elders* (pp. 3–27). San Diego: Academic Press.

Muurinen, S., Nuutinen, H.-L., & Peiponen, A. (2002). Omaisten mielipiteitä vanhusten hoidosta Helsingin ympärivuorokautisen hoidon yksiköissä 2002 . (Relatives perspectives in long-term care in the City of Helsinki 2002.) *Tutkimuksia 2002:2.* Helsingin kaupungin sosiaalivirasto, Helsinki.

Muurinen, S., Raatikainen, R., Silander, E., Tolvanen, A., Turtainen, K., Peiponen, A., & Valvanne, J. (2001). Asukkaiden tyytyväisyys hoitoon Helsingin vanhustenhoidon yksiköissä 2001. (Client satisfaction in long-term care in the City of Helsinki in 2001.) *Tutkimuksia 2001:2.* Helsinki: Helsingin kaupungin sosiaalivirasto.

Muurinen, S., Valvanne, J., & Mukkila, S. (2004). *Performance indicators for the long term care of older people. Indicators for professional quality.* http://www.carekeys.net

Nagatomo, I. Kita, K., Takigawa, M., Nomaguchi, M., & Sameshima, K. (1997). A study of the quality of life in elderly people using psychological testing. *International Journal of Geriatric Psychiatry, 12*(6), 599–608.

Øvretveit, J. (1998). Evaluating health interventions. An introduction to evaluation of health treatments, services, policies and organizational interventions. Buckingham: Open University Press..

Raatikainen, R. (1995). Hoitotyön kehitysvaiheiden luokitus. *Sairaanhoitaja, 68*(9), 31–34. (The model of phases in patient care).

Rantz, M., Jensóttir, A. B., Hjaltadóttir, I., Gudmundsdóttir, H., Sigurveig Gudjónsdóttir, J., Brunton, B., & Rook, M. (2002). International field test results of the Observable Indicators of Nursing Home Care Quality instrument. *International Nursing Review, 49*, 234–242.

Schroll, M., Jonsson, P. V., Mor, V., Berg, K., & Sherwood, S. (1997). An international study of social engagement among nursing home residents, *Age & Aging, 26*, (Suppl. 2), 55–59.

Subasi, F., & Hayran, O. (2005). Evaluation of life satisfaction index of the elderly people living in nursing homes. *Archives of Gerontology & Geriatrics, 41*(1), 23–29.

Veenhoven, R. (2000). The four qualities of Life. Ordering concept and measures of the good life. *Journal of Happiness Studies, 1*, 1–39.

Voutilainen, P., Isola, A., & Muurinen, S. (2004). Nursing documentation in nursing homes—state-of-the-art and implications for quality improvement. *Scandinavian Journal of Caring Sciences, 18*, 72–81.

Weman, K., Kihlgren, M., & Fagerberg, I. (2004). Older people living in nursing homes or other community care facilities: Registered Nurses' views of their working situation and co-operation with family members. *Journal of Clinical Nursing, 3*, 617–626.

World Health Organization (WHO) (1995). WHOQOL-100. Facet Definitions and Questions (WHO Division of Mental Health and Prevention of Substance Abuse, Geneva, Switzerland).

WHOQOL group (1998) Development of the World Health Organization WHOQOL-BFER quality of life assessment. *Psychological Medicine, 28*, 551–558.

10
Quality of Life and Dementia

Andrew Sixsmith, Margaret Hammond and Grant Gibson

Introduction

Cognitive impairment due to age-related dementia such as Alzheimer's disease will present considerable challenges to health and social care services as populations age worldwide. As well as expanding services to meet increased numbers of people with dementia, the challenge will also involve providing care that will ensure a good quality of life (QoL) for people who are vulnerable and dependent. Dementia also presents considerable challenges in terms of developing frameworks for evaluating the quality of care. The Care Keys approach emphasises the need to incorporate measures of QoL and well-being in the evaluation of care, while also 'giving a voice' to the client by eliciting their views on their own well-being and satisfaction with the services they receive. However, this is problematic with cognitively impaired people who may be unable to comprehend questions, formulate coherent answers and articulate and communicate their views. This has often resulted in people with dementia being excluded from research into QoL (cf. Balcombe, Ferry, & Saweirs, 2001). Recent research on QoL in dementia has attempted to address this situation (Torrington, 2006), arguing that the views and responses of people with dementia should still be taken seriously. However, there are limits to this when the severity of the dementia may prevent meaningful verbal communication and, in these situations, alternative approaches are required.

Unfortunately, approaches to assessing QoL for people with dementia remain conceptually and methodologically weak. A traditional biomedical perspective generally frames the experience of dementia in terms of cognitive decline and associated functional impairment. However, alternative perspectives suggest that QoL in dementia is more than just cognition (Banerjee et al., 2006) and that a wider perspective encompassing aspects of the person, context and care (Sixsmith & Gibson, 2006) need to be considered. As far as the concept of crQoL is concerned, a number of key theoretical and methodological issues need to be resolved. Firstly, are the concepts underlying the crQoL model appropriate to people with dementia? Secondly, are ideas of subjective well-being that have been developed particularly in respect to non-demented people, applicable to people with dementia? Finally, can care make a difference to the QoL of people with dementia? In this context, this chapter presents some of the results of work carried out within the Care Keys project that specifically addressed the needs of people with dementia.

The Challenge of Dementia

The term 'dementia' is associated with a range of diseases and disorders that affect the structure and function of the brain leading to deterioration in cognitive function. Common symptoms of dementia include loss of short-term memory, reduced vocabulary (aphasia), impaired motor functions (apraxia), a failure to identify and recognise objects (agnosia), and increased difficulty with planning, ordering or abstracting tasks (American Psychiatric Association, 2000; Thomas & O'Brien, 2002). There may also be behavioural and personality changes such as emotional outbursts or mood disturbances. Symptoms in most cases are progressive and terminal, although usually a person will die from other factors, exacerbated by the dementia. In some cases dementia-like symptoms may be caused by other health problems not classified as dementia, including depression and alcohol dependency.

Dementia is used as a general descriptive term for over 100 different specific illnesses and disorders. The most common type of dementia is Alzheimer's disease, accounting for approximately 50% of all cases (Thomas & O'Brien, 2002; Wattis & Curran, 2001). Alzheimer's disease is associated with the presence of amyloid plaques and neurofibrillary tangles throughout the brain, leading to the death of brain cells. No single known factor has been identified as causing Alzheimer's disease, although a range of general factors including age, diet, general health and environmental factors may possibly contribute to its onset. Other common types of dementia include vascular or multi-infarct dementia, caused by damage to the vascular system (such as stroke or progressive small blood vessel damage); and Dementia with Lewy bodies, associated with the deposition of protein in nerve cells, which may inhibit chemical messengers in the brain.

Although dementia is not exclusive to older people, its prevalence, and particularly the prevalence of Alzheimer's disease, rises with age. Prevalence rates appear to rise exponentially, doubling every 4.5 years beyond age 60 (Wattis & Curran, 2001). Epidemiological studies indicate a dementia prevalence of 1.4% for people aged 65–69 rising to over 20% for people aged 80–85 (Hoffman, Rocca, & Breteler, 1991). Although there is much debate as to the causes of dementia, it is important to note that even in extreme old age, dementia is not a natural part of the ageing process, and that the majority of people at these ages will not suffer from this illness. Nevertheless, dementia is a major and growing challenge to health and social care providers, at national and international levels of governance, as well as to wider society.

European and many countries worldwide are currently undergoing significant demographic shifts, characterised by ageing of the population. The numbers of people with dementia across Europe are rising as a result of demographic ageing, so that 4.9 million people over the age of 60 years were estimated to have dementia in 2001, a figure estimated to rise by 43% to 6.9 million by 2020, and by 102% to 9.9 million in 2040 (Ferri et al., 2005). Within the UK, an estimated 750,000 people currently have some form of dementia. These rates are forecast to rise to 840,000 by 2010, and 1.5 million by 2050 (O'Malley & Croucher, 2005). As a result of this shift, increasing attention is being paid to dementia and its effects. The growth in the prevalence of dementia raises major concerns for the design and implementation of health and social care policies across the European Union, and future research on the development of effective treatments.

If the challenge of the growing numbers of people with dementia illustrates the scale of the problem, a further challenge relates to how this challenge is met, namely in the provision of health and social care services that can meet the complex, intensive and economically expensive care needs of those suffering from the illness. People with dementia can face a wide range of problems within their everyday lives. Work arising from the social model of disability, such as in the work of Kitwood (1997) has illustrated that while many of the problems faced by people with dementia arise from the cognitive impairments symptomatic of the disease, these are often exacerbated by health and social care practices, and indeed by general ageist perspectives and attitudes within wider society (Blackman et al., 2003; Bond, 1999). Increasingly, research is attempting to understand how people with dementia create and understand their own social worlds, part of which requires people with dementia to be viewed as active participants with a 'voice' to be engaged with, rather than research subjects as seen within many forms of biomedical research into dementia (Bartlett & Martin, 2002).

As noted, providing effective care services for the growing numbers of people with dementia will be a significant challenge to health and social care provision at an EU wide level. Developments such as the Dementia Care Mapping observational tool (Thornton, Hatton, & Tatham, 2004) and a growing awareness of the specific health and QoL needs of people with dementia have contributed to the development of more effective care and support services. In particular, increasing attention is being paid to the development of care practices that can enable people with dementia to live independently for as long as possible, delaying or even removing the need for admission into residential care or other services. As numbers of people with dementia rise alongside Europe's ageing population, such strategies may become the mainstay of social care provision for these groups.

Recently, an increasing focus in dementia care is being paid to QoL for people with dementia. An implicit part of this focus is that, although the impairments resulting from dementia have severe impacts on people's ability to participate in the taken for granted activities of everyday life, they can gain pleasure, and a sense of achievement and purpose from participation in activities (Bond, 1999; Sixsmith & Gibson, 2006). Further research has demonstrated that people with dementia in the milder stages are able to make judgements about their QoL, and can have a positive QoL with the assistance of effective support strategies from formal and informal carers (Katsuno, 2005).

Finally, it is important to consider the theoretical and methodological challenges facing researchers in examining QoL of people with dementia and its relationship with care. The discussion of the theoretical background to crQoL in earlier chapters in this book provides a general perspective on the QoL of frail older people. However, researching this area becomes even more challenging when considering people with dementia, whose life experiences may undermine conventional ideas about well-being and QoL; the difficulties in communicating feelings, ideas and attitudes may further complicate this (Thompson, 2005).

Theoretically, the issue of dementia and QoL is of considerable interest. A very naïve perspective may dehumanise the experience of dementia and even question whether ideas of QoL and well-being are applicable to people who may be severely confused about where and when they are, who they are with, what they are doing or even who they are. Indeed, it was discussed in Chapter 4 that the traditional biomedical view characterises dementia in terms of the deterioration of the brain and consequent decline in the person's social and personal capabilities. The characterisation has had implications for the concept of care for people with dementia, which has often amounted to little more than basic support for personal activities of daily living (ADL) and making the person 'comfortable'.

More recent perspectives, especially the work of Tom Kitwood (1997) has re-evaluated the concept of QoL of people with dementia and developed care concepts that have been framed by social–psychological theories and models. This alternative perspective argues that many people with dementia can experience a reasonable QoL, despite their condition, and focuses on the 'personhood' in terms of a sense of personal worth, agency, confidence and social reciprocity. While the dementing illness can undermine aspects of personhood, some or many other aspects may remain intact. The role of care is to facilitate the maintenance of personhood (a coherent self), through providing care and support that encourages and supports the person in their everyday lives.

A further important aspect of the re-evaluation of dementia is an emphasis on 'ecological' perspectives of QoL (Fig. 10.1). From this perspective (Torrington, 2006), a person's activities and well-being are seen to be influenced by a number of factors, such as attributes of the person (functional ability, cognitive ability, psychological factors, etc.) and attributes of the context (formal support network, social network, physical environment and cultural context). Everyday activities can be seen to be either facilitated or constrained by these personal and contextual factors. How a person derives meaning from their everyday activities is central to their well-being. Positive well-being (e.g. happiness, life

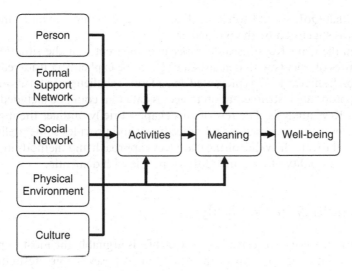

F_{IG}. 10.1. Ecological model of well-being and dementia (Torrington, 2006).

satisfaction) derives from being involved in activities and situations that are personally meaningful and valued, whereas negative life experiences derive from being unable to be involved in these.

It is important to evaluate the varying theoretical perspective on QoL and dementia in terms of their relevance to the CareKeys concept of crQoL. There are strong similarities between the models suggested by Kitwood and Torrington and colleagues and some of the key theoretical concepts underlying crQoL. Lawton's idea of person–environment fit (Lawton & Nahemow, 1973) has clear parallels. This suggests that increasing frailty in old age leads to a reduction in the ability to perform ADL and that people with reduced personal capacities are more vulnerable to environmental demands compared with people whose capacities remain intact. In this context, environmental factors become very important in terms of their everyday tasks of living and QoL. Lawton (1991) extended his model by introducing subjective well-being and described QoL in terms of four overlapping sub-domains: behavioural competence – the capacity to deal with the demands of everyday life; objective environment – physical and social context within which a person lives; perceived QoL or the subjective evaluation of their function and circumstances; psychological well-being – well-being, happiness, and so on.

The above theoretical discussion has two clear implications for the CareKeys research into crQoL. Firstly, the discussion has emphasised the importance of context and that care inputs are likely to have a significant impact on the client's experience of dementia and on their QoL. Secondly, the subjective – 'perceived quality of life' is crucial. Although this may be the outcome and conditional in part upon situational and person-related factors, it is highly unlikely that QoL should solely be dependent upon cognitive and functional abilities, as suggested by the biomedical model.

Within the Care Keys research it became apparent that the situations and perspectives of clients with dementia needed to be explicitly considered within the crQoL framework. This presented considerable challenges in terms of developing appropriate instrumentation to access data that could be included within the Care Keys analysis. The rest of this chapter briefly outlines the methodological approach (instruments and procedures) and provides some preliminary results to illustrate the value of the Care Keys approach and methods in exploring issues of quality of care and QoL for people with dementia.

Methodology of the Study

While the subjective 'perceived quality of life' is arguably the most important from the clients' perspective, at the same time it poses the greatest challenge to meaningful assessment of persons with severe dementia. In CareKeys a specific aim was to incorporate the 'voice' of people with dementia into the assessment of crQoL. As noted in Chapter 2, the key approaches adopted in Care Keys were self-reports and proxy accounts. Chapters 2 and 3 provide detailed accounts of the approach and methodology adopted in the Care Keys survey. This section provides a brief overview of aspects of methods as they are specifically related to people with dementia.

Self-Reports

The Care Keys' client interview instrument CLINT incorporated two standard and well-validated outcome measures of QoL and well-being. The WHOQOL-Bref (WHOQOL Group, 1998) provides an interview-based measure of general QoL. In addition, psychological symptoms of depression and anxiety were measured indirectly using the Philadelphia Geriatric Center Morale Scale (PGCMS-Lawton, 1975). Information on the client's subjective evaluations of their care was also elicited. However, it was clear that a very significant proportion of older people using social and health support services will have some degree of cognitive impairment and that there will be a substantial number of those who will be unable to give meaningful responses to WHOQOL-Bref and PGCMS.

Third-Party Informants

For clients who were unable to provide responses to the self-report questionnaires, the views of a key informant were elicited. Two instruments were used (see Chapter 2, this volume). The QUALID–instrument (Weiner et al., 2000) is answered by an informant who may be either a family member or professional caregiver in regular contact with the client. QUALID uses five point scales to measure aspects such as appearance of sadness, discomfort, vocalising discontent, irritability and enjoyment of contact and activities. A sum score of responses indicates relative well-being in a range 11–65, with lower scores representing higher QoL. The Cornell Scale for Depression in Dementia (Alexopoulos, Abrams, Young, & Shamoian, 1988) is answered by the relative or care person who knows the client well. Three-point scales are used to measure items such as mood, behavioural disturbance, physical signs, cyclic functions and ideational disturbance. A sum score indicates overall depression with scores also for the different sub-components. An evaluation of the quality of care provided to the client was also elicited using the Relative's Information questionnaire of Care Keys (RELinfo), adapted from the client satisfaction questions in the CLINT.

Assessing Cognitive Capacity

It was also important to define cognitive capacity in order to determine which approach to instrumentation was appropriate. The Standardized Mini-Mental State Examination (SMMSE) (Folstein, Folstein, & McHugh, 1975; Molloy, Alemayehu, & Roberts, 1991) covers aspects such as orientation in time, place, memory and attention. Scores are commonly categorised into three groups: no/mild impairment (score 19–30); moderate impairment (score 16–18); severe impairment (score < 18). The cognitive performance scale (CPS) (Morris et al., 1994) is derived from the RAI assessment procedure and uses five items to assign the person to one of seven categories. The CPS categories are highly related to the SMMSE and it is possible to map them onto the MMSE categories.

Care Keys Survey of Care and QoL of People with Dementia

One of the aims of the CareKeys survey approach (see Chapter 1) was to ensure that the instrumentation and procedures for people with dementia matched as closely as possible those for people without dementia in both homecare and institutional care settings. The general approach was identical with data collected using the CLINT, InDEX and ManDEX instrumentation.

A key initial task at the beginning of the CLINT was to record the CPS score or the SMMSE score. Respondents were then categorised into three groups, according to CPS/SMMSE scores:

• The cognitively intact, borderline, or mildly impaired, who have SMMSE scores of >18, or CPS scores of 0, 1 or 2
• The moderately impaired, who have SMMSE scores of 16, 17 or 18; or CPS score of 3.
• The severely impaired, who have SMMSE scores of 15 or less, or CPS scores of 4, 5 or 6.

The survey protocol suggested that: respondents in Group 1 then completed the normal CLINT (HC or IC); respondents in Group 2 had the normal CLINT (HC or IC), plus CORNELL and QUALID completed for them by a third-party informant; respondents in Group 3 had CORNELL and QUALID instead of the PGCMS and the WHOQOL-Bref. The client satisfaction questions (HC or IC) were completed by the clients' relatives where available. However, in practice there was more flexibility in who answered the self-report questions, as the SMMSE and CPS categories were not always good indicators of wether a person was able to effectively respond.

Results

The results of the analysis of a sub-sample of people with dementia in the Care Keys dataset are presented below, focusing on two issues: differences in well-being in the five participating countries and predictors of well-being for people with moderate to severe cognitive impairment.

Well-being in the Different Countries

There were 394 people in the total survey group for whom QUALID and CSDD data were collected. Of these, 292 (72.1%) were women and 89 (22.6%) were men (cognitive score data were missing for 13 (3.3%) respondents). The mean age of the respondents was 83.86 (SD 8.37), mode 84 years (minimum age 49, maximum 101 years). Three hundred and twenty were living in residential care (81.2%) and 74 (18.8%) were living in their own homes. Of the 313 (79.45%) classified as having moderate or severe cognitive impairment (Table 10.1), the mean SMMSE score was 5.4 (minimum 0, maximum 18); mean CPS score 4.18 (minimum 3, maximum 6). Data were categorised into two of three categories according to SMMSE/CPS score.

There was a difference between countries regarding the living place of the respondents: all respondents from Sweden and the UK lived in institutions (e.g. nursing or residential homes), while 79% of Finnish participants, 74% of German participants and 53% of participants from Estonia lived in institutions. (It should be noted that this does not necessarily reflect the patterns of

TABLE 10.1. Care Keys sub-sample of people with cognitive function scores, categorised as moderate and severe.

	Estonia	Finland	Germany	Sweden	UK	Total
Moderate	3	51	6	33	6	99
Severe	28	66	97	20	3	214
Total	31	117	103	53	9	313

care provision in the different countries, rather this reflects different sources of participants that were available for the study.)

The overall scores for the QUALID was a mean of 22.89 (SD = 7.9), median value of 23 and a range of 53 (minimum 11, maximum 25). For the CSDD, the mean score was 8.72 (SD = 4.8), a median value of 8 and a range of 25 (minimum 0, maximum 25). However, it is interesting to examine patterns in the five countries, and QUALID and CSDD results are presented in Table 10.2, differentiated by country, gender, care type and level of dementia.

Using Kruskal–Wallis analysis of variance, significant differences were found between countries. For the QUALID scores, there was significant difference between countries (Kruskal–Wallis ANOVA, Chi-square 11.2, d.f.= 4, asymp sig. = 0. 024). Tamhane's T2 test found Finland to have significantly better QoL scores than Estonia (mean diff. =−3.97, p = 0.03) and Germany (mean diff. =−3.05, p = 0.04).

There was a highly significant difference between countries for CSDD scores (Kruskal–Wallis ANOVA, Chi square 23.5, d.f. = 4, asymp sig.= 0.000). Estonia had significantly worse scores than Finland (mean diff. 3.57, p = 0.002), Sweden (mean diff. = 2.9, p = 0.028) and the UK (mean diff. = 5.84, p = 0.034). Germany had significantly worse scores than Finland (mean diff. = 2.0, p = 0.017).

Relationships between gender, care type, cognitive impairment and QoL and depression were examined within each country (except UK because of small numbers) using Kruskal–Wallis ANOVA. No significant differences were found between CSDD or QUALID and gender, place of residence, or cognitive function in Finland or Germany. However, significant results were detected in Sweden and Estonia.

In Sweden, significant differences were recorded in QUALID scores between gender, with women having significantly higher scores, and therefore a lower QoL (male mean QUALID score 19.03; female mean QUALID score 23.37. Chi square 8.490; df = 1; p < 0.01). Significant differences were also detected between CSDD scale scores and level of dementia, with lower CSDD scores being recorded among those with severe impairment (moderately impaired

TABLE 10.2. QUALID and CSDD scores for each country.

	Estonia (n = 45)	Finland (n = 120)	Germany (n = 107)	Sweden (n = 113)	UK (n = 9)
QUALID (Lower score = better QoL)	25.4 (8.0)	21.4 (5.9)	24.5 (9.2)	22.1 (7.8)	21.2 (6.2)
	23	21	23	21	20
	13–43	11–41	11–54	11–48	11–31
CSDD (Lower score = less depressed)	11.2 (5.6)	7.6 (4.2)	9.6 (5.2)	8.3 (4.6)	5.4 (4.3)
	11.2	6.9	8.8	7.5	5.4
	0–27	0–22	0–25	0–22	0–11

Mean (SD), median, minimum–maximum

CSDD score 9.10, severely impaired CSDD score 6.98. Chi square = 4.186; d.f. = 1; $p < 0.05$).

In Estonia, significant differences were noted between CSDD score and care type, with higher scores on the CSDD, and therefore higher levels of depression, for those living in institutional care when compared to home (homecare mean CSDD score 13.02, institutional care mean CSDD score is 25.54. Chi square = 5.026. d.f. = 1; $p < 0.05$).

Significant differences were also found between the QUALID measure and levels of dementia, with a lower mean score recorded for those with moderate impairment, indicating a higher QoL (moderately impaired mean QUALID score 18.00; severely impaired mean QUALID score 26.69; Chi square = 4.316; d.f. = 1; $p < 0.05$).

It is important to qualify the results of the above analysis. Firstly, the sampling procedures varied to some extent between the countries (see Chapter 3). Secondly, the recruitment of the study participants with dementia in the various countries varied based on a 'convenience' approach, depending on involvement of particular care-providing organisations. Thirdly, data collection procedures were not entirely congruent, although a basic protocol for data collection was observed. These limitations make it difficult to make direct comparisons between the different countries and it is not possible to claim that the samples are 'representative' of their respective countries. However, there is no reason to think that the samples are not reflective of their national situations, especially in relation to the macro-welfare context. Generally speaking, the key trend in the data was that the CSDD and QUALID scores were lowest in Sweden and Finland (i.e. indicating better QoL) and highest in Estonia (excluding the UK, because of the very small sample). While these differences were not large they do reflect similar patterns found in other studies that have found significant differences according to the prevailing macro-level welfare regimes in European countries. For example, Wilson (2006) has found relatively high levels of depression in former Eastern-bloc countries (Hungary and Latvia) compared with countries in Western Europe. The generally poorer living conditions and standards of social care and support of older people in the transitional economies in the east may lead to a reduction in well-being.

Predictors of Well-Being of People with Moderate to Severe Cognitive Impairment

The crQoL model suggests that QoL is influenced by a range of personal and contextual factors, including physical health, physical functioning and social support; and that care service provision will modify the influence of these. Data relating to people with moderate to severe cognitive impairment living in institutional care was used to examine the relationships between QoL as measured by the QUALID and a number of variables recorded in the Care Keys InDEX instrument. Characteristics of the individual, such as their documented need for help in ADL, need for help relating to physical health conditions, care provided and the relationships of these with scores from the QUALID instrument were examined, using independent t-tests and one-way ANOVA. A probability level of <0.05 was considered significant. Where the significance level of Levene's Test was <0.05, results not assuming equal variance were used.

Background variables: There was no significant difference between genders for QUALID score ($t = -1.1$, d.f. 379, $p = .3$). Whether the person received care in their own home ($n = 74$), or in an institution ($n = 320$) did not determine differences in QUALID scores.

Social network and social contact: Informal networks, rated as the existence of none, one, or two or more persons, was significantly associated with QUALID score ($F = 2.2$, $p = 0.03$). Frequency of informal contacts or supply of volunteer help were not significant predictors. Participation of informal supporters in supply of care for basic ADL and personal care was not significantly associated with QUALID score.

Need for help in ADL: The need for help in selected ADL were rated as: no need, low need, medium need, high need, or intensive need, according to information from care planning documents. The ADL items were analysed for their association with QUALID scores. The need for intensive help in ADL tended to predict a lower QoL than needing no help. Requiring help with oral care ($F = 1.9$, $p = .04$), toileting ($F = 1.9$, $p = 0.05$), and especially getting up and going to bed ($F = 3.1$, $p = 0.002$) were associated with differences in QUALID scores.

Physical and psychological health: Among the care outcome variables, QUALID scores were predicted by the occurrence of pressure ulcers ($t = -3.29$, d.f. = 262, $p = .001$, 95% CI -6.6 to -1.6), and the client suffering from pain ($t = -3.53$, d.f. = 132.3, $p = .001$, 95% CI -5.9 to -1.7). The occurrences of falls, nosocomial infections, loss of weight not due to illness or diet, and the use of sleeping tablets, were not significant predictors. Requiring treatments for wounds or pressure ulcers ($F = 2.7$, $p < 0.000$), and needing support for visual impairments ($F = 2.5$, $p < 0.000$) influenced QUALID scores. There were significant differences for people with diabetes ($F = 1.6$, $p = 0.05$), delirium ($F = 1.6$, $p = .03$), hearing deficits ($F = 1.8$, $p = 0.02$) and special communication needs ($F = 1.6$, $p = .04$), as well as need for care with dehydration ($F = 2.3$, $p = .001$). There was a trend towards significance in people with cardiovascular conditions ($F = 1.6$, $p = 0.06$). Having respiratory conditions, or special nutritional needs, did not influence QUALID scores. Among the binary variables relating to health care, requiring pain management was significantly associated with a reduction in QoL ($t = -2.3$, d.f. = 132, $p = 0.001$, 95% CI -5.9 to -1.7). Requiring palliative care and a need for fall prophylaxes made no significant difference. For those clients documented as requiring support due to depression, there was a significant difference among groups ($F = 1.6$, $p = 0.05$), with QoL decreasing with increasing need for depression support. Need for support due to memory impairment was significant ($F = 2.1$, $p = 0.004$).

Environmental factors: Having individual toilets or bathrooms made no significant difference to QUALID scores; nor did having access to a balcony or garden. However, people observed as living in well-lit and spacious rooms ($n = 171$) had significantly lower QUALID scores (mean $= 23.4$) than those who did not ($n = 20$, mean $= 19.35$) ($t = 2.28$, d.f. $= 189$, 2-tailed significance $= 0.024$, 95% CI 0.54–7.48).

Psychosocial elements of care: Psychosocial support was documented as binary variables. The provision of psychological counselling was significantly associated with better QUALID score ($t -2.9$, d.f. $=134$, sig. 2-tailed $= 0.004$, 95% CI -15.8 to -3). The documented supply of emotional support and encouragement to independent daily care, social advice or legal counselling were not associated with QUALID scores. The documented supply of individual leisure activities inside the care home was significantly associated with improved QUALID score: ($t = 3.2$, d.f. $= 197$, sig. $= 0.002$, 95% CI 1.4 to 6), as was the documented supply of recreational events inside the care home ($t = 2.5$, d.f. $= 81$, $p = 0.01$, 95% CI 0.63 to 5.6). There was a trend towards significance for the supply of group hobbies ($t = 1.9$, d.f. $= 227$, $p = .06$, 95% CI -0.1 to 4.1). Other elements of social participation (recreational events outside the home, contact with people outside the home and religious activities) were not significantly associated with QUALID. The documented participation of informal supporters in psychosocial support and access to activities was not significantly associated with QUALID.

Quality of care planning documentation: Quality of care planning documentation was taken as an indicator of quality of care delivered. Independent *t*-tests were used to examine the significance of characteristics of the documentation in the prediction of QUALID scores. Significant predictors of QUALID score were 'Does care plan include information which methods of care and help will be used, the times when they will be used and their frequency?' (mean diff. $= 2.4$, $t =1.98$, d.f. $= 92$, $p = 0.05$, 95% CI $-.005$ to -4.7). There was a trend towards significance with the care plan making reference to important preventative measures ($t = 1.9$, d.f. $= 82$, $p = 0.07$, 95% CI -0.16 to -4.8), and 'Does the regular evaluation consider the adequacy of involvement of informal carer?' (mean diff. $= 3.47$, $t = 1.9$, d.f. $= 136$, $p = 0.06$, 95% CI $-.21$ to -7.14). All other items (explicit consideration of four goal dimensions, interventions to support autonomy, review and update of care plan, consideration of preferences and lifestyle, evaluation of goal attainment, reference to need for or use of external services, information about informal carers, strategies for team work, evidence of team work, evidence of involvement of informal carer, changes from care plan due to staff absence, named cooperating physician) were not significant predictors.

All of the variables that were found to be significant predictors of QUALID score in the separate parts of the INDEX were entered into stepwise linear regression analyses, with probability of *F* to enter $<=0.05$, and to remove $> =0.10$. In ADLs, the need for help in getting up and going to bed was the only significant predictor of QUALID score (standardised b $= 0.19$, $R^2 = 0.03$). Among variables relating to health, the best model consisted solely of 'Does the client suffer from pain so that it interferes with daily activities? (b $= 0.23$, $R^2 = 0.05$,

$F = 8.9, p = 0.003$). Both of the two social participation care supply variables, supply of recreational events (b= −0.17), and individual leisure needs (b = −0.15) were significant in the model ($R^2 = 0.06$, $F = 6.8$, $p = 0.001$). The following variables were included in the final stepwise linear regression analysis (for theoretical model behind the selection, see Chapter 4):

Block One, person and environment variables influencing QUALID score:

• Size of social network
• ADL: need for help getting into and out of bed
• Suffering from pain
• Need for depression support
• Need for support with memory impairment

Block Two (mediating variables) included in the analysis:

• Environment: well-lit and spacious rooms
• Care service: provision of recreational events
• Supply of individual leisure activities
• Provision of counselling
• Care planning documentation: Does the care plan include information of which methods of care and help will be used, the times when they will be used and their frequency?

'Well-lit and spacious rooms' and the care planning documentation item were excluded in the analysis. In this analysis, only the supply of psychological counselling was significant in the prediction of QUALID score ($R^2 = 0.23$ (SE 6.9), F = 6.7, b = 0.52, $p = 0.02$). However, as the number of cases of people receiving psychological counselling was extremely small ($n = 6$), the analysis was repeated without this variable. In this model, pain and the social network were significant, but there was a further significant contribution from the provision of recreational events inside the care home (see Table 10.3).
To summarise, the key findings from the regression analysis were

• Pain appears very important in determining well-being. However, this result needs to be viewed with caution, as the well-being outcome measure used (QUALID) incorporates expressed discomfort as its first factor, accounting for 22% of the total variance in the scores.
• The presence of a social network consisting of more than one person is also important, and confirms other findings within the Care Keys research.
• The influential contribution of psychological counselling, even though the numbers receiving it were exceedingly small, suggests that there is value in providing this kind of care and support to people with dementia.
• The supply of recreational events within the care home had a substantial influence on the QoL scores to an extent that is difficult to explain as an artefact of measurement. Of the 320 cases, 31% of the data were missing. Of the remainder, three quarters (166) were recorded as having recreational events, while one quarter ($n = 55$) did not. It is difficult to say whether the supply of recreational events in itself is directly influential on well-being, or

TABLE 10.3. ANOVA of QUALID scores for people with moderate to severe cognitive impairment.

Model	Sum of squares	Degrees of freedom	Mean square	F	Significance value
Regression	593.446	1	593.446	10.675	0.001[a]
Residual	8005.267	144	55.592		
Total	8598.712	145			
Regression	869.248	2	434.624	8.041	0.000[b]
Residual	7729.465	143	54.052		
Total	8598.712	145			
Regression	1235.455	3	411.818	7.942	0.000[c]
Residual	7363.257	142			
Total	8598.712	145	51.854		

[a] Predictors (constant) Does the client suffer from pain?
[b] Predictors (constant) Does the client suffer from pain? Informal network
[c] Predictors (constant) Does the client suffer from pain? Informal network, recreational events inside – supply

TABLE 10.3. ANOVA results and coefficients from stepwise linear regression identifying predictions of QUALID scores for people with moderate to severe dementia.

Coefficients

Model	Unstandardised coefficients		Standardised coefficients		Significant values
	B	Std. Error	Beta	t	
1. (constant)	20.547	0.742		27.695	0.000
Does the client suffer from pain	4.366	1.336	0.263	3.267	0.001
2. (constant)	24.393	1.853		13.163	0.000
Does the client suffer from pain	4.392	1.318	0.264	3.333	0.001
Informal network	−2.354	1.042	−0.179	−2.259	0.025
3. (constant)	26.916	2.048		13.140	0.000
Does the client suffer from pain	4.386	1.291	−0.264	3.398	0.001
Informal network	−2.372	1.021	−0.180	−2.323	0.022
Recreational events inside – supply	−3.499	1.317	−0.206	−2.657	0.009

whether this is more generally reflective of the culture of the home. However, both illustrate the potential impact of care and support on the well-being of people with dementia.

• Interestingly, the analyses indicated that well-being in dementia was not associated with either functional or cognitive abilities

Discussion and Conclusions

The discussion of the challenge of dementia highlighted the necessity of countries worldwide to respond to growing levels of need within the population. However, the response has to be about the nature and quality of services as much as the quantitative level of care provided. It is important that care and support is provided to people with dementia living at home and in residential and nursing homes does more than just focus on basic needs, but will also afford a good QoL.

The aim of the Care Keys project was to provide a suitable methodology that would allow care managers and planners to evaluate the services they provide, in particular incorporating the clients' perspective on services and well-being into models of performance evaluation, effectively giving a 'voice' to the client within this process. However, this ambition is problematic in the case of people with dementia, who may be unable to formulate or articulate their ideas and opinions. Moreover there has always been a danger that people with dementia are excluded from user research because of their cognitive disabilities. This is in part because of methodological challenges in determining QoL for this group, but is also reflective of a biomedical perspective that has marginalised issues of well-being, depression and QoL among people with dementia. In response to this, the Care Keys project utilised alternative approaches based on third-party informants where appropriate, specifically the QUALID and CSDD scales, and this paper has reported some of the key findings based on data from five European countries.

While comparisons between the participating countries need to be treated with care, the lower CSDD and QUALID scores in Finland and Sweden indicated better QoL while the relatively higher CSDD and QUALID scores in Estonia indicated lower levels of well-being, matching trends indicated in other research (Wilson, 2006). This may reflect macro-level circumstances in the transitional economies of former eastern-bloc countries. Disparities in the health and well-being of older people represent a major health and social policy challenge to establishing some level of parity between member states. For example, there is a need for appropriate health and social care responses to meet undiagnosed and untreated depression within those communities. There is also a need to develop wider social policies to address the key problems of social isolation, poor housing, low income, and so on of this vulnerable group of people. Unfortunately, the transition to free-market economies has tended to marginalise the needs of older people as the social policy focus has been on reforming basic economic and political structures within those countries, while economic change has undermined the financial status of many older citizens.

The research presented in this chapter also provides a strong indication that the general model of crQoL is appropriate to people with dementia and that their QoL was 'more than just cognition'. It was noticeable in the empirical analysis that neither cognitive nor functional abilities were predictors of well-being, while factors relating to context, such as social network and physical environment played a significant role. The theoretical discussion and empirical analysis also emphasised the value of using measures of subjective well-being, despite the methodological challenges that these may pose.

The variation observed between the various participating countries may also reflect micro-level aspects of care practice and the chapter presented a brief analysis of predictors of well-being, as measured by the QUALID scale. The analysis suggested a number of aspects of the care environment that appear to have an impact on the well-being of people with dementia living in care homes, notably psychosocial aspects of the care environment, such as the provision of counselling and recreational events. The analysis highlights the point that care can make a 'difference', contributing to a better QoL of people with dementia. Equally, neglect of these aspects of care can have a negative effect on well-being. There is a need to ensure that care provision, particularly in residential environments, is based on a model that emphasises a person's social and psychological needs as well as those relating to their medical and functional status.

References

Alexopoulos, G. S., Abrams, R. C., Young, R. C., & Shamoian, C. A. (1988). Cornell Scale for Depression in Dementia. *Biological Psychiatry, 23,* 271–284.

American Psychiatric Association (APA). (2000). *Diagnostic and statistical manual of mental disorders (4th edition)* Washington, DC: American Psychiatric Association.

Balcombe, N. R., Ferry, P. G., & Saweirs, W. M. (2001). Nutritional status and well being. Is there a relationship between body mass index and the well-being of older people? *Current Medical Research Opinion, 17*(1), 1–7.

Banerjee, S., Smith, S., Lamping, D., Harwood, R., Foley, B., Smith, P., Murray, J., Prince, M., Levin, E., Mann, A., & Knapp, M. (2006). Quality of life in dementia: More than just cognition. An analysis of associations with quality of life in dementia. *Journal of Neurology, Neurosurgery and Psychiatry, 77,* 146–148.

Bartlett, H., & Martin, W. (2002). Ethical issues in Dementia care Research. In H. Wilkinson, (Ed.), *The perspectives of people with dementia.* London: Jessica Kingsley.

Blackman, T., Mitchell, L., Burton, E., Jenks, M., Parsons, M., Raman, S., & Williams, K. (2003). The accessibility of public space for People with Dementia: a priority for the 'open city'. *Disability and Society, 18*(3), 357–371.

Bond, J. (1999). Quality of life for People with Dementia. Approaches to the Challenge of Measurement. *Ageing and Society, 19,* 561–579.

Ferri, C. P., Prince, M., Brayne, C., Brodaty, H., Fratiglioni, L., Ganguli, M., Hall, K., Hasegawa, K., Hendrie, H., & Huang, Y. (2005). Global Prevalence of Dementia: A Delphi consensus study. *The Lancet, 366,* 2112–2117.

Folstein, M. F., Folstein, S. E., & Mchugh, P. R. (1975). "Mini mental state": A practical method for grading the cognitive state of patients for the clinician. *Journal of Psychiatric Research, 2,* 189–198.

Hofman, A., Rocca, W. A., & Breteler, M. M. B. (1991). The prevalence of dementia in Europe: a collaborative study of 1980–1990 findings. *International Journal of Epidemiology, 20,* 736–748.

Katsuno, T. (2005). Dementia from the Inside: how people with early stage dementia evaluate their quality of life. *Ageing and Society, 25*(2), 197–214.

Kitwood, T. (1997). *Dementia reconsidered: The person comes first.* Buckingham: Open University Press.

Lawton, M. P. (1975). The Philadelphia geriatric center morale scale: A revision. *Journal of Gerontology, 30,* 85–89.

Lawton, M. P. (1991). A multidimensional view of quality of life. In J. E. Birren, J. E. Lubben, J. C. Rowe, & D. E. Deutchman (Eds.), *The concept and measurement of quality of life in the frail elderly* (pp. 3–27). New York: Academic Press.

Lawton, M. P., & Nahemow, L. (1973). Ecology and the aging process. In C. Eisdorfer & M. P. Lawton (Eds.), *Psychology of adult development and aging* (pp. 619–674). Washington DC: American Psychological Association.

Molloy, D. W., Alemayehu, E., & Roberts, R. (1991). Reliability of a Standardized Mini-Mental State Examination compared with the traditional Mini-Mental State Examination. *American Journal of Psychiatry, 148*: 102–105.

Morris, J. N., Fries, B. E., Mehr, D. R., Hawes, C., Phillips, C., Mor, V., & Lipsitz, L. A. (1994). MDS Cognitive Performance Scale. *Journal of Gerontology, 49*(4), M174–82.

O'Malley, L., & Croucher, K. (2005). Housing and Dementia Care – a scoping review of the literature *Health and Social Care in the Community, 13*(6), 570–577.

Sixsmith, A., & Gibson, G. (2006). Music and well-being in dementia: A qualitative study. *Ageing and Society, 27*(1), 127–146.

Thomas, A. J., & O'Brien, J. T. (2002). Alzheimer's Disease. In R. Jacoby, C. Oppenheimer, (Eds.), *Psychiatry in the Elderly* (3rd ed.). Oxford: Oxford University Press.

Thompson, L. (2005). Is it possible to conceptualise and measure quality of life for people with severe Alzheimer's Disease. *Generation review, 15*(1), 22–24.

Thornton, A., Hatton, C., & Tatham, A. (2004). Dementia Care Mapping Reconsidered: Exploring the reliability and validity of the observational tool. *International Journal of Geriatric Psychiatry, 19*(8), 718–726.

Torrington, J. (2006). What has architecture got to do with dementia care? Explorations of the relationship between quality of life and building design in two EQUAL projects. *Quality in Ageing, 7*(1), 34–49.

Wattis, J. P., & Curran, S. (2001). *Practical psychiatry of old age* (3rd ed.). Abingdon: Radcliffe Medical Press.

Weiner, M. F., Martin-Cook, K., Svetlik, D. A., Saine, K., Foster, B., & Fontain, C, S. (2000). The quality of life in late-stage dementia (QUALID) scale. *J Am Med Dir Assn, 1*, 114–116.

WHOQOL Group (1998). Development of the World Health Organization WHOQOL-BREF quality of life assessment *Psycological Medicine, 28*, 551–558.

Wilson, K. (2006). Private communication, 6th April 2006.

11
The Target Efficiency
of Care—Models and Analyses

Claus Heislbetz, Petteri Hertto and Marja Vaarama

Introduction

Care managers constantly face the question of how best to utilise scarce resources and how to avoid waste of resources. This is especially emphasised in the phrase "increasing needs versus decreasing resources". However, it is also currently widely agreed that the cost containment does not mean "as cheap as possible" but "achieving the best possible outcomes on available resources". Therefore, simple productivity measures are insufficient, as service providers, purchasers, governments, clients and customers require value for money also in the terms of quality and effectiveness of interventions. Thus, efficiency is not only a matter of economics, but also involves doing the right things in the right way and in the right time. Central questions are: How effectively the care meets the client's needs? How efficiently the resources are used and would some alternative way of using them provide with better outcomes? To what extent the available resources are adequate to satisfy the assessed needs? How equal is the resource distribution among the needy groups? It is clear that to be able to answer to these questions is a matter of efficient care management, and moreover, it also helps the managers to defend their resources against cuts or to claim for new resources. Because resources are inevitably limited compared with needs, the use of the resources has to be considered carefully, but the allocation of care cannot be based only on principles of conventional economical efficiency but also on principles of quality and equity. For example Knapp defines efficiency as a combination of equity, economy and effectiveness (Knapp, 1984, 70–81; Vaarama, 1995).

As described in Chapter 1, the fourth pillar of Care Keys research is the concept of Target Efficiency of Care (TEFF) (Bebbington & Davies, 1983; Davies, Bebbington, & Charnley, 1990; Kavanagh & Stewart, 1995). The concept involves two target efficiency measures: (i) Horizontal target efficiency, which is the proportion of people who have been assessed as being in need and who receive the service, or the extent to which those deemed to be in need of a particular service actually receive it. Thus, it measures the efficiency of care in meeting the client needs, and on the other hand, also the unmet need. (ii) Vertical TEFF, which is the proportion of recipients of a service who satisfy the criteria of a priority need, or the extent to which the available care resources are received by those deemed to be in need. Thus, it measures the efficiency of resource allocation against the need being satisfied (Bebbington & Davies, 1983; Davies et al.). The basic idea of TEFF is that people should receive the service and care that they are in need of, and the resources should be allocated efficiently to meet these needs in an equitable way (see Chapter 1).

The TEFF concept was selected for use as the measure of efficiency of care in the Care Keys project because it sets not only economical but also social and ethical objectives of care as the criteria of the efficiency of care. An aggregated-level TEFF evaluation model developed by Vaarama, Mattila, Laaksonen, and Valtonen (1997) offered a practical starting point for the development of the TEFF measures in the Care Keys project, especially because the model demonstrated a high reliability and validity also in a further exploration by Hertto and Vaarama (2005) on a representative data of older Finnish long-term care clients. In Care Keys, we first tested the usability of the aggregate-level model, after which we developed two new TEFF measures for use at the individual client level. These were then implemented in the software program named MAssT (Mini-evaluation Tool for assessment of care quality, see Chapter 13 and http://www.carekeys.net). This chapter describes briefly the development of these measures and shows how they are implemented in the MAssT.

The Group-Level TEFF Model

The group-level TEFF has its focus on the match between the need, supply and equity of care at aggregated client group levels. The initial TEFF model developed by Vaarama et al. (1997) was developed using the Finnish RAVA-dependency scoring, which is an ADL-based dependency scoring system with little attention to cognitive or psycho-social needs and no attention to the IADL needs. The RAVA classification was originally developed for monitoring of the correctness of allocation of clients on different "care stairs", that is with increasing levels of care service needs. Used in this way also with TEFF measures, the model gave encouraging results (Vaarama et al.), and was selected as a topic of further development in Care Keys.

As indicated already, the group-level TEFF model calculates the results for different dependency groups. For calculation of the TEFF values, each dependency group has to be assigned with a quantified need and supply of optimal services (care package, service type, etc.), and when both are defined in similar terms, the correct allocation can be defined and achievement of it can be evaluated. In the group-level TEFF model, horizontal target efficiency (H) describes the ratio between the number of clients who receive a particular service package and the number of clients who are deemed to be in need of this very package. Vertical target efficiency (V) is the ratio between the number of clients who are deemed to be in need of a particular service package and who also get it, related to the number of all clients of that service. In other words, H measures the extent to which the clients receive the service package they really need (and the proportion of those who need it but do not get, i.e. unmet need), and V measures the proportion of correctly (against the need) allocated resources (and simultaneously also misallocation of resources). The ratio between H and V reflects the degree of efficiency and equity of the resource allocation against the priority need and the sufficiency of the available resources, that is whether current resources are sufficient to satisfy all the assessed needs and whether they are allocated correctly. The results that are calculated with costs give the most meaningful results with least interpretation problems. Using the cost as measurement units renders also possible to calculate over-targeting or under-targeting of care in monetary terms (surplus or deficit), and see how equitable the allocation has been, and whether it would be possible to improve the situation by reallocation of resources, and how much money would be needed for the care system to be able to meet all the assessed needs (Vaarama et al., 1997). However, a big hindrance for use of the cost-based TEFF model is the poor availability or quality of the information of costs.

In the Care Keys project, the group-level TEFF was tested in all project countries on diverse databases, and with expert evaluators to rate the usability, practicality and utility of the model. In addition, these results were encouraging as the testing on different data sets by different researchers gave sensible and constant results, and the model was very much desired by care managers. Testing results indicated also that the group-level TEFF model is very flexible in terms that it gave reliable results on any aggregated database (e.g. survey data, register data) where the need and the supply were measured in a comparable manner. However, the precondition of the need and supply being measured in similar terms was and is also a serious weakness of the group-level TEFF model as the currently poor documentation of need and supply of long-term care rarely follows this rule. A number of practical limitations for the application of the group TEFF model were found during the piloting of the model in the six project countries:

1. The lack of appropriate data in general.
2. The discrepancy between the data needs of TEFF and the existing data collection and documentation practices.
3. Needs-assessment procedures were highly variable and were not always based on validated instruments.
4. Care planning procedures were not standardised, they were nontransparent and the link between dependency grouping and service packages was often lacking.
5. The diversity of service types, products and packages was high in the project countries, as were the concepts of care implemented in the care practices.
6. Problems of how to link time or costs to service packages and these to the dependency groups were apparent.
7. The needs assessment and the documentation of care supply were not clearly separated, resulting at a biased picture, in which need and supply were seemingly highly congruent.

Some of these problems were specific to national care systems and policies, but most were common to all countries. The most important limitation was that the current care documentation practices are poor and rarely contain all the data necessary for detailed TEFF calculations. Even though the group-level TEFF model is able to tolerate a wide variation in data quality, this also leads to difficulties with the interpretation, lowering the validity of the results. In Care Keys, we tried to solve the problem by directing the further development of the TEFF model towards providing a range of TEFF measures and (sub) models that would be able work in a valid and reliable way in different care systems with varying quality of care documentation. The development resulted at two TEFF models, which are working at the individual client level but the results can be aggregated also in diverse groupings. The two models, the "Care Package TEFF" and the "Dimensional TEFF", are implemented in the MAssT application developed in the project (see http://www.carekeys.net). The dimensional model sets the least demands on the documentation quality, whereas the Package model requires more exact data, but gives also additional information for example on costs. All in all, the Care Keys project provided three models for evaluation of the TEFF, which not only meet the restrictions of the quality of data, but also the needs of care managers at different management levels who need different kinds of TEFF information. Client-level care management benefits best from individual-level TEFF information, whereas the higher-level managers may be more interested in aggregated TEFF results (see http://www.carekeys.net).

The Care Package TEFF Model

Whereas the group-level TEFF model gives aggregated results only, the individual-level TEFF models calculate them for a single client. The name of the "Care Package Model" is derived from the fact that it works with flexible mixes of individual service types or "products" (e.g. Meals-on-Wheels, sitting service, toe nail cutting, cleaning and helping in diverse daily activities). The model renders possible combining individual care packages from the variety of single service types at an individual client level. For each single package, the individual TEFF values for n clients ($i = 1,2,...n$) can be calculated with these formulae:

$$H_i = \frac{A_i}{N_i} = \frac{\min(N_i, S_i)}{N_i} \text{ (Horizontal target efficiency or needs responsiveness)}$$

$$V_i = \frac{A_i}{S_i} = \frac{\min(N_i, S_i)}{S_i} \text{ (Vertical target efficiency or supply efficiency)}$$

$$(H/V)_i = \frac{H_i}{V_i} = \frac{S_i}{N_i} \text{ (Over- and under-targeting or resource availability)}$$

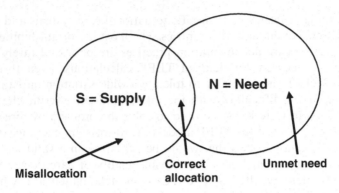

FIG. 11.1. The need–supply–comparison: correct allocation, misallocation and unmet need.

with N_i and S_i as the individual need and supply (see Fig. 11.1; also Chapter 1). These three TEFF values will be completed by a fourth TEFF value for relative equity (see later).

Basically, individual TEFF values can be calculated for the achievement of whatever goal given to the care, provided that both the goal and the achievement are expressed numerically and can be treated using a similar scale (measured e.g. by quantity, time or costs). But this is seldom the case as we learnt from our explorations in six project countries. Therefore, we had to pursue flexibility without compromising the validity in the further development of the Care Package TEFF. The solution was to adapt the instrument to the different care and documentation systems by rendering possible for a single provider/unit or other care organisations to freely combine individual care packages from an adjustable number of up to 20 care products or service types, and specify the amount of need and supply by each individual client in terms of hours or times (visits) per week or per month. In addition, the unit costs can be given in different currencies. Figure 11.2 illustrates the section of the MAssT configuration, where all these adjustments can be set.

active:		in hours or times	per week or per month	cost per unit in [EUR]	active:		in hours or times	per week or per month	cost per unit in [EUR]
☑	Only Home nursing	⦿ h ○ t	⦿ w ○ m	22,50	☑	Bathing service	⦿ h ○ t	⦿ w ○ m	10,00
☑	Only Home help	⦿ h ○ t	⦿ w ○ m	25,00	○	Other service	○ h ⦿ t	⦿ w ○ m	10,00
☑	Alarm service	○ h ⦿ t	○ w ⦿ m	26,00	○	Other service	⦿ h ○ t	⦿ w ○ m	0,00
☑	Ambulatory rehabilitation	○ h ⦿ t	○ w ⦿ m	27,00	○	Other service	⦿ h ○ t	⦿ w ○ m	0,00
☑	Meals on wheels	○ h ⦿ t	⦿ w ○ m	10,00	○	Other service	⦿ h ○ t	⦿ w ○ m	0,00
☑	Transport / taxi voucher	○ h ⦿ t	○ w ⦿ m	15,00	○	Other service	⦿ h ○ t	⦿ w ○ m	0,00
☑	Laundry	○ h ⦿ t	⦿ w ○ m	5,00	○	Other service	⦿ h ○ t	⦿ w ○ m	0,00
☑	Help with shopping/banking	○ h ⦿ t	⦿ w ○ m	10,00	○	Other service	⦿ h ○ t	⦿ w ○ m	0,00
☑	Accompanying / escort service	⦿ h ○ t	○ w ⦿ m	15,00	○	Other service	⦿ h ○ t	⦿ w ○ m	0,00
☑	Recreational activities	○ h ⦿ t	○ w ⦿ m	10,00	○	Other service	⦿ h ○ t	⦿ w ○ m	0,00

FIG. 11.2. Configuration of care packages in the MAssT for the TEFF calculations.

When the configurations are done, the results are displayed in an evaluation window (Fig. 11.3), and they are also contrasted with other MAssT results (Dimensional TEFF, the Quality of Care indices and the Quality of Life indices). As Fig. 11.3 illustrates, each service type or "product" in the care package is numbered from 1 to 20, and (in the configuration stage) the defined need and supply values for each are shown by the length of the horizontal bars, whereas monetary values for a service type are given for a period of 1 week. With "Met Needs" (needs responsiveness), "Supply Efficiency" and "Resource Distribution" (resource availability), the H-TEFF, V-TEFF

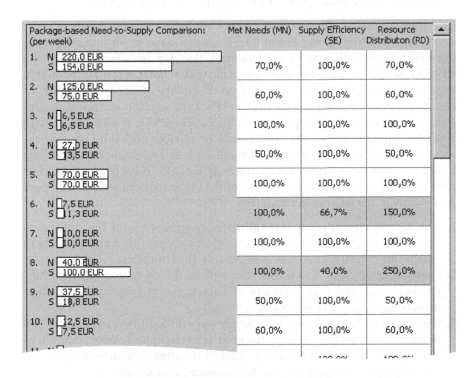

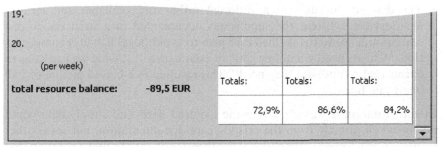

FIG. 11.3. Window for the evaluation of TEFF values of an individual care package in MAssT.

and *HI V*-TEFF results are displayed for each single care activity or product included in the individually tailored care package of a client. There is also a figure of total resource balance which shows how much additional money would be needed (or is spent too much) for this particular client in order to satisfy all his needs (under the precondition of correct allocation). It is also possible to aggregate all these individual results at any kind of client grouping.

The Dimensional TEFF Model

Development of Dimensional TEFF Model Using Care Theories

To ensure good and effective care it is crucial that care meets the client's true needs. The piloting of the initial TEFF model made it very clear that the current data collection and care documentation practices in long-term care of older people seldom were able to provide with reliable information on this, especially regarding the four dimensions of quality of life (see Chapter 4). Due to the poor documentation, the Care Package solution was not accessible for many managers in the project countries. Therefore, it was necessary to find also another model that still would be reliable and valid, exploit the available data and minimise requirements for any extra documentation or data collection. But as described in the following list, also this effort was facing a number of practical obstacles because of the incomplete information on need and supply in the five project countries:

1. The care documentation was rather heterogeneous with big differences between providers and different care organisations; this was the fact both within one country, and especially between the countries.
2. Care documentation was mostly incomplete, failing to account especially psychological and social aspects of care properly (physical or medical aspects were generally better documented).
3. Comparisons between need and supply were difficult because of time lags between the documentation of the need assessment and documentation of the supply, and because need and supply were often measured in categories that were barely comparable (scales, variables, indices, etc.).
4. The defined "needs" often reflected rather the available and refundable services, whereas the supply was documented in a strict one-to-one correspondence to the defined care plan to avoid (legal liability) compensation. "Clients need what they get!" or even worse: "… what we can offer to clients (get refunded!), they need!" This resulted in a biased picture of "all being just fine".

In this situation it was clear that the required need and supply data could not be taken directly from the existing care documentation, but some other solution was necessary. We checked the theories of care to find a solution that would allow a more qualitative interpretation of the available information, and allow definition of need and supply independently. A crosswalk between acknowledged care theories (see Chapter 5) resulted in a definition of 11 major dimensions of the long-term care (Table 11.1). All project countries were unanimous of these, so the model was named as "Comprehensive long-term care model", implicating the diversity of the needs the care should meet. To diminish the number of dimensions, and ideally to end up with a model corresponding the four dimensions of QoL, that is physical, psychological, social and environmental (see Chapters 4 and 5), we continued by defining first a six-dimensional model based on the current division between disciplines in care, which we named as the "Care Domain Model". In pursuing the four-dimensional model we used much iteration, but could not find one solution that had been satisfying all five countries. Instead, we ended up with two four-dimensional models: a Lawton-orientated care model (c.f. Lawton, 1991; Chapter 4) and an activation-orientated care model. These are in many dimensions similar and both are driving towards enhancing the QoL of older people, but the models differ in how they approach the IADL and ADL needs. In the "Lawtonian Model", ADL help is seen as belonging to the body, that is physical care, and to behavioural competence, whereas IADL help is seen as environmental support; thus, the model corresponds to the four-dimensional model of care-related QoL (Chapter 4). In the "Activation Model", the needs for help in daily living are seen as a central task of care of older people,

TABLE 11.1. Models for classifying the care needs and care responses in dimensions.

Quality of care dimensions

Comprehensive long-term care model according to the care theories	Care domain model	Care model corresponding to Lawton's QoL	Activation orientated care model
1. Medical care and cure	I. Medical	I. Physical	I. Medical
2. Assistance in sensory functions and verbal communication			
3. Memory, cognition/dementia			
4. Personal care/ADL	II. Personal		II. Daily activities
5. IADL	III. Instrumental	IV. Environmental	(I/ADL)
6. Environmental and technical aids	IV. Environmental		IV. Environmental
7. Need for counselling/social work			
8. Psychological care (involving others)	V. Psychological	II. Psychological	III. Psycho-social
9. Emotional (within care relationship), spiritual and existential support			
10. Support for identity and social networks	VI. Social	III. Social	
11. Support for participation and activities			

and also IADL help is seen as an integral part of care and not "only" as environmental support. The philosophy behind this is that care must meet the everyday needs of dependent people, and not only aim at support but also at activation of the older people themselves to use their own resources and develop self-efficacy in daily living, where doing the IADL tasks together with a care professional is seen as a means to realise this goal. The Lawtonian Model was seen as adequate for the German care system, while the Activation Model was favoured by the Nordic countries and UK. The two models are not reflecting any disagreement of the goal of long-term care (to provide comprehensive support and maximise QoL of the client), but the difference is rather in the care philosophy behind the concept of professional care.

The 11 care dimensions can be operationalised by an exchangeable set of indicators for each dimension (forming at the same time also a "minimum data set" for evaluation of the quality of long-term care by care dimensions). In MAssT, the care dimensions are operationalised by defining for each need and supply variable a set of empirical care situations. For example, in the dimension "1. Medical care and cure", the variable "Wound treatment/pressure ulcers" is operationalised by "bandage change, special wound therapies, secondary preventions"; and in the dimension "2. Assistance in sensory functions and verbal communication", the variable "Communication" is operationalised by "handle verbal and nonverbal forms of communication, agree on signals, help with phoning, speaking exercise, foreign-language understanding, provide more time". All pairs of need and supply variables use the same scale. In the pilot study in Care Keys, two types of scales were used; nominal yes/no scales and ordinal scales with five grades between "no need/supply" to "intensive need/supply". The goal has been to keep the data extraction as flexible as possible and to reduce the complexity of evaluation. The nicety of the solution is in that if one of these variables is missing in the care documentation, it can be replaced by some other within the same dimension. A well-trained data extractor (preferably a trained care professional) can use the dimensions also as guidelines to interpret the need and supply information in the existing care documentation.

The dimensional TEFF model allows the calculation of the TEFF indicators also at different aggregation levels. The most detailed analyses focus on each service type or care activity separately (e.g. medical treatment, bathing, toe nail cutting, laundry, psychological counselling), allowing a detailed evaluation of how well the client's needs are met in each pair of need and supply. This is mainly relevant for the client-level care management. For less detailed analyses, aggregation of the care activities (e.g. ADL/IADL support) at diverse care dimensions provides a useful solution. Which of these four models one chooses for the base of his TEFF evaluations depends on the purpose of evaluation and on the data availability. It is also important to note that the different models give equal weights to different dimensions, but this can be also changed by defining different weights to different needs and their responses prior to the calculation of TEFF values. In Care Keys, an approach was selected to assign equal weights in order to give psychological and social aspects a better representation than in the typical "medical" models that generally emphasise the medical and functional aspects in care.

Calculation of the Individual TEFF Values Based on Dimensions

To be able to calculate the dimensional TEFF values, need and supply variables have to be presented in linear transformations, so that all of them are scaled within the interval [0;1], with 0 indicating no need/supply and 1 indicating the highest degree of need/supply. Invalid need or supply information is marked outside this interval. Following this, the variables have been attributed to the 11 care dimensions (this defines need and supply variables n_i^j and s_i^j, with j for the care dimension and i for the variable within this dimension). Variable g_i^j can be computed with $\left(g_i^j = \begin{cases} 1 & \text{for} \quad n_i^j, s_i^j \in [0;1] \\ 0 & \text{else} \end{cases} \right)$, which indicates whether both variables are valid. The need in a certain dimension j with k need–supply pairs is then given by

$$N^j = \begin{cases} \dfrac{\sum\limits_{i=1}^{k} g_i^j n_i^j}{\sum\limits_{i=1}^{k} g_i^j} & \text{for} \quad \dfrac{\sum\limits_{i=1}^{k} g_i^j}{k} \geq \pi, \text{the corresponding supply by} \\ \text{invalid} & \text{else} \end{cases}$$

$$S^j = \begin{cases} \dfrac{\sum\limits_{i=1}^{k} g_i^j s_i^j}{\sum\limits_{i=1}^{k} g_i^j} & \text{for} \quad \dfrac{\sum\limits_{i=1}^{k} g_i^j}{k} \geq \pi \text{ and the amount of correct allocation among} \\ \text{invalid} & \text{else} \end{cases}$$

this by

$$A^j = \begin{cases} \dfrac{\sum\limits_{i=1}^{k} g_i^j \min(n_i^j, s_i^j)}{\sum\limits_{i=1}^{k} g_i^j} & \text{for} \quad \dfrac{\sum\limits_{i=1}^{k} g_i^j}{k} \geq \pi. \ \pi \text{ is the ratio of all need–supply} \\ \text{invalid} & \text{else} \end{cases}$$

variables that are necessary to get valid dimensional results. For theoretical reasons, the value can be set rather low, as all variables within a dimension are chosen so that they can substitute each other. If the ratio is higher than the chosen value for π, then a result for N^j, S^j, $A^j \in [0;1]$ (invalid dimension results are marked with some constant outside this interval) is derived for each dimension and TEFF indicators can be calculated with

$$H^j = \frac{A^j}{N^j} \in [0;1], V^j = \frac{A^j}{S^j} \in [0;1] \text{ and } \left(H_{/V}\right)^j = \frac{S^j}{N^j} \in [0;\infty].$$

It is also possible to aggregate the results at the next higher care domain level. The aggregation rules can be seen in Table 11.1. The 6 care domains are either a combination of 2 or 3 care dimensions (from the 11-dimensional set), or they are identical with 1 care dimension. Where necessary, the calculations for aggregation have to be done in the same way as described earlier for the 11-dimensional level. Again, a missing dimension can be substituted by the other(s) of the same domain as long as a certain ratio of dimensions per domain is not exceeded. The next aggregation step to the two alternatives for four-dimensional models (the Lawtonian Model and the Activation Model) follows the same logic.[1]

One particular methodological problem is associated with these calculations. It may happen that within one dimension or domain, a client's need or supply is 0, so that the formulae of the TEFF results lead to a division by 0 (e.g. a 0-need in dimension j leads to $H^j = \frac{A^j}{N^j} = \frac{0}{0}$). In fact, such a ratio is not

interpretable within the TEFF logic. Although H-TEFF provides information about the degree of satisfied needs, it is not possible to say how big this proportion is if a client has no need at all in a certain dimension. If H-TEFF is interpreted in terms of how "well" the situation of the client is regarding his needs, and V in terms of how "well" the given care meets the needs, then some justification is needed to call needs satisfaction and the supply efficacy as "perfect", when there is no need/supply at all. This provides a reason to set a value of 1 for H, V or H/V in this special case. But this has very problematic implications as in this case the TEFF reflects the performance of a care organisation. If a care organisation performs poorly in terms that it never satisfies the client's needs in certain care dimensions, then this organisation will get better values when the clients have no need in this dimension. It is therefore not the quality of care performance, but the discrepancy caused by hidden or latent needs and supplies that determines the TEFF values. This becomes even more problematic when (which is quite realistic) the client needs in a particular care dimension are not 0 in reality, but only 0 in the care documentation, because the poorly performing care organisation doesn't address client needs in this

---

[1] For the TEFF results used in this chapter, missing information in the need and supply variables were imputed (by EM-imputation procedure available in SPSS software package) before they were fed into the TEFF algorithm. This is statistically advisable, because, when variables are correlated, their sum-indices show less variance than the single variables. Hence, when we substitute variables by others within one dimension, we increase the variance of the TEFF results. This is especially problematic in the analysis using the TEFF results in probability calculations. The relevance of the described substitution lies more in the practical use of the dimensional TEFF calculations, where imputation procedures are not available.

dimension. Hence, H-TEFF (as well as V and H/V-TEFF) shall be marked as "not defined" for clients with no need (no supply). Such a note is then always a hint, to check from the needs assessment and in the care documentation whether the need and/or supply is really 0.

Relative Equity Measure

As the TEFF indicators inform on how resources are distributed among the care-dependent people, also evaluation of the relative equity of the distribution between the individual clients is possible introducing the fourth TEFF value and a clearly social and ethical objective. To be able to do this, first the group whose equity is concerned must be defined. For example, the equity evaluation may concern all clients under a certain administrative responsibility (such as a local community, care district or unit). A pursuit of equity is a task of the care management, and they should distribute the available resources or scarcity of them equitably among the clients but relative to their needs. In other words, resources are distributed relatively equitable when the clients face the under-targeting or over-targeting of care in a relatively same degree (whereas over-targeting of course shall be avoided to avoid a waste of resources). The amount of care resources allocated to each client in relation to their needs can be calculated as a ratio of (H/V).[2] Ideally, in an equitable situation, this ratio does not vary between the clients within one care organisation, and the standard deviation $s(H/V)$ in this case is 0. As the equity measure shall be independent from the level of resources, it has to be divided by the mean of the resource distribution (again in relation to the needs of each individual client) within the organisation. This results in an equity indicator based on the variation coefficient:

$$\text{Equity} \quad \frac{s\left(H/V\right)}{\overline{H/V}} \in [0;\infty) \quad \text{(relative equity of distribution of care resources)}$$

with small values indicating equitable and high values a non-equitable resource distribution.

Empirical Explorations of the Reliability and Validity of the TEFF Measures

The reliability of a measurement refers to its stability, asking whether the repeated measurement (with different data sets and by different researchers or data collectors) leads to similar results? In the Care Key pilot studies high Cronbach's Alpha values indicated a rather high reliability for all need and supply variables used in the TEFF models (Tables 11.2 and 11.3).

---

[2] The measure indicates relative equity of distribution of care resources. An alternative equity measure can be developed based on utility theory. A just distribution of resources demands then for each client an equal marginal utility induced by the last unit of care (see Chapter 6).

TABLE 11.2. Reliability (Cronbach's Alpha) of imputed need and supply variables in the dimensional TEFF model for homecare (HC).

	N	Number of variables	Cronbach's Alpha
Need variables	512	47	0.872
Supply variables	512	47	0.833

TABLE 11.3. Reliability (Cronbach's Alpha) of imputed need and supply variables in the dimensional TEFF model for institutional care (IC).

	N	Number of variables	Cronbach's Alpha
Need variables	435	47	0.899
Supply variables	435	47	0.876

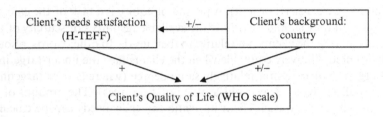

FIG. 11.4. Construct validity of H-TEFF results, a theoretical construct.

Another question is the validity of the measures, that is whether a scale actually measures what it intends to measure. This is analysed by methods of construct validity, where the scale in question has to be brought into some theoretical concept or framework, with well-founded (inter-) relationships. The Care Keys model suggests following theoretical concept (Fig. 11.4), which is explored statistically later.

The basic assumption is that satisfying the client's needs well has a positive impact on their QoL. Already in early Care Keys model explorations, the H-value was found to have a statistically significant connection with the subjective QoL of the clients, a high H-value impacting positively (significance in T-test 0.012; Hertto & Vaarama, 2005). The results of analyses of five project countries suggested also that the connection between H-TEFF and QoL may be influenced by country effects (see Chapter 7), and we will see later in this chapter that the TEFF results are influenced as well. Therefore, the analysis of the relationship between H-TEFF and the WHOQOL-Bref domains need to be controlled with the client's country of residence. In the testing of the validity of our theoretical model, we dichotomised the country variable to include all five countries in the analysis. Four of these dummy variables were used (the fifth was redundant) together with the dimensional H-TEFF values as independent variables in a multiple regression analysis (stepwise method with probability of F-to-enter 0, 05) to test their connections to the QoL of

TABLE 11.4. Connections between the WHOQOL-Bref domains, country of residence and the dimensional H-TEFF values in the Lawtonian model of homecare (HC). Linear stepwise regression analysis.

WHOQOL-Bref domain (dependent) variable	N	Dimensional H-TEFF values and country, (independent) variable/s	Adjusted determination coefficient (R^2_{adj})	Standardised coefficient (Beta)	T	F
Physical	345	Estonia	0.150	−0.175	0.003	
		III. Social		0.212	0.000	0.000
		IV. Environmental		0.146	0.010	
Psychological	345	Estonia	0.134	−0.313	0.000	
		I. Physical		0.127	0.014	
		Sweden		−0.124	0.016	
		II. Psychological		0.109	0.031	
Social	345	Estonia	0.104	−0.326	0.000	0.000
Environmental	345	Estonia	0.169	−0.322	0.000	0.000
		IV. Environmental		0.156	0.005	

the clients. Table 11.4 presents the results for the Lawtonian Model in the case of home care (HC).

Except the social domain, the dimensional H-TEFF values have a positive connection to each of the WHOQOL-Bref dimensions. At the same time, each of the H-TEFF dimensions is important in at least one of the models. It is interesting that meeting well the needs in the physical dimension is influenced by social and environmental aspects of care. As assumed, country of residence has some impact; living in Estonia has a rather negative impact, as was demonstrated also in the analysis of QoL variation in five project countries (Chapter 7).

A positive impact of H-TEFF on QoL was found also in the institutional care (IC) (Table 11.5). According to the model, every WHOQOL-Bref dimension was impacted by H-TEFF to some extent. The most significant connection was found between the environmental TEFF dimension (in the Lawtonian Model including IADL) and QoL. Again, living in Estonia had negative impact on many QoL-domains, reflecting the situation of a transition economy. That UK had such positive values is probably connected to the fact that their data did not really represent an institution but a service house, where both clients are usually better off and the care arrangements more individual.

These findings are in correspondence with the results of early piloting with H-TEFF and QoL on a different database (Hertto & Vaarama, 2005). The results described in Tables 11.4 and 11.5 indicate acceptable validity of the TEFF measures, especially when keeping in mind that data were derived from two different sources: Quality of Life data from the clients and the TEFF data from the care documentation.

TABLE 11.5. Connections between the WHOQOL-Bref domains, country of residence and the dimensional H-TEFF values in the Lawtonian model of institutional care (IC). Linear stepwise regression analysis.

WHOQoL-Bref domain (dependent) variable	N	Dimensional H-TEFF values and country of resi-dence, (independ-ent) variable/s	Adjusted determination coefficient (R^2_{adj})	Standardised coefficient (Beta)	T	F
Physical	312	Estonia	0.037	−0.144	0.011	0.001
		IV. Environmental		0.133	0.018	
Psychological	312	Estonia	0.071	−0.162	0.004	0.000
		UK		0.130	0.027	
		IV. Environmental		0.117	0.040	
Social	312	I. Physical	0.084	0.219	0.000	0.000
		UK		0.154	0.006	
Environmental	312	Estonia	0.194	−0.282	0.000	0.000
		UK		0.236	0.000	
		IV. Environmental		0.109	0.041	

Pilot Results

Due to the limited space, it is not possible to reproduce a comprehensive picture of all TEFF results from the pilot study. Therefore, we present only the most important findings with the Lawtonian Model of homecare.

Figure 11.5 shows that the best H-TEFF results are achieved in the pilot countries in the psychological dimension of care, where all countries seem to meet the needs almost thoroughly. In the physical and environmental dimensions such results are achieved only for the two Nordic countries Finland and Sweden, whereas clients in other countries are in a relatively inferior position. Biggest differences between the pilot countries are in meeting the client's needs in the social care dimension, which seem to be in general the dimension where no country performs very well. Especially poor results are found for Estonia and Germany.

According to Fig. 11.6, all countries have near to 100% supply efficiency, which means that they use their resources efficiently to meet the client needs. According to this, a waste of resources is not a problem in these countries. Most notable misallocation of resources seems to be in the environmental dimension of care (including IADL), especially in Sweden and in Finland.

Figure 11.7 suggests that most of the care dimensions have insufficient resources compared with the needs, and especially this affects the social dimension of care (indicated by values below 1). On the other hand, Sweden and Finland seem to have used a bit more resources than needed in the environmental care domain (values above 1). When comparing the Swedish and Finnish results against their supply efficiency (V-TEFF) results (both clearly under 100%), the result suggests that Sweden has sufficient and Finland almost sufficient resources to meet the environmental needs of the clients, but due to misallocation of resources, the clients are not getting enough help in this

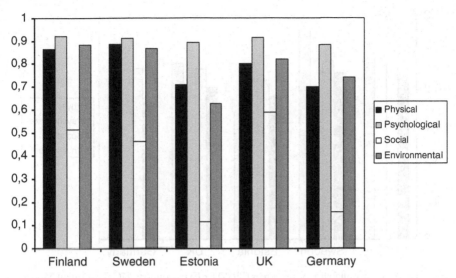

FIG. 11.5. Average needs responsiveness (H-TEFF) by country (HC, Lawtonian Model).

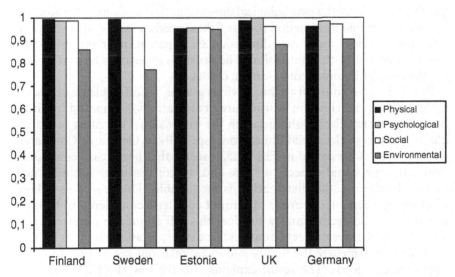

FIG. 11.6. Average supply efficiency (V-TEFF) by country (HC, Lawtonian Model).

dimension, and the situation could be improved by reallocation of resources. On another hand, as there was not any great over-targeting of resources in any dimension, the result may refer also to that, in fact, the resources are scarce, and due to this, there may have been prioritisation of care dimensions, leading to savings in the environmental dimension (such as in the IADL help). Regarding

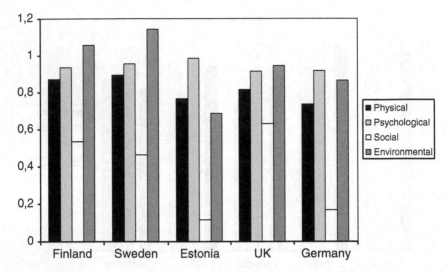

FIG. 11.7. Average availability of resources (H/V-TEFF) by country (HC, Lawtonian Model).

the TEFF values of the psychological dimension, the values may be too good because of the underestimation (bias) of these needs in care documentation. The poor values in social care dimension are apparent, referring to a widespread disregard of this dimension. The situation appears to be particularly problematic for Estonian and German clients.

In Fig. 11.8, in contrast to the previous graphs, a preferable result (equitable resource distribution within care organisations) is marked by short bars. Comparing the results between the dimensions, the most inequitable situation is in the social dimension, especially in Germany. Compared with the results presented in Fig. 11.5, it seems that home care commonly disregards the social aspects of care and, where resources are allocated to this dimension, the distribution is inequitable. This leaves us asking whether the social needs are in all project countries considered to be least important in homecare, and what does this tell about the philosophy of homecare in the five project countries? One interpretation suggests (Chapter 6) that in homecare the family and social relations are assumed to take care of social needs. The result explains also the low H-TEFF results in general, but it can also be connected with the poor quality of homecare documentation, which was stated in Chapter 8. The German homecare seems to deny most strongly the needs of care in social dimension—maybe because their supply is not refundable by care insurances. Figure 11.9 supports these interpretations.

In the IC, we find indeed a much more equitable distribution of resources within the social dimension. Furthermore the social need satisfaction (H-TEFF) is good to excellent in all countries (results not displayed here). Social care

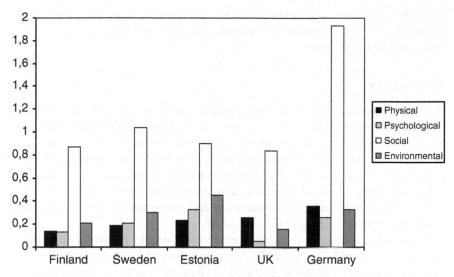

FIG. 11.8. Average equity of resource distribution by country (HC, Lawtonian Model).

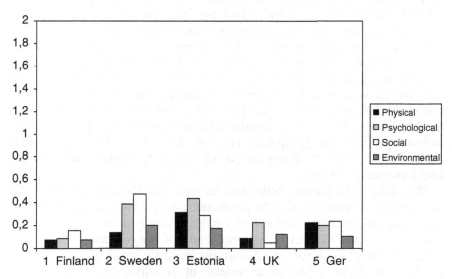

FIG. 11.9. Average equity of resource distribution by country (IC, Lawtonian Model).

aspects are clearly more valuated and satisfied in the IC. Regarding the other care dimensions, there appears to be an especially equitable distribution of resources in Finland, both in the community and in the institutional settings. This is quite understandable, given the Finnish welfare system, with its common standards provided under the unifying responsibility of the local authorities. However, it is rather difficult to interpret the generally less equitable distribution of care resources in Sweden (especially in IC) where a rather similar welfare system is in place.

Discussion

One of the goals in the Care Keys project was to specify reliable and valid measures for evaluation of the efficiency of the long-term care of older people, which would be based not only on the criteria of conventional economy but also takes the social and ethical objectives of care into account. The project adopted the concept of TEFF as the measure to be used, and took the earlier developed pilot model of TEFF as a starting point from which to proceed further. The testing and expert evaluation gave encouraging results, suggesting a high potential of the measure.

A special challenge in the Care Keys project was to be able to develop a measure that would be applicable in five project countries with different care systems. A major problem was caused by the poor quality of care documentation in all project countries, especially regarding homecare. As a solution, three different models for evaluation of the TEFF were provided: a group-level TEFF model for higher-level care managers, a "Care Package model" and a "Dimensional TEFF model", which are intended on client-level quality management, but also give aggregated results. The models are adjusted to different data availability and to different information needs at different management levels. The data requirements are defined in the Care Keys Minimum Data Set (Chapter 13), with the aim to be as highly as possible congruent with the existing documentation systems to avoid extra documentation or data collection. This solution rendered it possible to use at least one of the TEFF models in each of the project countries. The models are implemented in two software packages: the group-level TEFF model and the MAssT application (Mini-evaluation Tool to assess the quality of care, for both applications, see http://www.carekeys.net).

The piloting and testing results demonstrated that the measures give valid and sensible information, and the results remain stable with different studies. There is a clear evidence on that better targeted care is connected with better QoL of the clients. Further, the piloting results of five countries demonstrate some scarcity of resources in all countries compared with the needs to be satisfied, and there is even some evidence of misallocation of resources in the environmental dimension. This may rather be due to the prioritisation of certain needs as the resources are not sufficient for meeting all of the needs. The fact that resources were used very efficiently and no waste of resources was identified speaks for this interpretation. It was a remarkable result that homecare on all countries largely denies the needs of old people in the social dimension of care (and QoL). In the light of these results, the Nordic countries had a better balance of needs and resources, whereas Germany and Estonia were performing worse and especially poor in the social dimension of care.

This type of information is very important for the care managers, politicians and older people themselves. Still, a question remains whether the results really reflects the real situation in the pilot sites, or are they due to the poor documentation of care needs and supply?

Somewhat problematic is that the individual TEFF measures are not always easy to understand, and it may be advisable to choose terms that are closer to practical usage in each language. In addition, a number of other tasks remain to be solved, one of the biggest still dealing with the fact that although the dimensional TEFF model can be used also with poor care documentation and data availability, the more exact Care Package TEFF model (including costs) is not applicable in these contexts. Where such poor documentation exists, too many missing values prevent the calculation of TEFF results with costs, or the data may exist but be biased, and cannot produce reliable results.

This leads to another potential obstacle for the acceptance of the TEFF models, namely the *willingness* of care practitioners to provide the information the TEFF evaluation requires. In principle, it should be in the interest of care managers to recognise inefficient use of resources to be able to improve the situation, but they may also be reluctant to use any tool that may bring their inefficiencies to the surface. Furthermore, the inequalities may originate from regulations or reimbursement systems, and in these situations, care management cannot do much to improve the situation. Why then evaluate if nothing can be changed? It is also possible to imagine situations in which care providers may benefit from ineffective and/or inefficient delivery of services, for example when necessary services are not reimbursed (but must be delivered in the client's interest) and other financed services are documented (but not provided), or, particularly challenging or stressful (but necessary) care activities are avoided and/or easier (but not necessary) services are provided instead. In such situations, it may not be possible to expect the care practice to be always interested in reliable TEFF indicators.

The best use of the TEFF tools would be in using them to help in identification of directions towards which the care provision should and could be developed. There may be many different opportunities for reallocation of resources in order to improve the equity of distribution of care resources and meeting of the clients needs, and a tool such as TEFF can make them visible. This way the TEFF evaluation procedure can at best be a common learning process, where the managers and the teams evaluate how they are performing and find out together the means on how to do better.

As said earlier, the TEFF results are vulnerable for biased data and misinterpretations. To ensure the credibility of the information, the TEFF results should be contrasted with the results of the evaluation of Quality of Life, Quality of Care and Quality of Management, using at least partly other sources of information. The first version of an instrument providing such a concise picture for higher-level managers is the Q-MAT instrument developed in the Care Key project (see Chapter 13), whereas the MAssT instrument allows comparison of the individual-level TEFF results with the results of analyses of the subjective QoL and the subjective and documented quality of care which the tool includes (see www.carekeys.net). The Care Keys Toolkit offers also sets of key indicators of the client quality, professional quality and management quality of care, and these together with the TEFF values are able to give a more comprehensive picture of the situation. And finally, even the results presented here are very encouraging, they are still explorative, and further research on well-documented care is necessary for further validation of the measures.

References

Bebbington, A., & Davies, B. (1983). Equity and efficiency in the allocation of the personal social services. *Journal of Social Policy, 12*, 309–330.

Davies, B., Bebbington, A., Charnley, H., & colleagues (1990). Resources, needs and outcomes in community-based care. A comparative study of the production of welfare for elderly people in ten local authorities in England and Wales. PSSRU, University of Kent at Canterbury.

Hertto, P., & Vaarama, M. (2005). Palvelujen kohdennustehokkuus ja elämänlaatu (Target efficiency of care and quality of life). *Terveystaloustiede 2005.* Helsinki: Stakes.

Kavanagh, S., & Stewart, A. (1995). Economic evaluations of mental health care. In M. Knapp, (Ed.), *The economic evaluation of mental health care. PSSRU. CEMH.* (pp. 27–60). Aldershot: Arena.

Knapp, M. (1984). *The economics of social care. Studies in social policy.* Hong Kong: Macmillan education.

Lawton, M. P. (1991). A multidimensional view of QoL in frail elders. In J. E. Birren, J. E. Lubben, J. C. Rowe, & D. E. Deutchman (Eds.), *The concept and measurement of QoL in frail elders* (pp.3–27). San Diego, CA: Academic Press.

Vaarama, M. (1995). Vanhusten hoivapalvelun tuloksellisuus hyvinvoinnin tuotanto -näkökulmasta (Performance Variation in the Care of the Elderly. A production of welfare-analysis of the public care system in Finnish municipalities). Jyväskylä: Gummerus <http://www.carekeys.net>

Vaarama, M., Mattila, V., Laaksonen, S., & Valtonen, H. (1997). Target efficiency of care. Report on development and piloting of the target efficiency indicators and model. Deliverables of the European PLANEC-project. Helsinki: Stakes.

12
Quality Management and the Care Keys Quality Matrix

Richard Pieper, Claus Heislbetz and Mona Frommelt

Introduction

Theoretical and empirical research on the effect of management strategies and service organisation on the quality of care and on the quality of life of clients is still developing. In view of the growing importance of the provision of care in an "ageing society" this state of the art should raise concern and induce enhanced research efforts. The Care Keys project tried to make a contribution to the theoretical and empirical issues, even addressing practical concerns by developing tools for quality management in long-term care. The theoretical framework for management has been presented elsewhere (Chapter 6), and the reader might like to refer to this discussion for more detail. The objectives for the following analyses focus on empirical issues. We will investigate the effects of elements of "good" management strategies on the quality of care and care outcomes for the client. Drawing on the theoretical background, the concept of management will be put into operational terms by a set of indicators, which may guide quality management. The aim is to demonstrate the empirical significance and impact of the indicators in order to provide at least preliminary empirical support both for the indicators and for the structure and comprehensiveness of the strategy employing them. The practical aim of developing a matrix of quality indicators into a tool for quality management will, thus, be supported by a first evidence base.

The contribution will proceed in the following steps: first, the theoretical background will be sketched out. The aim is to clarify basic concepts of "good management" and to provide a model of management impacts as a basis for the empirical theses to be investigated. Second, the aim is to define and to structure the set of variables and to discuss some issues about the indicators, data and methods used in the following analyses. Third, the results of first analyses are shown focusing on the reconstruction of management styles from the data by cluster analysis, and the investigation of causal impacts by regression analyses. Finally, the results will be discussed and some conclusions drawn for further research.

Research Objectives and Theoretical Framework

The basic inquiry of Care Keys is into the relationships between quality of management (QoM), quality of care (QoC), and quality of life (QoL) of clients as "final outcome" of a production of welfare process. The basic assumption certainly is that "good" management supports "good" care, which in turn will generate "good" QoL. As discussed in the chapter on management quality, the concept and strategy of Total Quality Management (TQM) is designed to facilitate this flow of quality through the service process, and it aims to produce quality services by focusing on quality (i) in each phase of the production process (input/structure, process, outcomes), (ii) from the perspective of all stakeholders involved in the process, in the present case from the perspective of management, of staff, and especially of the client, and (iii) by including all relevant aspects or dimensions of quality. We will approach the issues primarily from the perspective of management treating "good" care as an intermediate output, which is to be promoted by the selection of favourable conditions and strategies. In turn, "good" care is expected to produce positive "final outcomes" for the QoL of clients. In line with TQM, the focus is on identifying conditions and management options that can be operationalised into a set of goals and key indicators for quality of performance and outcomes. The strategic task of management is then to implement the goals and indicators of their achievement into practice. A well-known methodology for this approach is the Balanced Scorecard (Fridag & Schmidt, 2004; Niven, 2003), which can facilitate good performance as well as innovative change.

A characteristic of the management perspective especially in the realm of social and health care will be that it is or should be "client oriented", but not only in the interest of the individual client as "customer". The manager has to consider the interests of staff (often underpaid or volunteers), who will produce QoC only in favourable work conditions, where they can realize their own professional and personal concepts of "good" care, and the interests of the broader community, which will expect equitable, effective and efficient care provision. Notably the "just" distribution of the always scarce resources in care services will not necessarily coincide with the interests of specific clients. And the public interest will also put high priority on cooperation and integration of care (including sharing of scarce resources), which will not always be easily consolidated with interests of a given service organisation and its clients. The QoM and QoC has to be specified within a framework of a "philosophy" or "vision", which is oriented (also) towards a "common good", not (only) towards preferences of individual clients.

To learn more about the concrete determinants of successful management it is helpful to look more closely at the conditions and characteristics of strategies, which result in more or less "good" outcomes for clients. The size (clients, staff) and the resources (finances, technology, care environment) can be expected to be influential, but also the structure of the organisation and the welfare regime that determines management options (Currie, Harvey,

West, McKenna, & Keeney, 2005; Görres, 1999). The context may be a welfare regime, which provides comprehensive social and health care services in often large municipal organisation (e.g. in the Scandinavian system), or in a fragmented system of different private or non-profit providers of social services and health care services with little coordination and cooperation (e.g. in the German system). Thus, the tasks and responsibilities for teamwork and integration will vary widely, as will the strategies for integration (Pieper, 2005).

It is also important to distinguish between levels of management, since the criteria of performance will be different. On the first level, there is the *process of care*; here management tasks consist especially in determining the autonomy to be given to professionals in their work. Next, a level of *care process management* may be distinguished that structures, monitors and evaluates the care processes and is typically the tasks of senior professionals still themselves engaged in care. On a third level of *care service management*, the care process is seen in the context of supporting services and management tasks such as resource management, marketing, personnel management and quality management. In larger organisations this level may not be in the responsibility of a professional carer anymore, in small homecare services all three levels may collapse into one level of partners sharing the work. Managers of small services typically have to coordinate their services with services from other agencies. They have to be "networking" managers, since the success and quality of their service usually will depend on the quality of the work of their partners and the quality of the integration of care services. In a "mixed economy" of public, non-profit and for-profit providers, networking and integration are demanding, and unfortunately often neglected tasks. (Evers, Haverinen, Leichsenring, & Wistow, 1997; Vaarama & Pieper, 2005). Especially in large organisations providing social and health care services, managers have the tasks of integrating diverse services *within* their organisation. On a fourth level of *care system management* (e.g. in a social and health care department of a municipality) management will be quite remote from the level of care and the focus will be on general tasks of organisational management.

In smaller service organisations and on lower levels of management, therefore, we will find a closer integration and interdependence of management and care tasks. The management of care processes and the management of care services will strongly interact, and the special character of care as a service for frail older persons will have a stronger influence on management strategies. Management has to be sensitive to the affordances of care, the quality of other management tasks (e.g. supporting services, personnel management) and the environmental setting, and it will have a decisive impact on the QoC and care outcomes. For example, the manager designing and managing a care institution that strives to realize a "home" situation with clients, staff and management forming a "care community" (Owen & NCHRDF, 2006) will have to be more responsive in his strategies, then the manager administrating a care service system of a municipality. Especially in a TQM perspective and on levels close to the care process, "good" management will be quality management, and the factors and determinants of successful management (QoM) will be at the same time elements of quality management. This is also the level and scale at which the indicators developed and analysed in the Care Keys research are primarily aimed to apply.

Besides these conditions, the elements of "good" management have to be considered. Or in a somewhat different perspective, we should look for the elements of successful management of innovation, since care services are recently experiencing a process of rapid change and innovation—not necessarily by their own liking, but under the pressure of demographic trends, new market conditions and restrictions of public finances. For services in general, not specifically for social and health care services, Reichwald (2006) has made an extensive review of the literature and identified four important determinants of success of innovation and service re-engineering:

1. High benefit of the innovation for the client — which implies a strong client orientation in all phases of service development, that is, the invention, conceptualisation, development and marketing and delivery of the service.
2. Systematic strategies of development — including methodological, goal-oriented and evidence-based approach for controlling effectiveness and efficiency.
3. Adequate resources — which includes the right mix of qualified staff, technology, support services, environmental setting and access and finances to carry the innovation through
4. Personnel development — focusing on motivation, work climate, teamwork, cooperation and involvement of partners and the wider community.

In the present context, it is important that the search for factors of a "good" management of innovations re-produces the four dimensions of management quality as discussed in more detail in Chapter 6, namely, the "concept dimension" (I) of client-centred care, the "procedure dimension" (II) of systematic and evidence-based goal-achievement, the "resource dimension" (III) of resource utilisation, technology and environment, and the "integrated care dimension" (IV) of cooperation, integration and motivating work atmospheres. Actually, client-orientation, cost-benefit and cost-effectiveness control, and staff qualification proved to make the difference between success and failure in Reichwald's review. Systematic procedures and strategies were somewhat less important. However, considering that we are concerned with services including health care, we propose that all four factors are equally important and formulate the following theses:

1. The quality of health care services affords systematic, evidence-based and risk controlling strategies of innovation. Professionalism of procedures and risk management should be expected to play an important role in care. In general we should expect that medical services and risk management should have a larger influence in institutions, because clients will typically

be more dependent on (the quality of) health care: Successful management will have strategies of risk management in place (dimension II).

This introduces a differentiation between the care setting of institutional care (IC) and homecare (HC), which will be a focus also in the present analyses (see Chapters 8 and 9 for more detailed analyses of HC and IC).

2. The tradition of health care and the "medical model" of care is assumed to be more influential in institutional care (IC) than in homecare (HC), where a "socio-cultural model" and a broader concept of client needs should guide the practice. This should be somewhat less the case in a "mixed economy" and fragmented systems where IC and HC tend to be less specialised as to the degree of dependency of their clients (see Chapter 6). Still: Successful management will implement a comprehensive client-oriented quality management in IC and HC (dimension I).

3. In IC, the institutional context is assumed to have a more direct impact on the QoC and QoL outcomes. The causal chain or production function of input, process and outcome should be expected to be closer in IC than in HC, because in IC management will have more influence on the whole process, especially on the interaction between management, staff and clients: Successful management will have a larger impact on QoL in IC.

4. In HC, a "mixed care model", that is, the cooperation of different services in the provision of care is more likely, and it may involve "case management" for the coordination of services for specific clients. Basically, the household and informal carers will be responsible for many care tasks and they might also choose to combine services from different agencies (e.g. health care and meals on wheels). Successful HC will often have the character of "community care" utilising the resources of the broader community: Successful management should utilise not only internal, but also external resources including informal care, in HC (dimension III).

Commenting on theses four assumptions, we may add that — following the distinction of approaches to care (see Chapter 5; Bowers, Fibich, & Jacobson, 2001)—"care as a service" should be a more frequent orientation in HC than in IC, since HC is in most cases given as an additional support (e.g. IADL home help) to specific health services and will be experienced as such by the client. Somewhat paradoxically we should expect that, on the one hand, a specific HC service will have less influence on the social aspects of QoL, because the client will be expected to have some social relations taking also responsibility for care—if they are missing, institutionalisation is likely. On the other hand, the importance of social relations and activities implies that HC has a high responsibility to support social relations. Still, in HC the service quality of a given service will have less influence on the QoL of clients and its effectiveness will depend on the integration of other sources of support. The subjective *evaluation* of care by the client, the subjective QoC (sQoC) may reflect the impact of care quality on their QoL better than the "final outcome" of life quality, the subjective QoL (sQoL).

5. The fact that HC strongly depends on other services to assure QoL for clients should be expected to produce a stronger impact of cooperation with partners on intermediate outcomes (sQoC) and final outcomes (QoL) in HC than in IC: Successful management will implement strategies of cooperation and integrated care, especially in HC (dimension IV).

This leads to a final and summarising thesis:

6. In successful management with positive care outcomes, all four quality dimensions are expected to have significant impact: client-oriented quality concepts (I), professional procedures (II), utilisation of resources (III) and cooperative strategies (IV).

These factors specify four dimensions of *input*, structures and conditions of "good" quality management. *Process* or performance management will have to attend to the same dimensions to assure that the input will be effective: Concepts of client-oriented quality assurance have to be applied in quality strategies (I); systematic, evidence-based methods have to structure the management process (II); resources have to be utilised efficiently (III); communication, cooperation and teamwork have to be facilitated (IV). Finally, *outcome* measures are central for management, they have to be specified, and their achievement has to be controlled in all four dimensions.

Performance Evaluation and the Quality Matrix

Following the production of welfare approach, the performance of management was evaluated in Care Keys by the target efficiency of care achieved in the care provision (see Chapter 11). The concept of target efficiency (TEFF) comprises four concepts and their measurement which together specify management goals and outcomes: equity, need-responsiveness, supply efficiency and resource availability

1. Equity (E) is an indicator for the concept dimension of quality management referring to the goal of just distribution of services and resources over the clients.
2. Need-responsiveness (H) is a measure of effectiveness of allocation, that is, the degree to which the needs of a client are satisfied by appropriate services. In this sense, H is a suitable indicator of client orientation of management. However, for our purposes we used it as an indicator for the contribution of services to QoL employing H as a measure for client outcomes of care, that is, the QoL as described in the care documentation (docQoL).
3. Supply efficiency (V) is a measure of efficiency indicating that there is no "waste" of resources or services on clients who do not need it. This implies good work organisation, and the indicator can and will be used as an outcome indicator to measure the quality of procedures as centred on correct

allocation. (Alternatively, H could be used, but in the research design it was rather used as a client outcome measure.)

4. Resource availability (H/V) is a measure of resource management and utilisation (over- and under-targeting of resources) and indicates the goal to have enough resources available for a (more) just allocation among the clients, to have the resources to satisfy all needs, and to make external resources accessible.

The target efficiency values (TEFF-values) as measured in CK provide, therefore, outcome measures for quality management in three of the four dimensions: Client-oriented and "just" provision of services (E, H), systematic goal-oriented procedures (V) and good resource management (H/V). They are calculated on the basis of information on assessed needs and delivered supply extracted from the care documentation by the InDEX instrument. While most of the other management indicators employed in the following analyses are based on information from ManDEX, that is, on an interview of the manager and possibly biased, these outcomes are measured independently are in that sense, more objective indicators (see Chapter 2 and 13). For the fourth dimension of cooperation an additional measure was developed which focuses on the existence (input), handling (process) and outcome evaluation of cooperation (COOP) with partners in a strategy for integrated care. For this purpose, ManDEX contained a checklist of nine typical cooperation partners (input) and the evaluation of the cooperation (outcome). (The teamwork aspect of this dimension was, instead, included in the measurement of QoC). As described in chapters on the theoretical framework of Care Keys (Chapters 1 and 6), all measures may be summarised in a quality matrix. The matrix contains three basic dimensions:

1. Dimension 1: production—input/process/documented outcomes/subjective outcomes
2. Dimension 2: stakeholders—perspectives of client/professional staff/management
3. Dimension 3: quality—four sub-dimensions for quality evaluation.

Dimension 1 follows Donabedian's (1969) distinction of structure quality, process quality and outcome quality, differentiating additionally objective outcome indicators as documented in the care documentation and subjective outcome indicators as obtained by interviews from stakeholders (clients, staff, managers). Dimension 2 introduces the perspectives of the three basic stakeholders following Ovretveit (1998). In the present context, the management perspective is the point of reference; staff and client aspects serve as dependent variables.

Dimension 3 adds the four (sub-) dimensions of "good" quality as described above for the case of management quality. Corresponding dimensions were defined for all three perspectives (with roman letters I–IV in Fig. 12.1).

In the management perspective, the matrix yields 4 × 4 cells (production × quality; see Fig. 12.1). These cells define the basic concepts or variables to be

Q-MAT	Quality	Input	Process	Outcome subj.	Outcome obj.
Client	Dim.I				
	Dim.II				
	Dim.III				
	Dim.IV				
Professional	Dim.I				
	Dim.II				
	Dim.III				
	Dim.IV				
Management	Dim.I				
	Dim.II				
	Dim.III				
	Dim.IV				

Client input		*Client* process		*Client* outcome documented	*Client* outcome subjective
		Professional input	*Professional* process	*Professional* outcome documented	*Professional* outcome subjective		
Management input	*Management* process		*Management* outcome documented		*Management* outcome subjective

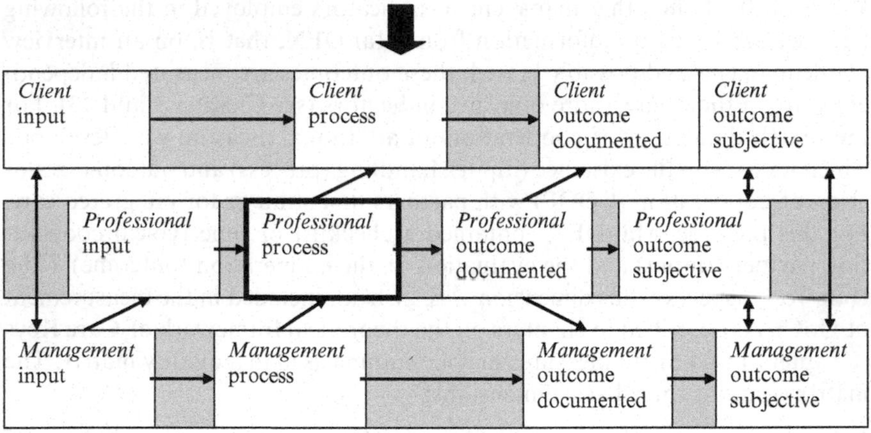

Fig. 12.1. The quality matrix Q-MAT and implied causal impacts.

considered as management factors in the following analyses. A similar 4 × 4 matrix can be constructed for the client and for the professional perspective adding up to the "magic 48" cells of the comprehensive quality matrix Q-MAT of the CK Toolkit (see Fig. 13.1 in Chapter 13). The four dimensions are introduced as "social" (dimension I), "physical/functional" (dimension II, "environmental/services" (dimension III), and "psychological" (dimension IV) in the concept and measurement of sQoL (see Chapter 4). They apply to care quality as reflected in the care documentation (docQoC) by distinguishing similar to management between "client oriented concepts" (dimension I), functional methods and "procedures" (dimension II), supporting "resources/ environment" (dimension III) and "psycho-emotional" aspects (dimension IV). The basic framework for the generalisation of the four quality dimensions to the professional and client perspective, especially to QoC and QoL, is provided by social systems theory (see Chapters 4, 5 and 6).

As Fig. 12.1 shows, the quality matrix can be interpreted as a causal impact model (the quality dimensions being left out in the causal model). In this view, also the central importance of client input as a condition and client outcome as the goal is specified, but also the importance of professional care processes, since low quality at this point will have the most effects on outcomes in the scheme (assuming equal weights for all effects): There is "no way around good care".

The objectives of the empirical analyses are (i) to provide evidence for the quality matrix as a meaningful framework to define and to organise key indicators for quality management and (ii) to inquire into the causal dependencies implied in the production dimension. Following the TQM approach we would expect positive influences "flowing" through the matrix from management to care and to care outcomes and from input variables to process variables and outcome variables as indicated in the model in Fig. 12.1. A lack of empirical effects would basically imply that the indicators have to be substituted by more valid ones. The TQM approach would exclude on theoretical grounds that a "box" in the matrix does not have an effect as indicated.

Research Results

Because of the complexity of the matrix a wealth of possible interdependencies would have to be checked. This is not feasible within the present context and will require also more research on the data. Actually, part of the relationship is investigated in other chapters of this volume, for example, the research on the client perspective (Chapter 7), and on QoC in homecare and in institutional care and their effects on measures of QoL (Chapters 8 and 9). Although the variables and scales used are sometimes differing from the ones suggested here (e.g. varying sQoL measures), from a practical point of view they could be introduced in the Q-MAT as alternatives (Chapter 13). We will present some first results and focus on management indicators as provided by the ManDEX instrument and on a selection of indicators and scales for QoC and QoL as dependent variables.

In the first step, we will introduce and discuss briefly the data, indicators and scales we used, and focus on the evidence for the four-dimensional quality structure. In the second step, the indicators for the management perspective are analysed by cluster analyses to identify patterns or "management styles", which can than be evaluated according to their effects on QoC and QoL. In the third step, we will look independently at the causal influences of key indicators to gain a better understanding of the effects of management strategies on care outcomes. A special focus will be on the differences between homecare and institutional care, since — as stated above—we will expect the strategies of management to be different in those care settings.

Indicators, Scales and Methods

The database has been described in detail elsewhere (Chapter 2 and 3). The following analyses will employ the international pooled database. The sample includes 37 homecare services (HC) and 30 institutional services (IC) and makes use of the same variables (64 and 63 variables, respectively; only the variables for the environment of HC and IC are obviously different). Basically, at least 48 variables are needed to include at least one indicator for each concept in the matrix and the model (Fig. 12.1).

Considering the dependent variables QoC and QoL, the quality matrix contains variables for all cells, but in the present analyses we have not investigated the client input (e.g. socio-economic status, age, gender, health, preferences) and the job satisfaction among professionals. The former specifies conditions, which have been analysed in some detail in other chapters (Chapter 7–9), and for the latter we do not have data, since data on subjective job satisfaction of professionals have not been collected. Professional quality of care (docQoC) was analysed in Care Keys by using the InDEX instrument. It contains a checklist for the evaluation of QoC as documented in the care documentation. The checklist was designed to cover the professional perspective on input, process and outcome (except for job satisfaction). Unfortunately, the documentation systems were not always sufficiently detailed and complete, thus, the information from the checklists was incomplete. Therefore, we have collapsed the matrix and the causal model in the professional perspective using all items to evaluate docQoC in the four dimensions of quality, while eliminating the distinction between input, process and outcome in the production dimension of care. A first important result from the analyses was that the items, in fact, revealed a structure of four dimensions (by confirmative factor analysis) for IC and HC. The factors were identified as "client oriented care concept" (dimension I), "care procedures" (dimension II), "care resources" (dimension III) and "teamwork" (dimension IV) and the factor scores were used to measure docQoC for each client.

Similarly, for sQoC as evaluated by the client the scales in the client interview (CLINT instrument) were analysed. Again, a satisfactory four-dimensional solution could be extracted corresponding to the theoretical framework. The factors were identified as "client centeredness" (I), respecting "client autonomy" (II), supporting "environment/resources" (III) and "client satisfaction" (IV). The client process factor was represented by scores for each of the dimensions of sQoC arguing that the perception of the client should reflect the quality of the care interaction. The factors correspond also to the four-dimensional description of sQoL in the CK model and its measurement by the WHOQoL-Bref (see Chapter 4).

Finally, docQoL has been analysed, as mentioned above, using the need and supply information assessed in a four-dimensional profile following the "Lawtonian model", that is, social (I), physical (II), environmental/IADL (III) and psychological (IV) needs (see Chapter 11). The TEFF-value H describing for each individual the needs-responsiveness of care was used to indicate a documented care-related (improvement of) QoL (docQoL). In this case, the four-dimensional structure could be confirmed by the empirical data only for

HC, because the psychological items did not produce an own factor for IC. This is an interesting effect in itself, since it indicates the lack of systematic support in this dimension, or at least its documentation. However, for the calculation of H for docQoL in four dimensions, not the factor scores were used, but scores provided by the TEFF-module (calculating also the TEFF-values for management outcomes; Chapter 13). Here psychological items are included on the basis of expert evaluations of the care documentation.

The empirical confirmation of the four-dimensional quality structure for QoC and QoL follows not necessarily from the fact that we tried to construct the scales and questionnaire items in concordance with the theoretical framework. Thus, it provides important validity to the theoretical approach. Altogether 16 indicators — QoC and QoL, both subjective and documented, in four quality dimensions — were eventually selected as dependent variables. An overview is included in the tabulation analysed in the next section (Tables 12.3 and 12.4).

The 16 indicators for the management perspective were selected from different sources. One problem was that the data from ManDEX—as indicated above—were not complete or not satisfactory. Still, indicators could be selected and scales be constructed obtaining indicators (at least one) for each cell, most of which turned out to be significant in the analyses.

For the *input* cells two indicators for each dimension were selected: "concept general" is a factor score derived from the checklist on quality standards including care-related standards, "QM-concept" comprises standards of quality management (both dimension I); a checklist of standards for procedures of risk management produced a factor for medical standards ("risks medical") and for care standards ("risks social") (both dimension II); resource information was largely incomplete, therefore, the indicators focus on environmental features (single room, email use in IC; safety technology, infrastructure in HC) (dimension III); the scale for cooperation partners yielded also two factors distinguishing medical care (coop medical) and social care partners (coop social) (both dimension IV).

For the *process* factors, two items for compliance with quality management standards could be selected for the concept dimension (one indicating teams/case conferences, the other staff surveys/external counselling (dimension I); the items were not the same for IC and HC due to missing data). For the quality of process procedures we used different scales for (i) measuring the frequency of missing items in the care documentation (docu complete), and (ii) measuring whether the items were missing in special parts (e.g. anamneses) or evenly over the documentation (docu unbiased) (both dimension II). The scales were calculated for each of the four dimensions in the TEFF-module separately, but only two scales were significant in HC *and* IC and selected. The measure for resource utilisation (dimension III) is only a proximate measure to be interpreted with care, since it reflects only the subjective estimate of the manager that resource goals were achieved (resource utilisation). For the cooperation dimension (IV), again, two items — combined into one indicator (coop activities)—were available to indicate cooperation and conflict management with staff and informal carers.

Finally, we used as documented *outcome* the TEFF-values of equity (I), supply efficiency (II) and resource availability (III) (calculated in each of the four dimensions of needs, but selecting only two common indicators for IC and HC for the analyses) together with two cooperation scales (IV) (medical/social partners). For subjective outcome we used the answers of managers to questions on subjective evaluation of their performance (satisfaction with effectiveness (I), efficiency (II), resource availability (III), cooperation (IV)). Altogether, 26 management indicators (out of 63) were selected for the 16 cells that were analysed for their impact on 16 dependent variables (see Tables 12.3 and 12.4).

Some comments on the variables used in this research analysis are necessary: First, the process dimension implies a temporal order, which renders the causal impact interpretation meaningful. However, it is a problem that the time of information collection and documentation was determined by the care documentation. For instance, assessments of client background and health status may be conducted only at the entrance to the service, and different time durations may have elapsed for different clients at the time of documentation analysis. The Care Keys database does not systematically control for time, but uses information extracted from the documentation over a period of up to 6 months. Second, client input is also important as a management input factor, since the mix of clients should be controlled by management to assure that there is a fit between the service capacities and the client's affordances. "Easy" clients will make successful care easy, but may lead to a waste of resources; "risk clients" will lead to "poor" performance measures, if this selection is not adequately reflected in the evaluation of outcomes. Third, the management indicators had to be revised after the pilot study and they clearly need more research. Especially, the input indicators for resources proved to be difficult to study because the services have already their own and quite different indicators in use and not all of them were prepared to provide the information for the pilot study. From a practical point of view this is not necessarily a problem, because the Q-MAT — especially in the management part — may be filled with own indicators. From a research perspective it was a problem, because the investigation of reliability and validity of Care Keys indicators was restricted to available common indicators of services from five countries.

Keeping the limited validity and reliability of the selected indicators in mind, there are still significant and interesting results, which certainly have to be further analysed and checked. To gain a first insight into the rather complex data structure, we invite the reader to abstract from the particular indicators used and to look at the more theoretical variables identified by the cells of the quality matrix. The indicators were chosen, after all, to represent these more theoretical concepts, and the dimensional structure — generally supported by the empirical analyses—provides an orientation for the analyses and interpretations. Thus, we will focus on patterns of significant relationships between dimensions in the quality matrix rather than on single indicators (and their causes or effects).

Results 1: Management Styles and Cluster Analyses

To identify "styles of management" (patterns of management indicators) in the Care Keys database we performed a cluster analysis—separately for HC and IC—on all 63 management indicators clustering the services according to their similarity. The WARD method was used and compared with alternative methods to establish the stability of the solution. Only few variables had to be omitted because of missing values or because of high correlations with other included variables (not desirable in cluster analysis). Thus, a set of indicators covering all 16 cells and dimensions could be identified (32 for HC; 37 for IC) to describe the clusters (differences tested by analysis of variance). In Table 12.1 and Table 12.2, an overview is presented for HC and IC, respectively, which shows only one indicator for each dimension selecting those indicators that were obtained in the IC *and* HC analyses (or proved to be significant in

TABLE 12.1. HC clusters with 4 × 4 management dimensions and dependent quality indicators.

		Cluster 1 "Scandinavian"	Cluster 2 "German"	Cluster 3 "mixed"
Cluster indicators				
Input	I. Concept (QM-strategies)	−	+	
	II. Risk procedures (care)	−	−	+
	III. Ressources (infrastructure)		+	−
	IV. Cooperation (not sig.)			
Process	I. QM-strategies (formal)		−	+
	II. Documentation quality	+	−	
	III. Ressources (not sig.)			
	IV. Cooperation activities		−	+
doc. Out-come	I. Equity	+		−
	II. Efficiency (V)	+	−	−
	III. Resource availability (H/V)	+		−
	IV. Cooperation (medical)	+		−
Subj. Out-come	I. Effectiveness (satisfaction)	+		−
	II. Efficiency (satisfaction)	−	+	
	III. Resources (satisfaction)		−	+
	IV. Cooperation (not sig.)			
Dependent indicators				
sQoL	Subjective QoL	+		−
docQoL	Documented QoL	+		−
sQoC	Subjective QoC		+	−
docQoC	Documented QoC		−	+

Distribution of clients (*n* = 223) by cluster and country

Frequency

		Cluster			
		1	2	3	Total
Country	1 Finland	32	0	3	35
	2 Sweden	49	0	0	49
	3 Estonia	2	6	40	48
	5 Germany	0	70	21	91
Total		83	76	64	223

TABLE 12.2. IC clusters with 4×4 management dimensions and dependent quality indicators.

		Cluster 1 "other"	Cluster 2 "Finnish"
Cluster indicators			
Input	I. Concept (QM-strategies)	+	−
	II. Risk procedures (medical)	+	−
	III. Resources (single beds)	+	−
	IV. Cooperation (not sig.)		
Process	I. QM-strategies (formal)	−	+
	II. Documentation quality	−	+
	III. Resources (not sig.)		
	IV. Cooperation activities	+	−
Obj. Out-come	I. Equity	−	+
	II. Efficiency (V)	−	+
	III. Resource availability (H/V)	+	−
	IV. Cooperation (medical)	+	−
Subj. Out-come	I. Effectiveness (not sig.)		
	II. Efficiency (not sig.)		
	III. Resources (not sig.)		
	IV. Cooperation (not sig.)		
Dependent indicators			
sQoL	Subjective QoL	−	+
docQoL	Documented QoL	−	+
sQoC	Subjective QoC	−	+
docQoC	Documented QoC	−	+

Distribution of clients (*n* = 223) by cluster and country

		Cluster		
		1	2	Total
Country	1 Finland	0	42	42
	2 Sweden	44	0	44
	3 Estonia	49	0	49
	5 Germany	88	0	88
Total		181	42	223

subsequent regression analyses). In the table, "+" signifies that a cluster has a relatively high value in that dimension, "−" signifies that a cluster has a relatively low value, no entry signifies a middle position or that the dimension is not distinguishing significantly. The clusters were then considered as independent variables to investigate their effect (by variance analysis) on the dependent variables of sQoL, docQoL, sQoC and docQoC.

The *cluster analysis for HC* suggested three clusters. As the addition to Table 12.1 shows, the first Nordic or "Scandinavian" cluster contains Finnish and Swedish services, the second "German" cluster contains German cases and the third "mixed" cluster combines Estonian, German and some Finnish cases. Looking first at the effects of the clusters, the "Scandinavian" cluster has better care outcomes for QoL, while the QoC indicators are (slightly) better for the other clusters. Inspecting the four dimensions of QoL and QoC (not shown in Table 12.1), the clusters have a significant effect on all four subjective and documented QoL dimensions (social, physical, environmental, psychological). In addition, three dimensions of sQoC (except client control) and three dimensions of docQoC (except client orientation) show significant differences between the clusters.

Interestingly, the "Scandinavians" are less claiming to apply quality standards (input), but have a better care documentation and clearly better documented management outcomes (i.e. equity, efficiency, resource availability and cooperation with medical partners). The "German" cluster has a medium performance, but claims the application of more quality standards, whereas the "*mixed*" type seems to combine the low performers from all countries. Strangely enough, this type also shows a better profile of docQoC. In HC, the "soft" conceptual input and process factors from the manager interviews (cluster 2 and 3) tend to go along with better care, but not with better care outcomes (cluster 1). This contrasts with IC (see below), where the more formal (and medical) qualities of management correspond with better QoC *and* better care outcomes. In HC the management style does have an impact on QoL, although different clusters show positive outcomes for QoL and QoC, the effects do not correspond. Finally, it is surprising and not easily interpreted that the "Scandinavians" see themselves as effective (subjective outcome), but not very efficient; the "Germans" see themselves as efficient, but in lack of resources; and the "mixed" group believes to have enough resources, but sees itself as relatively less effective. Perhaps even more interesting is the fact that the subjective evaluations of managers of their own performance do play a role in HC, while they are non-significant in IC. It supports a tendency in the data that "management matters" more for outcomes in HC and rather independently from QoC, while in IC we find a strong effect of QoM on QoC.

The *cluster analysis for IC* (Table 12.2) suggests distinguishing only two groups, the "Finnish" and "Others". (A three cluster solution did separate the Finnish services from the Swedish ones, but this solution was not confirmed sufficiently by alternative clustering methods.) Looking first at the dependent effects again, it is obvious that the "Finnish" have the better outcomes including QoC. However, the effects are not so prominent as in HC, because only one dimension (environmental) is significant in subjective and docQoL, only one dimension in sQoC (psychological), and only two dimensions of docQoC (procedures, teamwork) (not shown in Table 21.1).

Again, the "Finnish" do less claim to apply quality standards, but have better management outcomes in equity and efficiency. The cooperation indicators are worse, but this may be due to the fact that the Finnish care system is differentiated more internally within organisations of the municipality and requires less cooperation across boundaries. As noted already, the subjective evaluations of performance by managers do not distinguish between the clusters, which may correspond to a less pronounced effect of management styles on outcomes and a higher impact of QoC in the case of IC (see below).

Comparing HC and IC we note that the Finnish services have in both cases better outcomes, although the effect of management on outcomes appears to be larger for HC. Analysing the dimensions responsible for the good performance, the cluster profiles suggest that better values on "hard" indicators obtained from the care documentation (documentation quality, docQoM outcomes) produce favourable outcomes, while better values on "soft" interview items obtained from managers (input) do not ensure good performance.

There is an important effect in the results, though, which speaks for the high quality of the Finnish care system. Not only the quality of the documentation is better, but also the values for the achievement of equity in all four dimensions, both in HC and IC (except for the psychological dimension of HC in cluster 2 as Figs. 12.2 and 12.3 show). It is also interesting to note that the social dimension appears to be the least equitable, and that especially the "German cluster" has unfavourable equity values in the social dimension in HC. This would correspond to the fragmented German system, but this clearly needs more inquiry into the relationships and impacts, especially since the "German cluster" claims to realise more quality standards than the Finnish one.

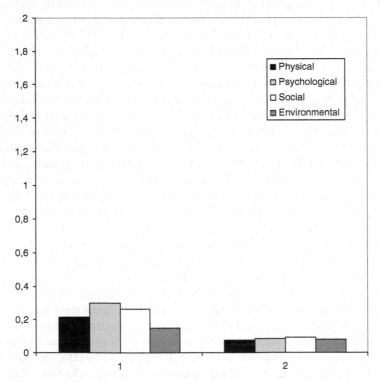

FIG. 12.2. IC "Finnish cluster" (2) and "Other cluster" (1) and their equity (TEFF-values) (note that lower values indicate higher equity).

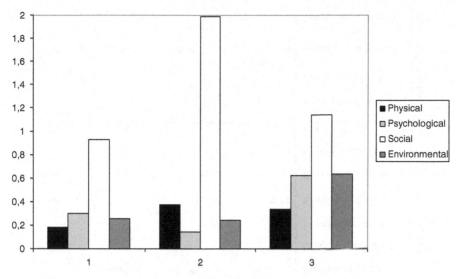

FIG. 12.3. HC "Finnish cluster" (1), "German cluster" (2) and "mixed cluster" (3) and their equity (TEFF-values) (note that lower values indicate higher equity).

Results 2: Impact Analyses in the Quality Matrix

A practical method in quality management for the analysis of relationships and impacts of a large number of variables is to present them in a matrix tabulating variables against each other. Analysing the number of impacts *of* a given variable, the number of impacts *on* a given variable, and clusters of relations provides a first insight into the complexity of interrelations. In the following analysis we make use of this method. The impacts will be characterised by significant independent effects (significance at 0.05 level, established in a multiple stepwise regression analysis introducing all variables considered in the present quality matrix). Rather than combining all variables in one large table, we will utilise our causal model and look at the effects of management factors on QoC and on QoL, and, in turn, of QoC factors as intermediate causes on QoL outcomes (see Tables 12.3–12.5). As stated above, only significant relationships are depicted and marked by a letter "P" for a positive independent impact and by "N" for a negative impact. For the present, we have limited the variables to (one or) two indicators for each of the four management dimension and selected variables, which were included in the cluster analyses above. Since each entry marks a significant relationship, there are many effects to be considered, but we will discuss—in this first analysis—only especially interesting patterns, and focus on a comparison of HC and IC. We should keep in mind that — given the chosen significance level — we should expect in any part of the matrix about 5% significant entries, both positive and negative, by chance alone.

TABLE 12.3. Impact analyses for home care (HC).

Impact on:	QoM-Input								QoM-Process						QoM-Obj. Outcome								QoM-Subj. Outcome			
	Concept general I	QM-concept I	Risks medical II	Risks social II	Environ. Technology III	Environm. Infrastr III	Coop medical IV	Coop social IV	QM-teams I	QM-formal I	Docu-complete II	Docu-unbiased II	Resource utilisation III	Coop activities IV	Equity physical I	Equity environmental I	Efficiency physical II	Efficiency environm. II	Resources physical III	Resources environm. III	Coop medical IV	Coop social IV	Effectiveness subj. I	Efficiency subj. II	Resources subj. III	Cooperation subj. IV
docQoL-social	N										P				N		P		P	P					P	
docQoL-physical	N															N			P	P					N	
docQoL-environmental					P	P																				
docQoL-psychological											N		N	N									P			P
sQoL-social						P		P												P	P					
sQoL-physical					P	P		P				P						P		P	N				N	
sQoL-environm.					P	P		P												P					N	
sQoL-psychol	P										P					N										
sQoC: Cl. Orient		P			N	P			P					P	P					N	P					
sQoC: Cl. Control			P			P			P	N	N											P			N	
sQoC: Environm.			P	N	P																					
sQoC: Psycholog.					P																			N		
docQoC: Cl. Orient.	P			P			N	N		P	P	P			P	N	P			P	N	P	P	N	N	
docQoC: Procedures								P		P	N	P			P	N	N		N			P			N	
docQoC: Environm.								N			P									P					N	
docQoC: Teamwork					N									N		P				N					P	N

TABLE 12.4. Impact analyses for institutional care (IC).

IC / Impact on:	QoM-Input — Concept general I	QM-concept I	Risks medical II	Risks social II	Environ. single beds III	Tecnlogy (email) III	Coop medical IV	Coop social IV	QoM-Process — QM-staff survey I	QM-case conference I	Docu-complete II	Docu-unbiased II	Resource utilisation III	Coop activities IV	QoM-Obj. Outcome — Equity physical I	Equity environmental I	Efficiency physical II	Efficiency environm. II	Resources physical III	Resources environm. III	Coop medical IV	Coop social IV	QoM-Subj. Outcome — Effectiveness subj. I	Efficiency subj. II	Resources subj. III	Cooperation subj. IV
docQoL-social	N	N	P	N	N	N	N		P	N	N		N	N	P		P		P					N	P	
docQoL-physical		N			P	N			P		N	N	N	N				P	P	P		N	N	P		
docQoL-environmental				N	P	N				N				N				P	P	P				P		
docQoL-psychological									P															P		
sQoL-social			N		P														N					P		
sQoL-physical									P			P							N					P		
sQoL-environm.			N		P										P											
sQoL-psychol.																						P	P			
sQoC: Cl. orient.		N	P	N																	N	P	N	P	P	
sQoC: Cl. Control																										
sQoC: Environm.			N																							
sQoC: Psycholog.					P							P	N						N							
docQoC: Cl. Orient.	N	N	P	P	P	N	P	N	P	N	P		N	N	P			P	P		N	N		P		
docQoC: Procedures		N	P	N	P	N		N	N	N			N		P	P			P		N			P	P	
docQoC: Environm.		N	N	P	P	N					P					N			N			P		P	P	
docQoC: Teamwork		N	P	P	P	N						P	N						N	N			P	P		

TABLE 12.5. Impact analyses for documented QoC (docQoC).

Documented QoC Impact on:	IC				HC			
	docQoC: Client I	docQoC: Procedures II	docQoC: Environm. III	docQoC: Teamwork IV	docQoC: Client orient. I	docQoC: Procedures II	docQoC: Environm. III	docQoC: Teamwork IV
docQoL-social	N		P				P	
docQoL-physical	P	P	P	P		P		
docQoL-environmental		P	P	P				N
docQoL-psychological	P	P	P	P				
sQoC: Client orientation	N	P	P			N		P
sQoC: Client control	N							N
sQoC: environmental								
sQoC: psychological		P		P				
sQoL-social		P	P	P				
sQoL-physical								
sQoL-environmental			P	P				N
sQoL-psychological		P	P	P				

Patterns consisting of predominantly positive or negative entries (or no entries) will call for an interpretation.

(a) Effects between factors of QoM

Following the TQM approach we first considered the influences of management variables on other management variables (e.g. the "flow" of influence in the management perspective of Fig. 12.1) by tabulating the variables against each other. In this table (not shown here) we find only few, scattered significant impacts, which we will leave for further and more detailed analyses. This holds for HC and IC. Certainly, in the framework of TQM we would expect more impacts than can be observed in the table. We have to conclude that indicators may turn out to produce some specific significant impacts, but are not strongly enough related to each other to represent a consistent management strategy producing concerted effects.

(b) Effects of QoM on docQoC and sQoC

Even a short glance at Tables 12.3 and 12.4 reveals that the impact of QoM variables on documented QoC is much larger in IC than in HC. There is a puzzling pattern of positive and negative impacts, but the frequency is much higher in IC, especially for QoM input and process (IC = 33 entries; HC = 14 entries). This result should be expected, since the impact of management on care practices should be stronger in the context of a residential institution than in homecare settings.

Looking especially at IC, we observe a quite consistent negative impact of QoM (except sQoM outcome) on docQoC in the dimension of care procedures ("how to do things right"), whereas the impacts on dimensions of client-oriented care, care resources and teamwork are positive. The dimension of procedures combines items, which quite narrowly refer to methods of care and might be expected to relate negatively to more comprehensive strategies of quality management. On the other hand, the self-evaluation of managers as "efficient" has a strong positive effect on all dimensions of docQoC (and QoL, see below). Then, we observe in IC that quality assurance standards (concept formal, case conferences), use of (email) technology, self-evaluated resource utilisation and cooperation with social partners (coop social) are negatively related to docQoC. Considering that QoM indicators have only moderate effects on care outcomes while docQoC has a noticeable influence (see below) this speaks for a somewhat independent and intermediate role of docQoC in IC with regard to management strategies, and an unaccepted role of quality management in IC.

In HC, the effects of QoM are much less pronounced and scattered with an interesting exception. Cooperation with social partners (vs. medical partners) relates negatively with the medically dominated aspects of docQoC (procedures, teamwork with physician).

For both HC and IC, the subjective QoM outcomes (self-evaluation by managers) has a surprisingly strong relation to docQoC. However, in HC, we find five negative (!) relations indicating that managers who evaluate their own performance critically are associated with better care performance as reflected in the documentation.

Comparing management effects on sQoC with docQoC the impacts are distinctly less frequent for sQoC. Interestingly, the effects are somewhat more pronounced in HC, again pointing to a higher impact of QoM in HC. Two effects might deserve special attention: (i) The indicators for environmental conditions and technology use show a high impact in HC, but are of little influence in IC, except for a somewhat puzzling strong effect of (email) technology use on docQoC (see above) and docQoL(see below). However, this effect is not substantiated in the subjective perspectives of QoC and QoL in IC. (ii) The relation of subjective QoM outcomes (self-evaluation) is rather negative in HC, which might speak again for the better performance of managers who see—especially the availability of resources (!)—rather critically. The pattern for IC renders itself not that easily to interpretation.

(c) Effects of QoM on subjective QoL and documented QoL

Following the theoretical framework, we would expect a larger impact of QoM on QoL in an institutional setting, since the institution affects the entire life of the residents. However, as Tables 12.3 and 12.4 show, there are stronger impacts on the docQoL in IC, but in HC we find more substantial impacts on sQoL than in IC. Looking more closely at specific patterns, it appears that the relations of QoM to sQoL in HC are to be found especially in the dimension of environment (safety technology, home environment), equity and resource availability (QoM input,

QoM outcome). This impact has to be interpreted with care, though, because the home environment cannot be influenced by management. Additionally, we find a strong impact of cooperation with social partners. Both findings confirm our expectations and correspond to the support services given in HC.

In IC, only the self-evaluation of managers as "efficient" relates clearly positive to sQoL (corresponding to the effect on most dependent variables). However, more puzzling is that most significant relations of QoM input and process to docQoL are, in fact, negative in IC. This corresponds to the frequent negative impacts we found on docQoC, while (see below) docQoC has a clear positive impact on docQoL. Management outcome measures, on the other hand, show a substantial positive impact in HC and IC.

(d) Effects of subjective QoM (self-evaluation) on QoC and QoL

A somewhat unexpected and puzzling result is that subjective evaluations of performance by managers do have a rather strong impact on all dependent variables, but very selective and different for IC and HC. In HC the self-evaluation of "having enough resources" appears to correlate negatively with docQoC and docQoL. In IC there is a surprisingly strong pattern of positive impact of the evaluation of "being efficient" as a manager on all dependent variables. Somehow a critical view towards the lack (?) of resources helps to provide good outcomes for clients in HC, whereas in IC managers with a self-image as efficient produce better outcomes.

(e) Effects of documented QoC

As indicated above, one important result influencing and mediating the impact of QoM appears to be the fact that in IC docQoC has a quite consistent effect on almost all dimensions of QoL, both documented and subjective, while it has much less influence in HC (Table 12.5). Only the subjective functional or health status of the client as captured in the "physical" dimension and the satisfaction with IADL/environmental support (sQoC environmental) seem not to be impacted by docQoC in IC. Puzzling are the negative impacts of docQoC teamwork on particularly the environmental dimensions of QoL, which point to a conflict between the medical character of the teamwork (with physician) and the social character of the environmental dimension (IADL services/environmental adaptations). The general finding supports our thesis about the impact of IC, since the QoL and the (importance of) QoC should be expected to depend less on care services in HC.

(f) Relations between docQoL, sQoL and sQoC

Subjective QoC and QoL are interdependent factors which should be interpreted as facets of a broader concept of care-related QoL (see Chapter 4). Their dependencies on care and their interrelations are analysed in more detail elsewhere (Chapters 8 and 9). To summarise the results in the four-dimensional framework employed in this management perspective (tables not presented here), we note that sQoC and sQoL are strongly related in (almost) all dimensions in HC and

IC. In both situations, life quality seems to be affected strongly by the way care is perceived, supporting the concept of care-related QoL, and the relationship suggests sQoC as a good proximate outcome indicator especially in HC. Between sQoL and docQoL more selective, but substantial relations are observed. In HC, the social dimension apparently is not affected by care contributions as documented—quite in correspondence to our expectations, since social relations are typically more independent from care in HC (in IC they might be reduced to other residents). In IC especially and surprisingly the support services (IADL and environment) have an impact on sQoL, which runs counter to our expectations that these services are more important in HC.

Discussion

There are differences between IC and HC, which go along with a more theoretical interpretation of the different settings of care suggested in the research theses above, and there are also results, which do not fit. The analyses of the management styles reveal the relative strong performance of the Finnish care system, both in IC and HC. However, the results also show the somewhat unexpected effect that professional and medical care-oriented styles appear to produce better performance for the client—this is disappointing in the sense that the Finnish performance is not better in terms of more "soft" indicators on quality concepts and cooperation and better with respect to "hard" evidence of professionalism as indicated by the quality of the documentation. However, it has to be emphasised, too, that among those "hard" indicators are also measures of equity, which consistently speak for the greater social justice realised in the Finnish care system.

As a kind of summary, it might be noted that the four-dimensional structure of the quality matrix receives substantial support by the analyses. Factors and effects in all four dimensions proved to be connected to significant relationships, even though a consistent TQM strategy does not appear from the investigations. The first theses suggested that successful quality management would include a good risk management, because of the special situation in health care. This could not clearly be established, since, on the one hand, standards of risk management are claimed to be in place by those services, which do not have the best outcomes. On the other hand, risk standards have a significant influence, especially in IC. But again, the effect is mixed with strong positive and negative effects. Taking into account that indicators of quality management tend to have a negative effect on QoC and QoL, while docQoC has a positive effect, one is tempted to conclude that QM-strategies are at odds with effective and efficient care in IC and of limited effect in HC. Still, the managers in IC who see themselves as very efficient do have good results.

A summary of the results of the impact analyses is provided in Figs. 12.4a and 12.4b. The expectation of a closer chain of effects in IC than in HC is

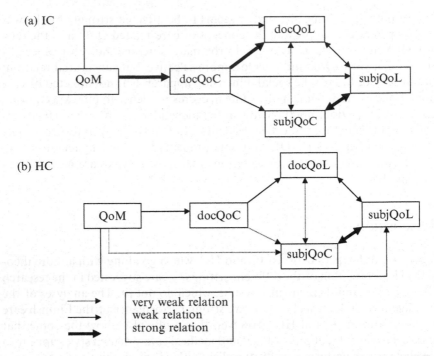

FIG. 12.4. (a) Impacts of Quality of Management (QoM) in institutional care (IC). (b) Impacts of Quality of Management (QoM) in home care (HC).

supported by the analyses. But again, the results are somewhat mixed. While in IC there is a clearly stronger influence of QoM strategies on docQoC and docQoL, the combined effects on the subjective measures of QoC and QoL tend to be stronger in HC. As Figs. 12.4a and 12.4b display, there are more independent direct effects of QoM on subjective care outcomes in HC than in IC. This may be due to the special situation of cooperation in HC, which we expected. It may also reflect the fact that HC services tend to be smaller organisations, which would enhance the direct influence of management on care outcomes. Or, the result may be due to the low response rate in the care documentation in HC. We also expected for HC that there is a stronger effect of cooperation with social partners, and a less prominent role of social aspects of the care itself because of the role of informal or family support (see also Chapter 8). Both effects are confirmed.

In IC, professional care appears to be mediating management strategies and have a more autonomous impact on care outcomes. This goes along with the expected larger role of medical teamwork and cooperation with medical partners. However, we need further research to understand why the more conceptual or non-material input by quality management in IC does not directly and positively relate to care quality as reflected in the care documentation, while on the other hand documented QoC has a strong positive impact on care outcomes for the client.

Conclusions

Clearly, the complexity of the interrelationships in the quality matrix and in the care process has to be further analysed. This has also been demonstrated by other contributions to this volume on the relation between QoC and QoL. The most important result of the analyses of QoM indicators and styles has been that there is, in fact, a demonstrable impact of QoM on QoC and QoL. The effects observed do not support a view that there is a consistent TQM strategy already realised in the more successful services producing good care outcomes. However, all factors or dimensions of successful management identified in the theoretical framework revealed significant impacts. Thus, the basic approach appears to be confirmed. The management situations in HC and in IC are quite different, and especially in IC, a "medical model" appears to be associated with better care outcomes, whereas in HC a "socio-cultural model" involving other social partners tends to have better outcomes for the clients. A finding that clearly needs further research is the precarious role of quality management in IC, which seems to be at odds with standards of good care.

Another important result consists of the confirmation of the four-dimensional structure of the quality matrix for QoM as well as for QoC and QoL measures. For QoM indicators this could not be established directly, but it certainly speaks for the validity of the framework, that indicators of all four dimensions proved to be significant in the cluster analyses and impact analyses. In a framework of TQM, this result was to be expected, but under the varying conditions in HC and IC and in different countries this result was not self-evident.

References

Bowers, B. J., Fibich, B., & Jacobson, N. (2001). Care-as-service, care-as-relating, care-as-comfort: Understanding nursing home resident's definition of quality. *The Gerontologist,41,*(4), 539–545.

Bruhn, M. (2003). *Qualitätsmanagement für Dienstleistungen (Quality management for services)*. Berlin: Springer Publisher.

Bullinger, H.-J., & Scheer, A.-W. (Eds.). (2006). *Service engineering*. Berlin: Springer Publisher.

Currie, V., Harvey, G., West, E., McKenna, H., & Keeney, S. (2005). Relationships between quality of care, staffing levels, skill mix and nurse autonomy: Literature review. *Journal of Advanced Nursing, 51*, 73–82.

Donabedian, A. (1969). Some issues in evaluation the quality of nursing care. *American Journal of Public Health, 59*, 1833–1836.

Evers, A., Haverinen, R., Leichsenring, K., & Wistow, G. (Eds.). (1997). *Developing quality in personal social services. Concepts, cases and comments*. Aldershot: Ashgate.

Friedag, H. R., & Schmidt, W. (2004). Balanced Scorecard, Planegg bei München.

Görres, St. (1999). *Qualitätssicherung in Pflege und Medizin (Quality assurance in care and medicine)*. Bern: Huber Publisher.

Lawton, M. P. (1991). A multidimensional view of quality of life in frail elders. In J. E. Birren, J. E. Lubben, J. C. Rowe, & D. E. Deutchman (Eds.), *The concept and measurement of quality of life in frail elders* (pp. 3–27). San Diego, CA: Academic Press.

Niven, P. R. (2003). Balanced Scorecard—Schritt für Schritt, Weiheim.

Øvretveit, J. (1998). *Evaluating health interventions. An introduction to evaluation of health treatments, services, policies and organizational interventions*. Buckingham, Philadelphia, PA: Open University Press.

Owen, T., NCHRDF (Eds.). (2006). *My home life — quality of life in care homes*. London.

Reichwald, R., & Schaller, Ch. (2006). *Innovationsmanagement von Dienstleistungen—* Herausforderungen und Erfolgfaktoren in der Praxis. In H.-J. Bullinger, A.-W. Scheer (eds.). Service engineering. Berlin: Springer Publisher.

Vaarama, M., & Pieper, R. (2005). Managing integrated care for older persons. European perspectives and good practices. Stakes and European Health Management Association. Saarijärvi: Gummerrus Publishing Oy.

Veenhoven, R. (2000). The four qualities of Life. Ordering concept and measures of the good life. *Journal of Happiness Studies*, *1*, 1–39.

13
The Care Keys Toolkit

Richard Pieper, Marja Vaarama, Gunnar Ljunggren
and Thomas Emilsson

Introduction

The aim of the Care Keys project was to make a contribution to the
improvement of long-term care on the level of the theory of care and care-
related quality of life, on the level of empirical enquiry into the relationships
between care and care outcomes, and on the level of practical instruments
and tools for care quality management. The theoretical and empirical
results have been described elsewhere in this book, and this chapter
will briefly describe the practical outcomes of the research (additional
information and prototypes of the tools are available on the project website www.carekeys.net). The main objective was to develop a set of "key
indicators" that could be used to guide care quality management, and to
take the first steps in developing instruments and tools for practitioners
using these indicators.

Combining a practical approach with the research objectives was
motivated by two considerations. First, it is increasingly recognised that
research has to look into the prospects and problems of dissemination
and implementation of its results, if it wants to have an impact on practice. Simply to assume that good research results will find their way into
care practice and to leave matters of implementation to educationalists
or practitioners appears to be ineffective. At least the first steps towards
practical implementation have to be taken by practice-oriented research
to provide an "interface". Second, many of the partners in the Care Keys
project were directly involved in social and health care services and were
well aware of the pressing need for practical improvements within their
own arenas.

The pursuit of being able to disseminate the Care Keys research findings
to the practice resulted in development of a "Toolkit" intended for use primarily by care and quality managers in long-term care of older people, but
also researchers and consultants in the field may benefit of it. The Care Keys
Toolkit comprises a number of tools that were developed and validated within
the Care Keys research: data collection tools, key indicators and a number of

analytical tools. The different parts of the toolkit can be used at different levels: some at a locality or provider level, some at a community level and some at the national level. The Care Keys Toolkit will support efforts to monitor, plan and develop high-quality care for clients of long-term care in both institutional settings and homecare. The functionality of the toolkit aims at the evaluation and management of:

1. quality of long-term homecare and institutional care of older persons;
2. effectiveness of care in contributing to the quality of life of the clients;
3. comprehensiveness of care in contributing to diverse domains of the client's QoL;
4. efficiency of resource use in terms of meeting the client needs and targeting care resources according to their needs;
5. equity of distribution of the care resources;
6. quality management in facilitating the achievement of the goals already mentioned.

Currently, the toolkit is still under construction with some instruments being already tested in practical contexts, while others are developed further. This will be indicated in the descriptions below.

Objectives, Concepts and Contexts of the Toolkit

The practical objectives were guided by a number of basic orientations. First motivation was the idea that care practice needs a stronger orientation towards the needs and perspectives of the clients ("clients first"). In the context of developing tools for care, this implied that the "final outcome" of care, the subjective quality of life of clients, should be measured by practical procedures and instruments. However, it is also necessary to include the views of all relevant "stakeholders" in the care process, that is not only the perspective of the client, but also the perspectives of professional carers, of management and (whenever possible) the view of relatives or other informal providers of support for the client (see Chapters 5 and 6). The instruments need to collect information from all these sources, but recognising the relevance of information from different sources is not enough; it is also important that this information is used in a knowledge-based and goal-oriented way. Care should focus on the well-being of the client, but it must, at the same time, reflect on the appropriateness, effectiveness, efficiency and equity of care, which can be supported by quality standards, good care documentation and tools for evaluation.

In addition, the practical approach was guided by an orientation towards information technologies and their increasing role in care provision and management. The tools and instruments should be, in principle, implemented as software to support information processing and evaluation. However, it is vital that this is done in a way that reduces the information load to what is necessary for care and care management on different levels. The general objective was to specify a "minimum set" of indicators relevant for quality evaluation. Documentation systems in care already tend to be very comprehensive and demanding in their application. In the Care Keys project, the aim was to identify important information for quality improvement, but at the same time to avoid increasing the requirements for additional information collection by trying to exploit as much as possible the data that were already available. As it turned out, this was difficult to achieve because the existing documentation systems are generally inadequate for the type of a multi-dimensional care evaluation and quality improvements the Care Keys Toolkit is intended to support.

Any attempt to provide tools for management of the quality of care will encounter the doubts and criticism that care performance cannot adequately be monitored by standardised and formalised tools. The Care Keys project was well aware of the limitations of such tools, and certainly the proposed toolkit needs to be further developed and adapted to the everyday "realities" of care. But equally, we recognised the necessity to introduce more standardised procedures to improve the quality and performance of care in view of the growing demand for care, as well as to increase accountability, transparency and democracy of performance evaluations. More formal procedures and tools certainly need to be implemented in care practices to support the empowerment of clients and informal carers in participation in the decisions on care. As argued elsewhere (Chapter 6), there is no inherent conflict between knowledge-based procedures and "good care". The Care Keys approach places the toolkit, therefore, in the practical context of a "negotiated order" (Chapter 6) involving all stakeholders, and a Total Quality Management approach. This should ensure that implementation of the tools and procedures are carried out in a cooperative way that is appropriate and adapted to specific care settings.

As described in the theoretical framework (Chapter 1), the key concepts on which the Care Keys research was based were: the production of welfare approach, the target efficiency concept, and a multi-perspective quality evaluation as suggested by Övretveit (1998). The original quality matrix of Övretveit was reinterpreted in Care Keys, distinguishing (i) a production perspective (input–process–documented outcomes–subjective outcomes), (ii) a stakeholder perspective (client–professional carer–care management) and (iii) a four-dimensional quality perspective. The production perspective has to ensure that all relevant stages in the quality chain are represented among the quality indicators. The stakeholder perspective has to add the different interests of the partners in the "co-production" of care. The target efficiency measures provided central indicators for performance evaluation from the management perspective, in addition to those for evaluation of cooperation. The four-dimensional quality perspective introduces a framework—based on social systems theory—for a common differentiation of four quality aspects throughout the entire quality matrix, providing a basis for analyses of quality aspects along the production chain and across the stakeholder perspectives in the matrix (Chapters 4–6). This common quality framework forms a complete

Care Keys Quality Matrix (Q-MAT), which is especially designed to facilitate the communication between all stakeholders, and across issues of quality of life, quality of care and quality of management (see Table 13.1).

Since the goal was to produce a toolkit that would be flexible for use on different levels of care management and different contexts of care, corresponding requirements had to be recognised. Thus, the toolkit will incorporate tools and design features for different levels of care planning, monitoring and evaluation. On a basic operational level of providing care, the care process should be guided by a comprehensive assessment instrument with a good documentation system. The Care Keys Toolkit is not intended for this level, although it can be seen to incorporate a strategic assessment instrument and tools for planning, monitoring and evaluating different elements of care (see the MAssT module later). To fully exploit the toolkit, a good system for needs assessment and care documentation should be in place to provide necessary information for calculation of "key indicators" and for other Care Keys analyses. For the extraction of data from the existing documentation systems, the toolkit includes the InDEX instruments (see Chapter 2). In this sense, the toolkit can also be understood as a guide for the development and evaluation of documentation systems, since it specifies the essential information needed for a multi-actorial evaluation of the quality and performance of care. On the level of care processes, the toolkit endorses a more "strategic" process of planning, monitoring and evaluating individual care that focuses on "key indicators", periodic performance evaluations and experience sharing among staff. The Care Keys Mini-Evaluation Tool (MAssT) is especially designed to support this practice.

The Care Keys Toolkit is intended for use on diverse levels of quality management; (i) on the individual client level; (ii) at the levels of diverse client groups; and (iii) on the level of service organisation or on other aggregated levels in homecare and institutional care. The MAssT module is designed to provide information at the individual client level, but it allows also aggregation, whereas the Target Efficiency module (TEFF module) is especially designed to provide central performance indicators on aggregated levels. The Care Keys Q-MAT combines all relevant information in one matrix, rendering possible a comprehensive quality evaluation. The aggregated "key indicators", the TEFF module and the Q-MAT can also be used at higher levels of management within the care system, provided that procedures to aggregate the data are implemented. In particular, the efficiency and equity of service allocation, aggregated costs, average care performance and client outcome measures are emphasized in the toolkit. The "key indicators" are in most cases identical for homecare and institutional care, supporting the comparison of results across different service types. However, certain indicators, especially concerning the environmental aspects of care are obviously context specific. Nevertheless, the four-dimensional structure of the quality descriptions will allow rather comprehensive and comparative evaluations.

The Structure and Functionality of the Toolkit

Overview

The Care Keys Toolkit comprises instruments for data collection, a set of key indicators, and tools for data analyses in homecare (HC) and institutional care (IC) as follows:

1. The instruments for collecting data

   a. CLINT—an instrument for the interview of the client; CLINT-HC (Homecare) and CLINT-IC (Institutional care).
   b. RELINFO—an instrument for the interview of a relative or a close one.
   c. InDEX—an instrument to extract information from the individual's care documentation; also available for HC and IC.
   d. ManDEX—an instrument to extract information from the documentation system of the organisation and from the management.

2. A database (not implemented yet)

   a. CK-MIDAS—combining the data from all instruments and data calculated by analysing modules.

3. Five tools to analyse and evaluate the quality of care

   a. Key indicators—indicators on quality of life, quality of care and quality of management.
   b. TEFF module—for analyses of the target efficiency (TEFF) of care (effectiveness, efficiency, equity).
   c. MAssT module—for "strategic" evaluation of quality, effectiveness and TEFF of care at the individual client level and aggregated levels.
   d. MAssT-D—same tool but applied for cases of clients with cognitive impairment.
   e. Q-MAT module—the Care Keys Quality Matrix, combining all indicators for management.

The intended structure of the toolkit is illustrated in Fig. 13.1, but–as already noted–the instruments need still further development. Later, when the toolkit is implemented in a software, it will also comprise a database necessary to run the analyses.

The Instruments

CLINT

CLINT is the client interview instrument for use with the clients in homecare (CLINT-HC) and in institutional settings (CLINT-IC) to: (i) gain or to confirm background information that is typically contained in most care documentation systems; (ii) collect self-reports on the need and supply of care in

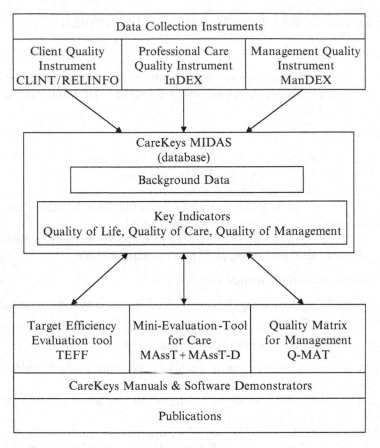

FIG. 13.1. The structure of the Care Keys Toolkit.

four dimensions (physical, psychological, social, environment); (iii) collect self-evaluations on the quality of care and (d) on subjective quality of life, using items from a set of scales (e.g. WHOQOL-Bref, PGCMS). Most of this information is not usually available in the care documentation, this implies that the interview has to be conducted on admission and at suitable intervals (e.g. 6 months) to monitor care performance from the perspective of the clients.

To collect information about quality of care and quality of life with cognitively impaired persons, Care Keys used instruments to collect information from third parties: the QUALID scale, the Cornell Depression Scale and the Care Keys RELINFO instrument. From these, RELINFO is developed for the toolkit, the others are available from the authors or organisations who have developed them (see Chapter 2). QUALID is also, with consent of its developers, included in the MAssT-D module of the Care Keys Toolkit.

InDEX

The instrument is designed to extract essential information from the existing care documentation of individual clients, and versions for HC and IC are available. Since the care documentation may not contain all the required items, it is also a guide for restructuring the documentation. The central parts of InDEX are: (a) background information including general health and functional status of the client, and environmental features at home or in the institution; (b) a list of key care service elements describing care needs and care supply to asses the target efficiency as documented; (c) selected care outcomes as documented; and (d) an evaluation (checklist) of the compliance of documented care to quality standards. Part (b) is essential for the analytical tools and, in effect, requires that care practice and documentation are structured in a way that a description of a client's needs (care plan) and supply (provision) are independently documented as element of a goal oriented care process. Part (d) is essential for performance evaluation and should not only be used as self-evaluation tool for the individual carer, but also as an instrument for "peer review" or supervision, that is integrated in practices of quality assurance among staff.

ManDEX

This instrument is designed to collect all information which characterises the service organisation, for example the homecare service or the residential care institution, rather than the individual client. Special scales address (i) quality concepts/standards in care services, (ii) cooperation with external partners, (iii) available resources, (iv) quality assurance practices and (v) scales for self-evaluation by managers. The instrument addresses the responsible manager(s) at a given level. Future development of ManDEX should provide several parts, containing also contributions from staff (e.g. feedback on job satisfaction) and compliance is the quality management procedures implemented. Since some of the information (e.g. information on personnel costs) may be available only at certain levels of the organisation, the instrument has to be adapted to the existing management structure. The instrument provides a structure for *types* of information to be used in quality management (rather than a fixed set of indicators validated by research), although some key indicators are suggested by the Care Keys, research, and by the MAssT and TEFF modules. Still, the Quality Matrix is open to the inclusion of an organisation's own indicators as implemented in existing quality management procedures (similarly to the Balanced Scorecard, see Chapter 6).

CK-MIDAS

The module is not yet implemented, but is intended to combine all data collected by diverse Care Keys instruments to build up a Care Keys Database for calculation of the "key indicators" and other Care Keys analyses, and to save the output of analyses (e.g. TEFF indicators of effectiveness, efficiency and equity) in the database. A special module that enables feeding the information into a comprehensive software version of the Care Keys Toolkit, and also providing user-friendly output functions (e.g. texts, graphs, tables) is not yet implemented, but would clearly be desirable. In particular, the InDEX and parts of ManDEX should be implemented as a software module that extracts the information (e.g. care needs and supply) directly from existing electronic documentation systems. However, given the restrictions of the Care Keys project in focusing on the empirical identification of "key indicators", the development of this comprehensive software was not possible, and will be pursued in future research projects. The scope of the database is determined, essentially, by the Care Keys Q-MAT (see Table 13.1), incorporating the general model of production of welfare and the target efficiency model (Chapters 1, 6, and 11).

Key Indicators

The key indicators are those that have been proved to be empirically valid, reliable and explanatory in the Care Keys research (see Part III). They can be used for routine evaluation of quality of long-term care of older people at different aggregation levels. As already stated, many of the indicators are common for both homecare and institutional care, and in addition there are context-specific indicators. The key indicators are partly constructed from scales or combining different items. At this stage the calculations are not (yet) supported by software available to users, but the relevant variables are listed in the chapters on empirical results (Chapters 7–12).

TEFF Module

The TEFF module is designed to support strategic planning and evaluation of the performance of the long-term care systems in terms of target efficiency of care. As described earlier (Chapters 1 and 11), the target efficiency concept involves three measures: (i) Horizontal target efficiency, that is the degree to which the client needs, are met (also a measure of unmet need); (ii) vertical target efficiency, that is the efficiency with which the resources are allocated against the priority needs, and (iii) equity of distribution of care resources among needy clients. The TEFF module in its present form is designed for use with any aggregated database that can differentiate between need and supply of care in corresponding terms. It can be used on aggregated data derived from care records, documentation or statistics and on survey data, but, as stated, on the condition that the need and supply information are documented in similar terms (see Chapter 11). The module is available as a demonstrator on http://www.carekeys.net.

MAssT and MAssT-D

The MAssT module is designed to support a goal-oriented planning, monitoring and evaluation of care on the client level, but analyses can be performed also at diverse aggregation levels. The module relies on the available

TABLE 13.1. The Care Keys Quality Matrix (Q-MAT).

Part 1: Client perspective

Quality dimensions	Input Conditions, preferences, life events	Process Subjective quality of care	Outcome	
			Objective Needs satisfaction	Subjective Quality of life
Client Background data: Age Gender Cohabitation Language/ethnicity				
Social	Social identity Care preferences Loss of social relationship	Client centeredness Social support	Social relations and participation	Life satisfaction Social relations
Physical	Functional abilities Health care needs Acute illness	Reliability and continuity of care Autonomy support	ADL functionality Autonomy Cognition scores	Competence/abilities Life energy
Environmental	Material resources Living environment Financial problems	Supportive services Availability, access	IADL functionality Environmental "fit"	Availability, access Service support Living environment
Psychological	Psycho-emotional characteristics Stress, mental health needs	Psycho-emotional support, interaction quality	Psychological well-being Depression score	Emotional well-being Loneliness Happiness

(continued)

TABLE 13.1. (continued)

Part 2: Professional care perspective

| | | | Outcome | |
	Quality dimensions	Input Structures/Conditions	Process Compliance	Objective Achieved targets	Subjective Job satisfaction
Professional	Care concept	Concepts/"visions" client centeredness care ethics	Compliance with care concept	Client centred outcomes	Satisfaction with work accomplishment and personal growth/ethics
Background data: Age Gender Ethnicity Work contract	Procedures	Procedures Care standards	Compliance with care procedures	Documentation quality Risk management of clinical outcome	Satisfaction with skill utilisation and work autonomy
	Personal and material resources	Qualification Time Care technology	Compliance with resource utilisation	Availability Accessibility of services	Satisfaction with material incentives and workload
	Atmosphere and teamwork	Informal care involvement Internal cooperation	Compliance with cooperation/team work	Participation in activities Absenteeism	Satisfaction with work atmosphere/teamwork

(continued)

TABLE 13.1. (continued)

| | | Part 3: Management perspective | | |
| | Input | Process | Outcome | |
Quality dimensions	Material/immaterial, structures and resources	Documentation of activities	Objective Goal achievement	Subjective Achievement evaluation
Management Background data Service type Client mix Organisation size Public/private ownership				
Quality concept	Quality management Concepts/"vision"	Quality management activities (weekly protocol)	Equity, efficacy and stakeholder benefits (TEFF values H, E)	Self-evaluation: efficacy and equity
Procedures	Procedures and risk management	Procedures (weekly protocol)	Supply efficiency (TEFF value V)	Self-evaluation: efficiency/ allocation
Resources	Material and immaterial resources, staff mix, technology, finances	Resource utilisation (weekly protocol)	Resource availability (TEFF value H/V)	Self-evaluation: resource availability
Integrated care	Cooperation concept/contracts with internal/external partners	Cooperation and conflict (weekly protocol)	Cooperation quality (cooperation scale)	Self-evaluation: care integration

needs-assessment and care documentation systems, and utilises the information on care needs and supply for each individual client in 11 dimensions of care combined into 4 quality dimensions (see Chapters 5 and 11). It evaluates the target efficiency of care at the client level, and relates it to measurements of (i) quality of care as documented (e.g. compliance with care standards), (ii) quality of care as evaluated by the client (e.g. client satisfaction with services), and (iii) subjective QoL of the client. All three quality aspects (documented care quality, subjective care quality and subjective quality of life) are measured in terms of four dimensions to facilitate comparisons across quality aspects and the introduction of the indicators into the quality dimensions of Q-MAT. Additionally, the module allows goals to be set in each care dimension and to monitor their achievement. The results are shown in bars and "smilies" to give direct feedback also to the care personnel and other stakeholders, not only to the care managers.

A MAssT-D module has been provided to adapt the tool to clients with dementia by employing appropriate scales. In MAssT-D, the QUALID scale (Weiner, Martin-Cook, Svetlik, Saine, Foster, & Fontain, 2000; see Chapter 2) is implemented in a way that allows also interpretation of results in the four-dimensional profile as central in the Care Keys approach. Both MAssT modules have been implemented as software demonstrators, and they have been available for free testing in the Care Keys web site (www.carekeys.net). Currently they are waiting for further development.

Q-MAT

The Q-MAT module forms up the Care Keys Quality Matrix, combining all relevant quality indicators from the perspective of the client, the professional care and management. The matrix renders possible analysing the quality of a service organisation, including the calculation of the indicators, and comparison of the results with previous measurements, with given standards, or with indicators from other organisations (benchmarking).

The Q-MAT has a structure comprising the "magic" 48 cells (4×3×4) as illustrated in Table 13.1 (see also Table 12.1). They include: (i) the *production perspective* (four elements: input–process–documented outcomes–subjective outcomes); (ii) the *stakeholder perspective* (three elements: client–professional carer–management) and (iii) the *quality dimension* (four elements: concept/visions–procedures/functional capabilities–resources/environment–cooperation/integration). Each cell may actually contain more than one indicator or alternative measures (e.g. the subjective quality of life (outcome) measured by WHOQOL-Bref or QUALID in case of dementia; the management resources (input) measured by staff mix, technologies and/or financial budget). To facilitate the orientation by, and recognition of the four quality dimensions, each dimension has been assigned a specific colour in the analytical tools. For example, indicators referring to environmental resources (light green), can be distinguished easily from indicators referring to concepts (light purple), functional capacities (light blue) or integration (rose).

The same colours are suggested to distinguish between the corresponding dimensions of care-related quality of life and quality of care (see Chapter 4 and Chapter 6). The choice of the colours was informed, if not based, by colour psychology, which tends to associate corresponding contents with similar colours (Heller, 2004; Welsch & Liebmann, 2004).

The Q-MAT information can be presented in two formats, enabling a quick overview or a deeper evaluation. The overview is given in form of a "traffic-light analysis", visualising the entire matrix (48 cells). In each cell, the status of indicators is reduced to "green" (good performance), "yellow" (check on performance) and "red" (poor performance), in relation to a pre-defined standard or average of performance for preselected indicators. The expanded matrix contains all quality indicators defined for a given cell of the matrix. In its present form the matrix contains selected key indicators, relevant background information of the client, the staff and the organisation and some additional indicators (suggested by the literature review) to complete the matrix in cases where the empirical research has not yet identified available and practical indicators. The module will be further developed to comprise an input/output interface; a module for searching and editing in the database; a module for monitoring quality control and goal setting on the basis of weekly protocols; a module for benchmarking (comparing a current status of indicators against previous states or values from standards or other services) and some basic tools for user's own data analyses.

Reliability and Validity of the Toolkit

Most parts of the toolkit have undergone tests for validity with several methods such as focus groups, interviews and statistical methods, being conducted within the participating countries and in comparison between the different countries. The first version of the TEFF module was tested at the beginning of the project in all partner countries, showing that the approach of target efficiency is basically applicable in a wide range of care settings and welfare regimes. However, the generally poor standards of care documentations create a problem in that not all the necessary information is available. The TEFF module was further developed in correspondence to the MAssT module to include the dimensional structure of care needs and supply (Chapter 11). In addition, the user groups in each country, consisting of social and health care professionals and care managers, evaluated the key indicators, TEFF, MAssT and Q-MAT modules, giving this way a first practice validation to the instruments. Their feedback was very encouraging as they saw the toolkit to be a very necessary and desirable tool to improve quality of long-term care and to support care managers to facilitate this task. Most validation research on the key indicators, Q-MAT and the TEFF module has been described in the previous chapters, so here we focus on the validation of the MAssT module, which uses the information from the data collection instruments and also contains basic features of the TEFF module.

Reliability and Validity of the MAssT

The Mini-Evaluation Tool (MAssT) is intended for evaluation of the quality of care outcomes, and it combines the information gathered from individual clients using the CLINT instrument, and the data extracted from the individual client care documentation using InDEX. This information includes: care needs and supply, individual TEFF indicators, documented professional quality of care measures, subjective quality of care as evaluated by the client, indicators of quality of life, and additional information on the client (dependency group, relevant care group, administrative classification).

The specification and design of MAssT was completed by the Care Keys research team in collaboration with the national user groups. The instrument was tested in all project countries several times, using standardised procedures and focus groups sessions. Kappa values suggest a relatively good reliability. The instrument was tested and refined further before submission for final testing and evaluation with users and implementation on the project website. To be able to calculate the Kappa values for the items in the MAssT, a dual-assessment study was undertaken and completed within a 2-week period. Clients were selected if they met all of the following criteria:

1. Sixty-five years of age or over;
2. Subject to either homecare or institutional care;
3. Client agreement (verbal or written consent, according to national rules) to participate in the study.

Two assessments were completed for 10 clients within 72 hours. Assessors in each country conducted a MAssT assessment on 10 clients (5 clients in homecare and 5 in nursing homecare). Two assessors conducted assessments on the same clients within a 3-day time frame. If information about the client was needed to be collected from other sources than by asking the client (e.g. documentation), the client had to provide consent. The assessors were required to collect the information independently (not together). Information on time consumed for filling in the MAssT was documented in an evaluation form after completing the MAssT evaluation. This form helped us to measure the time burden the assessment process placed on staff participating in this process.

For the 138 variables in the MAssT, it was possible to calculate Kappa or weighted Kappa values. If the variable had more than two alternatives in the answer, the weighted Kappa value was used, otherwise the ordinary Kappa value was used. There were 12 of the values below 0.40, considered to be the limit of acceptance. However, several of these were not practice relevant, but were instead variables on name, occupation, etc. that are difficult to make reliable; 41% of the variables had Kappa values of 0.70 or better, indicating a generally good outcome for this exploratory research (Fig. 13.2). Given the mix of both new and already established instruments included in the MAssT, this was more than acceptable for a first round of development.

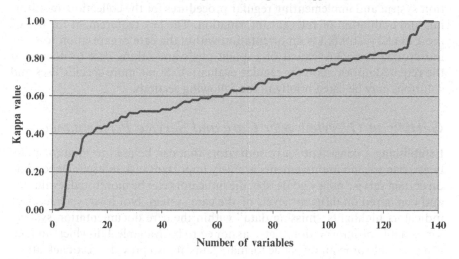

FIG. 13.2. Weighted kappa values of the MAssT module.

Face Validity of MAssT-D

Special attention from the users was received by the MAssT-D, the variant of the MAssT tool specifically for clients with dementia or other cognitive impairment. In general, users welcomed the move to include this client group, given their increasing numbers within the care system and the lack of appropriate instruments to include their perspectives. Doubts were expressed concerning the interview with the client's relatives for MAssT-D with a version of CLINT (RELINFO) adapted for this purpose to include especially scales on the perceived quality of care. For various reasons in the relative's "history" with the client, they might not always be an independent and trustworthy source of information on the client. To summarise the users' opinions, the MAssT-D with the inclusion of QUALID measuring client's quality of life as observed by carers was seen as having the potential not only to monitor and improve the well-being of people with dementia, but also to educate care staff and to draw attention to this special, highly professional care.

Some Insights into Using the CK Toolkit

The Care Keys Toolkit is still developing, but it can be used already to address a number of practical problems in care quality management. As indicated, the tools can be applied in homecare and institutional care settings and also, with the necessary cautions in the interpretation, across service types. On a general level, the tools provide some guidance for structuring the documentation system and implementing regular procedures for the collection, monitoring and evaluation of relevant information. The key requirement for use of the Care Keys Toolkit is an orientation within the care organisation towards monitoring the achievement of explicit goals and taking care to document the required information for regular evaluation. Some more specific uses and solutions may be listed briefly in the following sections.

Getting an Overview over Care and Service Performance

Establishing a consistent set of indicators that can be used to monitor practices, changes and improvements is a very important task in itself. Depending on certain service policy goals, specific indicators can be monitored, evaluated and compared on different levels of the care system. Not least, such a set of indicators highlights "missing data" within the care documentation system, for example of information that is assumed to be available, but which, in fact, is unavailable or in an unusable format. Thus, it also provides feedback about the quality of the documentation system.

"Strategic" Evaluation and Monitoring of Care Processes

Care documentation systems (when in place) are mainly used to monitor care itself, not for the evaluation of care. The MAssT module provides a tool for the professional carer by supporting care planning, monitoring and evaluation at regular intervals. Target efficiency and costs can easily be related to a set of quality criteria or to the documented compliance with care standards. A consistent profile of quality dimensions makes it possible to evaluate the comprehensiveness of care and care outcomes. This can be done for the individual client and for relevant groups of clients, for example all clients of a given carer, or all clients with diagnosed dementia. In particular, the aggregated information can be used in staff meetings or team sessions where the intention is to improve practice. The "smilies" illustrate the results and help in forming a more comprehensive picture of the performance and identifying problems. The standard elements of MAssT give also structures for the involvement of the client in care planning and evaluations, thus helping the practice in giving a "voice" to the clients.

Evaluating Target Efficiency

The efficiency of delivering and providing care as planned can be evaluated with both TEFF and MAssT modules. As stated earlier, the former works on aggregated data with a strict requirement of having the information on need and supply in identical terms, whereas the latter works at the level of the individual client, combining need and supply in four dimensions and tolerating a certain degree of missing data. Thus, monitoring and evaluation of the effectiveness, efficiency and equity of care provision at the levels of an individual client, client groups, service organisation and other aggregation levels are possible. On a care system level, especially interesting information is that on over-targeting (clients getting services they do not need) and under-targeting (clients not getting all the services they need) of care, which informs about the relative equity of the resource distribution, but also about the inefficiencies of resource use. Both mismatches will produce less benefits for the clients and additional costs for the care system, whereas increasing equity (clients get a "just" share of available services) enhances the effectiveness of the care system and contributes to its acceptability.

Quality Management and Quality Improvement

Although selected sets of key indicators can be used to evaluate specific service developments and policies, the Care Keys Q-MAT provides a consistent and comprehensive set of indicators that allows for a balanced monitoring of improvements. As described earlier, the matrix distinguishes between input, process and outcome indicators from the perspective of the client, professional carers and management and differentiates four dimensions or aspects of quality. As discussed elsewhere (Chapter 6), the quality matrix can be used similarly as the Balanced Scorecard, since the dimensions correspond to the dimensions of this widely used instrument within quality management. In combination with other analysis tools such as statistical packages (e.g. SPSS, DEA) or spreadsheet programs (Excel) the set of indicators supports more extensive analyses in research or for educational purposes.

Summary and Conclusion

The Care Keys project was based on an extensive review of earlier research covering instrumentation and studies on their validation and reliability, prior to any decision to develop new instruments. For instance, crosswalks between client assessment instruments such as the RAI (resident assessment instrument) and the Finnish RAVA were undertaken. This demonstrated relatively good correspondence between these instruments and the underlying principles and models within Care Keys, suggesting that the users of other assessment instruments can also use the toolkit with their information base. However, the review also demonstrated that the Care Keys approach, with its emphasis on the client perspective and the integration of the perspectives of the clients, professional carers and care management within a single framework, and its focus on key information, modular structure and flexibility in respect to different care settings, opens up promising avenues for the development of a new "Toolkit" for quality management.

Although the Care Keys Toolkit needs further development, it already provides a set of models and instruments not only for use within quality management of long-term care of older people, but also for research on care-related QoL of older people and for the training and education of personnel working in care provision. The toolkit is research based and comprises a number of components and prototypes that can be used alone or together. The components of the toolkit developed so far can also be seen as a basis for continuous modification and further development. The systematic evaluation of client needs and supply of services, supporting a better care documentation, will provide a more comprehensive evaluation of care practices that will enable a more equitable allocation of resources, and contribute towards enhancing quality of care and a better quality of life for clients.

Finally, it is necessary to point out the crucial importance of the quality of data on which the Care Keys instruments are used. To avoid any new and extensive data collection, the instruments are designed to rely on available care documentation systems and, thus, to accommodate different information. There are two sides to this coin. On the one hand, it implies that the instrument can be used with different data collected with different methods and adapted to existing care practices (within the general restrictions posed on data quality by the instrument). On the other hand, it should be recognised that the support by empirical research and the validation of indicators provided by the Care Keys research may no longer apply if data have been collected using different instruments. Regarding the indicators and instruments used and developed within the project, they have been shown to be quite "robust" in varying conditions, since the instruments were tested and developed in five European countries and translated in five different languages. Items sensitive to cultural contexts pose a challenge for qualitative standardisation, which has to be considered especially when using the Q-MAT, and surely, in future development of the toolkit.

References

Heller, E. (2004). Wie Farben wirken. Farbpsychologie-Farbsymbolik-Kreative Farbgestaltung. Reinbek bei Hamburg.

Øvretveit, J. (1998). Evaluating health interventions. An introduction to evaluation of health treatments, services, policies and organizational interventions. Buckingham: Open University Press.

Weiner, M. F., Martin-Cook, K., Svetlik, D. A., Saine, K., Foster, B., & Fontain, C.S. (2000). The quality of life in late-stage dementia (QUALID) scale. *Journal of the American Medical Directors Association, 1*, 114–116.

Welsch, N., & Liebmann, C. Ch. (2004). Farben: Natur-Technik-Kunst, München: Elsevier.

<http://www.carekeys.net> (CareKeys project website).

Part IV
Summary

14
Care-Related Quality of Life: An Overview

Marja Vaarama and Richard Pieper in collaboration
with Gunnar Ljunggren, Seija Muurinen, Kai Saks
and Andrew Sixsmith

The discussion presented in this volume has been multifaceted, looking at quality of life (QoL) in care-dependent old people in many ways both theoretically and empirically. The main purpose has been to examine the relationship between long-term care and QoL in frail older persons from theoretical, empirical, methodological and practical perspectives. Our key questions were

1. What are the determinants of QoL in older people receiving regular formal homecare or living in institutional settings?
2. How does formal long-term care contribute to their QoL, and what are the features of a good quality and effective care from the perspectives of the clients and professional care?
3. How does care management contribute to good client and professional outcomes, and how could quality management (QoM) be improved by evidence-based performance evaluation?

For a number of reasons the project was quite complex and ambitious. From the outset of the project it was clear that there was a lack of knowledge and scarcity of research on QoL of care-dependent, frail older people. In addition, there was criticism presented in previous studies on the general concept of QoL as not being able to take the situations of frail older people properly into account. Specific models should be developed, so the suggestion in the literature, maybe even models specific for types of care and for the diverse client groups. Thus, there arose a need for the development of theoretical concepts and models, and our basic approach was to favor a unified and generic concept of QoL to be further specified by empirically tested indicators.

Additionally, most of the available instrumentation for QoL-research was not designed especially for older people (WHOQOL-OLD was not yet available in 2003; Power, Quinn, Schmidt, & WHOQOL-OLD Group, 2005), and with a few exceptions, they were not designed for use with frail older people, and even more seldom with cognitively impaired people. Regarding the definitions and measures of quality of long-term care, there was a wealth of definitions on quality of nursing care in care institutions available, but less on quality of social care or homecare, and only few had any integrated features, even though for frail older people, medical care, nursing care and social care are all necessary. Moreover, measures of the quality of care (QoC) from the perspective of the clients were scarce. And finally, if measures were available, they tended to emphasize the physical dimension of care, and were either commercial products or their use was protected or regulated in some other way. As we wanted to develop a multi-dimensional "everyman's toolkit" based on valid instruments that were free of use in research and development, we had to look for other solutions. As a consequence, we had to add four more tasks in our list of research objectives:

4. To develop a theoretical model of "care-related" QoL that would take the special situation of dependent and frail older people into account, to guide our research
5. To develop an integrated model for the evaluation of quality and effectiveness of long-term care of older people, which would combine the perspectives of clients, professional care and management
6. To develop instrumentation for our research that would fit for use with frail and even cognitively impaired older persons, be as much as possible in line with the existing care documentation and management practices, and in addition, be able to collect information on issues that are important for the effectiveness of care of older people but which are currently not usually and regularly collected and documented (clients own perceptions being a good example)
7. To verify and validate our models and instruments through own research.

The complexity of the study was further enhanced by the comparison of five countries (Estonia, Finland, Germany, Sweden, UK), and the interdisciplinary character of research spanning from the issues of QoL to the issues of QoM, and bridging between social and health care. The study design was cross-sectional, including 67 service organizations of both homecare and institutional care with a total sample of 1,500 older clients of these services, and it employed an extensive set of instruments covering a broad range of variables on care and care outcomes. Finally, our goal was also to develop from our concepts, explanatory models, instruments and results a toolkit for use in research, development and practical care management, and this goal introduced additional challenges into our study.

The complexity of the study design called for a unifying theoretical framework. Hence we based our study on application of the production of welfare approach (PoW) (see Davies & Knapp, 1981; Knapp, 1984, 1995). As described in Chapters 1 and 4, we combined the PoW approach with multi-dimensional models of QoL (mainly from Brown & Brown, 2003; Lawton, 1983, 1991; Veenhoven, 1996, 2000); and with a model of evaluation of the QoC as a "quality chain" from Jon Øvretveit (1998); and finally we integrated management issues into our model by using social system theory. It was challenging to prepare a common research protocol, to agree on common concepts and systematic rules of data collection, and to create a pooled database using the most efficient imputation system (EM), but this all paid back as it was possible to compile a database of 1,500 cases from five countries with reasonable quality to enable looking at the care-related quality of life (crQoL) in old age from diverse perspectives.

Our results can be grouped into theoretical, methodological, empirical and practical ones. Further, we provide an overview of the contributions of different authors in this volume, and attempt at integration of the results in an emerging theoretical model of crQoL. It is worth to note that the authors of this volume had the freedom to apply paradigms of their own within our common theoretical framework and to produce independent chapters under this common umbrella. Therefore, the contributions vary in their argumentation and ways of applying the methods and interpreting and emphasising the results. This is according to our understanding not only unavoidable but also important in a multidisciplinary research project, and only on the basis of these different perspectives it is possible to aim at interdisciplinary interpretations.

The Three Models of Care-related QoL

Theoretical frameworks prove their validity by guiding and structuring research, and it should be emphasized that the PoW framework—even though the framework was not subjected to test in a strict sense—provided a very fruitful base focusing on the different objectives and tasks of the project. As a "meta model" it gave a systematic place to issues of crQoL as "final outcome" of care, and to issues of professional care and care management as "intermediate" outcomes (or outputs), as well as to practical development of instruments and tools.

Our starting point was an understanding of QoL as a multi-dimensional concept, but the question was whether we should rely on some general model of QoL, or develop specific models of QoL for different client groups. Along the lines of previous research, our own early explorations specified nine conditions and input factors important for the subjective QoL in old age, namely: demographic factors; socio-economic factors; physical-functional competence and subjective need of help; psychological well-being; social well-being, networks and participation; life style and leisure activities; housing and living environment; traumatic life events and acute illnesses; and care, including satisfaction with care (see Chapter 1, Fig. 3). Based on this, we assumed that also for care-dependent old people, the four dimensions of QoL as reflected in the WHOQOL-measure would apply, that is, we assumed the basic dimensions to be the same for all groups. However, we also assumed that within these common dimensions, the variables would vary, reflecting the circumstances and special situations of being dependent on external help, and depending on whether the person is living at home or in an institution.

To investigate the validity of this assumption, the QoL model by Lawton (1983, 1991) proved to be adequate theoretical starting point to capture the situation of frail older persons receiving care, and the special circumstances of cognitive impairment due to dementia. Lawton proposed four basic dimensions of life quality (functional competence, environmental resources, life satisfaction, psychological well-being), which correspond quite well with the dimensions of the QoL model of the WHO (physical, psychological, social, environmental; see Skevington, Lotfy, O'Connell, & The WHOQOL Group, 2004). These again were comparable with the "four qualities of life" of Veenhoven (2000), and could be generalized to develop a corresponding four-dimensional framework for the QoC and care management (see Chapters 4 and 6). To achieve this, the model had to be modified and elaborated by a more consistent interpretation grounded on social system theory, but the approach to search for a generic model to be adapted to specific groups and care settings was generally supported by the fact that "key indicators" could be organized in this four-dimensional model of crQoL, and that only more specific indicators distinguished between groups and care settings (in home-care and institutional care).

The theoretical discussions had to take up a number of issues, which plague the concept of QoL, and we suggest avenues of solving them in a compre-hensive model of care-related QoL (crQoL), which we differentiated into three sub-models, each mirroring the QoL in care-dependent and frail old people from different angles: a structural model, a production model and a normative model. One issue is also the distinction of subjective and objective QoL, frequently considered of basic theoretical importance and character-izing distinct approaches. Although the distinction of subjective and objec-tive aspects of QoL is certainly relevant, we suggest treating this distinction primarily as a methodological issue concerning access to information by way of self-reports (interviews) or professional assessments including behavioral observations. Subjective QoL is, then, seen as a "core" within a more compre-hensive concept of QoL, which integrates, moreover, emotions giving them a role in affective regulation and as indicators of QoL based on observation, again structured in the four dimensions of the model.

Another and related issue is pertaining to the distinction of conditions of QoL and factors or elements of QoL. Here we introduced a distinction between two sub-models (see Chapter 4): (1) The *structural model* is focusing on the factors important to the QoL in care-dependent old people, emphasizing the "person–environment fit" (Lawton), and incorporating the most relevant fea-tures of the environment in the model, since the environment is conceived as actively selected and influenced by the person and, thus, "internalized." With frail older persons, care has to be considered as a relevant feature of their physical and social environment, and care is, therefore, included in the con-cept of crQoL. Reflecting on the role of care management in facilitation of a good QoC to enhance the QoL in the older clients, the model of crQoL was further elaborated in an "onion model" to combine the objectives and tasks of care and care management in pursuing good care outcomes. In a different perspective, (2) the *production model* focuses on the role of care in the production of QoL or welfare in frail older persons. This model suggests taking into account conditions and compensation needs of an individual, the causal relations in the production chain, and the active role of the client in adjusting to life circumstances and in co-producing the effects of care by participating in care decisions and activities (e.g. cooperating in rehabilitation, compliance in medication, etc.). In this perspective, subjective QoL may take the role of the "final outcome" in the evaluation of care outcomes, although the continuous evaluation of care will make use of other information such as clinical results or observed client behavior as well (e.g. in case of dementia).

Another issue deals with the fact that any concept of QoL has to include a strategy to solve the normative aspects necessarily involved in the concept of quality and quality standards. The process of evaluating QoL has to respect the subjective view of the person, as well as the role of communication with other persons relevant for a validated definition or "social construction" of QoL in diverse care settings. Hence, we introduced (3) a *normative model* into the concept of crQoL to make aware of the normative issues involved, and to point to the prerequisites for the participation of clients in the process of "negotiation," and to provide some guidance for the development of procedures and methods for this. Essentially, the normative model identifies the "care triad," that is, the triadic relationship between client, professional carer, and informal carer (or a substituting reference persons and advocate) as the agency which has to negotiate and agree on the normative issues in care on the individual level.

Further, the interpretation of the concept of quality in the framework of social system theory—taking up a lead from Veenhoven (2000)—turned out to be not only of theoretical interest, but also practically relevant. It furnished a unifying dimensional structure, which could be applied to the concept of QoL as well as to the concepts of QoC and quality of management of care (QoM); and as indicated, the dimensional structure can be used to systematically structure and organize also practical instruments, such as the assessment of care needs and supply in the TEFF model and the quality dimension in the Care Keys quality matrix. Our theoretical framework may be challenged—and certainly the system theory approach is challenged, not only in gerontology—and we have discussed an alternative foundation of the QoL concept starting from the model of Ivan Brown (Brown & Brown, 2003). We suggested a theoretical foundation of this model on pragmatic social philosophy (following Charles S. Peirce and George H. Mead), and the theory of "social triads" in the tradition of Georg Simmel (see Chapter 4). Again, an interesting result was that we were able to derive the four-dimensional structure of QoL also as a reduced model in this more differentiated and "critical" conceptual model.

Originally, the objective in Care Keys was not to make a contribution to the theory of care itself, but rather to develop a framework in the context of the "meta model" of PoW to understand the role of care in the production of QoL, and to find empirically and practically relevant indicators that could inform the evaluation of practices in care and care management. The emphasis on the quality of documentation of care as important for an evaluation of professional QoC—often argued in nursing care theories—was clearly supported by the Care Keys results. Moreover, the advantages of a well structured and unifying approach to *all* aspects of QoM in care for older persons seem to be obvious, and one of the theoretical results was that the four-dimensional framework could be fruitfully applied to issues of care quality. Our review of theories and functions of long-term care (at home and in institutional settings) revealed that care can be conceptualized in a framework following the dimensions of the QoL model. Our empirical results are considered below, but on the level of theoretical models of QoC, it is important that according to our results, care can be conceived as a "layer" in an "onion model" of crQoL, structured by the same dimensions, which renders possible a comprehensive—albeit quite general—concept of care quality including the perspectives of the clients and professionals. Additionally, as indicated already, the concept of a "care triad" (normative model) makes us sensitive to issues of negotiation of different interests of stakeholders in care. On the one hand, it links the concept of QoC to the concepts of QoL and QoM and, on the other hand, it describes and respects the care triad as the basic agent of individual care. These issues become especially important in the case of dementia when the client cannot speak up for herself anymore and needs advocacy.

Similarly as in the case of QoC, the discussion of quality of management (QoM) in Care Keys did not aim at contributions to the theory of care management, rather the objective was to improve our understanding of the role of management in care, and to identify evidence-based indicators for improving the management quality in facilitating the production of QoL as "final outcome." Still, it became clear that adequate concepts and strategies are developed only quite recently, and are often imported from other realms into long-term care for older persons, most often from health care, without special considerations for the affordances of long-term care. In this situation, the objective turned out to be not only to improve the information base of management, or to develop practical instruments such as the Care Keys Quality Matrix (see Chapter 13). In addition, we had, on the one hand, to look for a systematic framework relating the concepts of QoM, QoC, and QoL, and to bridge the conceptual gap between these concepts; and on the other hand, we had to look at the strategies of QoM such as Total Quality Management for their benefits in the improvement of the performance of care systems. Two theoretical results may be pointed out: (i) the conceptualization of QoM as supporting or "setting the stage" for the "care triad" as an essentially autonomous agency responsible for the "social construction" of visions of life quality and for the "negotiation of order" in care, and (ii) the reinterpretation of innovative strategies in QoM in view of our four-dimensional approach. The first result provided a link to conceiving QoM of care as a "discourse" negotiating between different stakeholder interests, namely, of the client, the professionals, informal carers, and management itself. The normative model of the "tetrahedron of quality management"—expanding the concept of the care triad—was proposed to guide the analysis of negotiation of potential conflict of interests. And it is argued that special affordances of long-term care (e.g. mutual trust in care relationships, balancing the needs of clients and staff) have to be respected also in QoM to give to care and the care relationship their special quality. Our second result linked the theoretical concepts to practical strategies such as the Balanced Scorecard, and the Care Keys Quality Matrix, both centering on multi-dimensional information in performance evaluation. These theoretical results of QoM are at this stage of a rather tentative nature, but they seem to be promising starting points for more thorough theoretical and empirical analyses, and for better understanding of the role of care in the QoL of older persons dependent on external care.

Methodological Results

The aim of the Care Keys project was originally not to make substantial developments in methods and instrumentation, but rather to rely on instruments already established. As discussed in Chapter 3, three problems were responsible for embarking on more extensive methodological development. First, a review of instruments for the measurement of QoL in older people revealed that the available instrument were seldom designed for use with old and frail old people, and even less seldom for use with cognitively impaired people. For instance, the scales for QoL were not adapted to frail older persons (e.g. the WHOQOL scale; the WHOQOL-OLD was not yet available), or the scales were not covering all relevant dimensions (e.g. the PGCMS scale; Lawton, 1975.) Second, established scales were not freely available or not covering all aspects considered relevant for the measurement of professional QoC and QoC management. Additionally, no common instruments were used in the five countries. Third, the existing care documentation systems proved to be often unreliable and limited in scope. For the purposes of comparison, a common strategy and instrumentation had to be developed. We decided to as much as possible use accessible scales, and integrate them with the existing care documentation to avoid cumbersome extra data collection from other sources.

The set of instruments we used in the Care Keys research, and the characters of the samples have been described in Chapters 2 and 3, as have been the methods for constructing the pooled Care Keys database for our analyses. As discussed in the relevant chapters, the selection of services and clients could not follow in all countries our common protocol controlling for types of services provided, size, and organizational conditions (e.g., a sample of old people living in sheltered housing was substituting the sample of homecare clients in the UK). In spite of the limitations indicated, it is one of the results of the Care Keys research that a sufficiently valid and reliable dataset could be obtained for a broad scope of aspects of care and care outcomes. Currently, the Care Keys instruments are further analyzed to define a comprehensive and yet practical set of methods, indicators, and scales covering all aspects of the Care Keys crQoL model, and to be implemented in the Care Keys Quality Matrix. While new indicators still have to be specified and tested for some dimensions (e.g., management resources, staff perception of care quality), a substantial set of "key indicators" for strategies of improvement of care practices could be empirically identified and validated for home care and institutional care as discussed below (Chapters 8–12).

Relevant especially in a practical perspective, but also of theoretical interest, are our results concerning the concept and measurement of the target efficiency of care. As emphasized in the empirical analyses, the data in the care documentations for the assessment of needs and supply in corresponding terms was especially characterized by incompleteness and unreliability. This prompted us to develop a strategy and method to measure target efficiency in eleven categories of needs and supply to be aggregated over four dimensions in correspondence with the dimensions of crQoL. It is a remarkable result justifying further development of the instrument that these aggregated indicators still proved to have empirical significance for crQoL.

An issue still to be emphasized is the fact that in the light of our results, the documentation of long-term care needs to be considerably improved before QoM can be based on the information provided by documentation practices. Perhaps the most important need for change in current care planning and documentation practices is the introduction of a more conscious goal achievement orientation, which systematically supports a comprehensive and empowering process of needs-assessment, care planning, care interventions, and evaluation of the QoC outcomes in appropriate time intervals. This transparency of care planning and evaluation increases not only the capacities of staff to improve their practices by learning, but it improves also the possibilities of efficient QoM, and supports the autonomy of staff and their participation in QoM. With the improvement of care documentation, a limitation of the research results presented here can be overcome, namely, that it does not systematically allow for the analyses of time series and developments. The Care Keys data were collected from the records over the last six months, and basically the care inputs as described in the documentation preceded the measurement of the care outcomes as obtained in the client interviews, but especially in homecare, the quality of the documentation and the lack of a repeated measurement of QoL outcomes did not enable systematic analyses of causal impacts.

From a methodological point of view, it also has to be noted that the theoretical discussion suggested a combination of different information in a multi-dimensional profile of QoL, including both subjective evaluations by older people, information extracted from the care documentation on the status of the client and on certain theoretically important features of professional care, self-evaluations of care professionals and care managers, as well as information from third parties such as informal care. In Care Keys, we were able to combine most of these information sources, but at this point, commonly used procedures and models for such a "triangulation" of methods and the combination of information have not yet been developed. The evaluation tool MAssT presents information on target efficiency, documented QoC, perceived QoC by the client, and subjective QoL for each client in a four-dimensional profile (possibly also service packages and their costs), but the integration of the diverse information is left to the professional carer, and ideally, to the discussion or "discourse" of the results among client, staff, peers, and informal carers (see Chapter 4).

Empirical Results

As described Chapter 1, the empirical Care Keys research was guided by the production of welfare approach, conceiving care as an intermediate output to produce QoL as a "final outcome." Although alternative concepts and measures were explored, the QoL model proposed by Lawton was the basic framework of our study, and the WHOQOL-Bref instrument furnished the central scale measuring QoL in a four-dimensional profile as suggested by Lawton's model. The large and multifaceted database was subjected to first analyses presented in this volume, and focusing on the comparison of QoL in five countries, on production of QoL in homecare and in the institutional care, and on the role of care management in production of care outcomes, with the special case of dementia care, and the special question of the target efficiency of care (see Chapters 7–12). The results support the generic model of QoL to be usable also for care-dependent old people; demonstrate the important role of care in production of QoL in this group of people; suggest care management to have an influential role in facilitating good care; validate the concept of target efficiency to be a promising way to measure efficiency of long-term care; and give stimulus for further research. The main results of these first analyses are summarized in the following, and the database will be subjected to further analyses beyond this volume.

QoL in Five EU Countries

In Chapter 7, Saks and Tiit are looking at the differences in subjective QoL outcomes in five countries participating in the research. They found Estonia with lowest life quality, UK with highest, and Finland, Germany, and Sweden were very similar. The differences were assumed to deal with the developmental stage and the standard of living in the case of Estonia, while in the case of the

UK, alternative explanations are suggested, dealing with the questions of differences in care cultures, but also with a possible bias in the UK database due to the selection of the sample (see Chapter 2).

Comparison of QoL of persons living in care institutions (IC) in five EU countries with those receiving homecare (HC) revealed that the QoL profile over the four dimensions was quite similar for both care types in all countries. Functional status of clients and the care type also determine QoL, although the differences between countries again were mostly insignificant. Loneliness was greater in HC except, interestingly, in Estonia. Satisfaction with the "physical" (functional and health) life situation was higher in IC, although the actual health status was higher in HC. Still, differences between countries appeared only in this "physical" dimension, with Estonia and Germany showing significantly less satisfaction in HC. As expected, housing and physical living environment, combined with problems with indoor and outdoor mobility were important factors for QoL in HC in all countries. It did not pose similar problems for clients in IC, probably as the environments are already adapted to the needs of older persons with lowered mobility, but the pattern was similar in all five countries. There were also differences in attitude toward own ageing and loneliness between HC and IC and between countries, suggesting that at least Finnish and Estonian clients in HC had a more negative attitude toward own ageing, and HC clients—especially Finns—were also lonelier. These findings correspond to the assumption that homecare is more system- and culture-relative than IC, partly probably due to the different mixes of social and formal production of welfare at home. In general, the results support the assumption that there is a four-dimensional profile of subjective QoL, which may vary in its level with country specific conditions, but appears to be rather stable, and thus, can be used as a reference for the analysis of more specific influences.

QoL in HC

In Chapter 8, Vaarama and Tiit demonstrate that the dimensions of QoL in old people in homecare were broadly similar to those of the adult population in general, suggesting that frail older people living at home should not be seen as too "different" from the rest of the adult population. This is supported by the fact that background information (e.g., age, gender, country) had no significant effect. However, the results highlight a number of factors that are important only when one is frail and care-dependent. Acute illnesses, problems with daily functional ability connected with problems with the housing and living environment, restricted possibilities to participate in social life and hobbies outside the home, and a passive lifestyle (no hobbies or exercises outside or at home), all had a negative influence on the QoL in homecare clients. These results are in line with earlier research in the field (e.g. Birren, Lubben, Rowe, & Deutschmann, 1991; Cummins, 1997; Hughes, 1990), and were demonstrated already in early explorations in the Care Keys research (cf. Vaarama, Pieper, & Sixsmith, 2007).

One of the remarkable results was the strong relationship between subjective QoC and QoL in care-dependent people living at home. Homecare had a positive impact on QoL when the client was as clean as he would like, his home was as clean as he would like, he dressed as he would like, he went to bed and got up as he would like, and he felt that the care workers listened to and understood what he would like. Obviously, this is not just a matter of being clean and tidy and well-dressed, but rather it is about having a responsive care that reflects the personal preferences or the client. Further, the results suggested that responsive homecare had a positive connection with adjustment (accommodation) to old age. The results call for a more client-oriented approach in care and for psycho-social support as effective ways of improving care outcomes, and the authors suggest that corresponding quality measures should be used in addition to the usual clinical outcome measures.

Regarding the professional quality of homecare and its contributions to the subjective QoL in the clients, the results pointed to the importance of comprehensive needs-assessment and goal-oriented care plans based on these needs; goal-oriented team-working; use of prophylaxes especially to prevent falls; good pain management; and involvement of the clients and informal carers through the entire process of care, from planning to evaluation of results. However, due to the low response rate and missing values in the care documentation (especially the case in Estonia but also evident in the other countries), the results need further investigation. Even so, the results highlighted some positive connections between the QoC documentation and subjective care outcomes, suggesting that a good care documentation is connected with good care outcomes. As the same was even stronger realized in the case of institutional care (see Chapter 9), it seems that QoC documentation is one of the conditions of good professional long-term care.

Quality of management of homecare was clearly connected with the QoC outcomes as important structural and process factors. Most frequently, care concepts ("services support autonomy"), the degree of goal-orientation in care ("setting the goals for care"), accessibility ("services within agreed time"), and sufficient resources ("number of care personnel converted into full time equivalents") emerged as important features. In addition, structures and processes for proper pain management; participation by clients and informal carers in care planning; written QoM procedures; and a living contact between management and employees were connected with good homecare outcomes. These results highlight the role of management as facilitator of a good care. The impact of management was stronger on QoL than on quality of professional care (measured as the QoC documentation), but it is not possible to determine how much this was due to weaknesses in the data, notably the low response rate in care documentation. However, the results correspond well with the management concept used in Care Keys, but further research is needed to develop a comprehensive strategy.

As a summary, 71 "key variables" were identified as being connected and causing variation in the subjective QoL of old people in homecare. They range from 47 client-specific conditions to the 10 key-indicators of subjective quality of homecare, 19 key items important for the documentation of professional quality of homecare, and 10 key variables to document and evaluate the quality of management of homecare. Practical experience within the Care Keys project suggests that these instruments are easy to administer with frail older people and within care routines. These "key variables" are, therefore, suggested for inclusion into the Care Keys Quality Matrix (see Chapter 13). The authors suggest that a regular use of these client quality measures, together with measures of clinical and other professional care outcomes would give a more multifaceted picture of quality and effectiveness of homecare, would give clients a stronger voice and role within the management of their own care, and support the development of homecare in general.

QoL in IC

Saks and associates (see Chapter 9) analyzed QoL in old people in institutional care (IC), and found some results already established for homecare (HC), namely, that there was little impact of background variables (e.g., age, gender) or of the country, nor was the level of functional abilities (ADL–activities of daily life) or general health important among institutional residents. Significant effects turned out for life events (e.g. current illness, financial problems). However, the most important factor determining the QoL in people living in care institutions was—similarly to homecare—subjective satisfaction with care, which in turn was influenced by professional QoC and living environment. These results were quite expected, and described by many researchers (Bowers, Fibich, & Jacobson, 2001; Caris-Verhallen, Kerkstra, & Bensing, 1997; Coulon, Mok, Krause, & Anderson, 1996; DePorter, 2005). In IC, care satisfaction proved to be important for subjective QoL especially in the dimension of care as a service (cleanliness), but also with regard to possibilities for outdoor mobility. Moreover, social relations and opportunities for leisure activities were having an impact, speaking for the fact that the institution constitutes not only physical but also psycho-social environment for its residents.

Besides satisfaction with care, two factors were revealed, which had high importance and direct influence on QoL of clients in long-term care institutions—involvement of informal network and the QoC documentation. Persons whose informal network was involved into the care process according to the care documentations had better QoL. This suggests for further research to investigate how informal carers can be involved most effectively into care processes in care institutions to improve the QoL of clients without creating too much burden for informal carers. Concerning the effects of care documentation it has to be said that, like in HC, the documentation quality was generally not very good (although better than in HC), but still the positive effect of good documentation on QoL could be established. Sometimes care managers and social politicians argue whether it would be worth to put so much energy into care documentation instead of spending the same time directly helping and supporting clients. From our study we have now evidence that this opinion is not appropriate. On the contrary, those clients whose care documentation was conducted according to modern care theories and complying with good practices had better QoL. We can assume that if a care worker records all essential aspects of client's needs, care plans, and goal attainment, it helps to provide better targeted and more comprehensive care. The amount and structure of missing values in the care documentation can be a complex indicator characterizing the quality of professional care, and should be applied in care evaluation especially when electronic standardized care documentation is used.

Especially in a practical perspective, a valuable result of our study was defining a short and empirically validated list of key variables for perform-ance evaluation, covering subjective life satisfaction, professional QoC, and the care environment (management variables have yet to be analyzed, but see for first results Chapter 12). Long lists of variables potentially influencing QoL cannot be used in everyday practice. In the survey, Saks and associates selected the most important and not highly correlated variables from the long and comprehensive list using the Care Keys pooled database. These key indicators had the greatest predictive power for the QoL of clients, and are suggested by the authors for monitoring the care results, and to be included in the Care Keys Quality Matrix (see Chapter 13).

QoL in Older Persons with Dementia

A very important result of the Care Keys research certainly is that it proved to be possible and practical to include persons with dementia in the study, as demonstrated by Sixsmith, Hammond and Gibson (Chapter 10). Although severe cases were often excluded from the study by care managers and, therefore, the sample may not be representative, the study still rendered some interesting results. And it drew a lot of interest from professional carers, since this group of clients increases, and poses a great challenge to care not only in institutions. Several scales were considered and tested in pilot studies, and the QUALID scale by Weiner and associates (2000) turned out to correspond best to the theoretical framework of Care Keys (see Chapter 4), but also the PGCMS yielded a satisfying measurement of QoL for persons with mild and medium dementia.

The analyses focused on two issues: predictors of well-being for people with moderate to severe cognitive impairment, and differences in well-being in the five participating countries. According to the results, pain as observed discomfort was in negative connection with the well-being of older clients with dementia, while the presence of a social network consisting of more than one person had a positive connection, confirming other findings within the Care Keys research. The supply of recreational events within the care home had a substantial influence on the QoL scores to an extent that is difficult to explain as an artifact of measurement. It is difficult to say whether the supply of recreational events in itself is directly influential on well-being, or whether this is more generally reflective of the culture of the home. However, both illustrate the potential impact of care and support on the well-being of people with dementia. Interestingly, the analyses indicated that well-being in dementia was not associated with either functional or cognitive abilities; the scales on cognitive impairment and measures of functional abilities did not reveal an impact on QoL, again quite similar to non-dementia clients. While comparisons between the participating countries need to be treated with care, the results indicated better QoL with dementia in Finland and Sweden, and lower levels of well-being in Estonia, the latter matching trends indicated in other research, also in the case of non-dementia clients (see above). Perhaps the most notable result is the fact that psycho-social aspects of care quality did make a difference confirming the similar findings by Lawton (see Chapter 4 and 10). Clearly, these first results need further research and validation, but they are promising.

The Target Efficiency of Care

The concept of target efficiency (TEFF) and basic algorithms for calculating the set of TEFF indicators (Vaarama, Mattila, Laaksonen, & Valtonen, 1997) were already available at the beginning of the project, and in Care Keys, they were subjected to further testing and development as described in Chapter 11. Basically, target efficiency measures the responsiveness of care to needs of the clients, the efficiency of allocation of resources against the priority needs (Bebbington & Davies, 1983; Kavanagh & Stewart, 1995), and the equity of distribution among needy groups (Vaarama et al., 1997). An early evaluation of the TEFF model in the Care Keys project proved its high potential value for care managers at different management levels, for politicians, and last but not least for the clients and their relatives. The model does not only help to strive toward an effective, efficient, and equitable provision of care, but the target efficiency can also be shown to contribute to its final outcome, the subjective QoL of the clients.

The further development of the TEFF during Care Keys focused on finding ways of getting the model applicable in different care systems characterized by poor care documentation—a problem that turned out to be the greatest challenge for a practical use of TEFF. To produce a flexible solution with necessary standardization, different TEFF models were developed in correspondence to the different use contexts. A key solution was to higher the abstraction level from individual needs and respective supplies to the level of 11 need categories derived from modern care theories, and to aggregate them in four dimensions corresponding to the four-dimensional QoL model. A key challenge was to achieve a high congruence with existing documentation systems, but still keep also the currently neglected information included. The solution was successful as the dimensional TEFF model was applicable in all project sites even with very different documentation systems, and although the missing data had to be collected by the Care Keys instrument (see Chapter 2). Multivariate analyses demonstrated that the TEFF indicators, including indicators for equity of distribution among needy clients, did have significant relations (although generally low) to indicators of QoC and impacts on QoL. The authors suggest the target efficiency measures to be used as indicators of the outcomes of quality (performance) management, to be included in the Care Keys Quality Matrix (see Chapter 12 and 13). Consequently, the first demonstrator of a tool for evaluation of care needs, processes, supply and outcomes (MAssT, see Chapter 13) was developed and implemented in the Care Keys website for free tasting (http://carekeys.net). This tool will be further improved in view of the empirically identified indicators and on-going research. Another task was to develop TEFF models that meet the different information needs at different management levels, from strategic level to front-line managers. The solution was to provide two tools for TEFF-evaluations, (i) first ("TEFF-model") working with any aggregated data that register the needs and their supply in the same terms (e.g., need for homecare in hours/supply of homecare in hours), and (ii) another tool ("MAssT") working at individual client level and aggregating the results to higher aggregation levels (e.g. to diverse client group levels), and evaluating the results in four dimensions.

These models and tools are promising, and highly desired by the care professionals and managers, but the authors point out that the tools are currently still at a developmental stage, and in spite of the progress made in developing TEFF, there are still many problems to solve. One of them is the fact that even if the dimensional TEFF-model can be used also in care systems with poor documentation, good cost data are rarely available for TEFF evaluations, an option available in the tool and of great interest to management. Another possible obstacle for a practical implementation of the TEFF models may be the *willingness* of care practitioners to use the TEFF-models as they discover inefficiencies and inequities in the care practices. In principle, it should be in the interest of care persons to recognize inefficient use of resources, but there may be insecurities for using a tool that exactly points our not only desired but also not desired achievements. Third, the existing legislation, and financial and reimbursement systems may pose institutional hinders for the improvement of target efficiency, even if managers and care personnel would like to do it. A fourth and very important notion is that TEFF can lead to misleading decisions if used with unreliable data, but this of course applies to all tools where the quality of data is on the responsibility of the user. The authors remind us that for validity and reliability, the TEFF results should always be contrasted with information from other sources, including, for instance, measures of QoL and QoC. Thus, the TEFF module should be used in conjunction with other instruments of the Care Keys toolkit, for instance, the Q-MAT tool, which combines the key information of the Care Keys Quality Matrix in 48 "magic" variables (Chapter 13). Another Care Keys tool is the MAssT-instrument, which contrasts individual level TEFF results with subjective and clinical care outcomes on the level of individual client, and for selected client groups (see Chapter 13).

QoM in Long-Term Care and the Care Keys Quality Matrix

Evaluating the performance of management is a complex task, and research on the outcomes of care management is only quite recently developing. In the Care Keys project, a substantial number of service organizations (67) were included in the study, but as Pieper and associates demonstrate in Chapter 12, their comparison was difficult: the care systems in the five countries were very different, homecare and institutional care had to be distinguished, the organizational structure and size varied considerably, and many organizations were quite reluctant to provide detailed information especially on their resources (e.g., finances and staff). Additionally, there were no established procedures and scales available to measure the implementation and performance of diverse QoM strategies, and these instruments (measuring e.g., the implementation of QoM, cooperation in integrated care, or goal attainment) had to be developed from scratch. Only the target efficiency indicators could be accepted as well established in previous research, and were, therefore, employed as indicators of management outcome. Although a systematic benchmarking between comparable services was not possible, an attempt was made to specify relevant indicators for each of the cells of the Care Keys Quality Matrix, combining the three dimensions (*production dimension*: input/process/subjective and objective outcomes; *stakeholder dimension*: perspectives of clients, staff, and management; *quality dimension:* four-dimensional quality concept) in a table of $4 \times 3 \times 4 = 48$ cells. The pattern of indicators in the matrix was then interpreted as characterizing strategies or "styles" of management.

Perhaps the most important result is that the structure of the Care Keys Quality Matrix could be supported by empirical analyses, since some of the causal effects suggested by the production chain implicit in the matrix could be demonstrated to be significant, and the four-dimensional structure of the quality dimension could be reproduced from client level data not only for the QoL outcomes, but also for perceived QoC, for documented QoC, and for the target efficiency indicators. Moreover, indicators from all four dimensions of quality turned out to be significant in some explanatory model. Thus, the basic Care Keys approach of identifying key indicators from care information, and combining them for performance evaluation in a table structured by the theoretical framework, received considerable empirical support.

Some more specific results were also obtained. The Finnish services were of good performance on practically all outcome indicators, for instance, regarding the variation of equity of service allocation among care units, rendering some validity to the new equity indicator of the TEFF tool. Confirming theoretical expectations, the impact of IC on QoL indicators was clearly stronger than for HC. Also expected, but less obvious was the result that the management impacted more on QoC in IC than in HC; while in HC, management had a stronger direct effect on QoL outcomes than in IC. The latter was assumed to be due to cooperative practices within provision of care and support at home. Most effects were rather weak, but showed patterns when displayed in the Quality Matrix, thus having a potential to guide QoM strategies toward improvements to the benefit of clients. At this point, further analyses are needed to select the proper final key indicators to complete the Quality Matrix. New scales and indicators need to be developed for some parts of the matrix, especially, for a more detailed assessment of the QoC, and the compliance to care standards by professionals.

Practical Results: The Care Keys Toolkit

In the Care Keys research, essentially, the focus was on theoretical and empirical research, while methodological developments turned out to be necessary for research purposes, and the practical concern was oriented toward the identification of a set of "key indicators." Care documentation was seen as a central instrument for improving QoC, and it was to cover the assessment of competencies and needs of the clients, care planning, performance evaluation, and QoM.

A systematic starting point was the three-dimensional quality matrix as suggested by Øvretveit (1998), combining (in a matrix of $3 \times 3 = 9$ cells) the distinction of input, process and outcome indicators with three stakeholder perspectives—client, professional care and management. The task was "to fill in the boxes" with respective indicators confirmed to have empirical validity. In the course of the project, conceptual developments made further elaborations of the matrix necessary, such as a differentiation between subjective and documented ("objective") care outcomes, and a systematic structure for the quality dimension within the cells. The latter differentiation was motivated especially by the fact that both the concepts of QoL and the concept of management quality had to be conceived as multi-dimensional of its nature, which posed the question of a comprehensive set of indicators covering all relevant aspects of these concepts. Eventually, the elaborated matrix received a new interpretation in the context of the production of welfare approach, combined with the stakeholder perspective, and the four-dimensional quality concept based on social system theory.

As descried earlier and especially in Chapter 3, a set of instruments had to be designed to collect the required information, and the stakeholder perspective implied that the clients have to be addressed directly (by interview) to get their needs and preferences respected; the professional perspective as reflected in the individual care documentation was to be analyzed; and the management view on good performance and the conditions set by the service organization had to be included. The result was a set of data collection instruments (CLINT, InDEX, ManDEX), each addressing one stakeholder, and bringing together information from these different sources. Thus, this "triangulation" of methods was not only based on affordances of empirical research, but it also considered as practical information needs for performance evaluation. It should be noted that the instruments are not intended to substitute the care documentation, but rather are designed as instruments for processing information from the data from existing assessment instruments and documentations. Thus, ideally, the data collection process for the Care Keys tools could be programmed as a selection of information from existing sources for calculation of the Care Keys indicators. Unfortunately, no existing documentation does currently provide all the necessary information, and especially not in a digital format. It is obvious that this limits the practicality of the Care Keys Toolkit at this point. The promising result, however, is that it was possible to specify a limited set of key indicators for evaluation of effectiveness and quality of long-term care, which could and should be incorporated in a redesigned documentation system to support QoM without necessarily producing unbearable new workloads of documentation for staff. Furthermore, the indicators and instruments proved to be quite "robust" in the sense that they showed significant relationships to care outcomes, even though they were translated into five different languages, and tested in different care systems and care cultures.

The main components of the Care Keys Toolkit have been described in Chapter 13, this volume. Here we would like to point out that the application of the toolkit does not only depend on a sufficient documentation system, but also on corresponding practices of performance evaluation and QoM. The central notions of target efficiency and client-centered outcome orientation imply that the practices of QoM follow a logic of goal achievement, that is, of setting the care goals, specifying the care interventions and criteria of goal achievement, documenting compliance with planning, and regular evaluation of achievements. Such professional procedures and attitudes are not necessarily in conflict with more usual practices of "humanistic" client-centered care, as has been pointed out (see Chapter 6), but so far they are not commonly implemented and supported by corresponding information technologies.

Reflecting Back to Our Three Central Study Questions

One of the questions in the Care Keys research was whether the determinants of QoL and QoC differ between clients in homecare and in the institutional care, and some results answering to this question are reported already in the previous section. One assumption was that the dimensions of QoL (physical, psychological, social, and environmental) may not differ from those found as important for adult population in general, but that at least some key variables may be different showing the specific situation of care-dependent older people. Some differences between homecare and institutional care were assumed, since, for instance, the living environments (adapted physical environment in the institutions and professional production of welfare in the institutions vs. social production of welfare at home), and the support they give to QoL will differ. Further, we assumed management to have less impact in homecare as production of welfare at home is usually a coproduction on which management has only limited impact. And management impact was assumed to be stronger in IC as these services are more coherent professional organizations.

All these assumptions were largely confirmed, but not all expectations were met. The most important variables distinguishing long-term care clients from other older persons are care and the compensation and comfort it provides to older clients, as well as the critical importance of the physical living environment. Correspondingly, we expected physical-functional ability (IADL, ADL) to be an important determinant of QoL in our study population, but in our analyses it was not in direct connection with the subjective QoL, neither in HC clients nor in IC clients. As previous research has demonstrated older people with low subjective health and IADL/ADL problems to have lower QoL than older persons not having these problems, we concluded that the functional ability plays a role, but in old clients, the effects are mediated by care. In other words, lowered functional ability per se is not important as older people might have accepted it, but then it becomes important whether they get enough care compensation for their needs or not. Thus, care was the first important factor differentiating the QoL determinants between the older population in general and the older clients of long-term *care,* but this fact did not differentiate between clients in HC and IC.

Regarding functional competence, we saw it to pose much more problems for HC clients than clients in the IC, probably due to different living environments and different levels of help received. The environment was an important factor for QoL in both HC and IC clients, but the variables were clearly different. In HC, barriers for indoor mobility and problems with kitchen, bathroom, stairs, no lift, inadequate heating/cooling and damp were serious problems for everyday performance and subjective QoL. Moreover, problems with the barriers in living environment in terms of difficult access to transportation and local amenities lowered subjective QoL in HC. For clients in HC it was important that home was as clean as they wanted. In IC, the care home was to be clean, cosy and homely, the indoor air good, and the residents wished to get outdoors easier, but the environment did not pose problems for mobility (apparently as in IC, it was adapted to be barrier free). These special nuances of living environment were the second important factor differentiating the care-dependent old people from other groups, and differentiating the HC clients from IC clients. For both client groups, housing and living environment are important, but the variables describing problems in this dimension, and the interventions to improve this dimension of QoL are different.

Social networks and participation were important for both client groups, as for the adult population in general. Both in HC and IC, it was important that clients had someone to feel close to, but in HC it made a difference whether it was a relative or a care worker, suggesting that not having close relatives is not a good situation for old people living at home. In IC, getting along with carers and other residents in the care home turned out to be very important for the QoL of the clients. Regarding persons over 80 years of age, getting help both from formal homecare and informal care increased QoL significantly. It was also important in HC that someone close has been visiting the client during the past 2 weeks, so also the length of the periods older people are alone at home matters (see also Baldock & Hadlow, 2002). Further, for both client groups it was important to have an active life in terms of participation and meaningful activities. In HC, QoL was in positive connection with participation in clubs and leisure activities outside home, or at least with having individual hobbies and exercises at home. For IC clients, it was important that they had enough things to do. In this respect, the older HC and IC clients do not differ from the older or adult population in general, so they also need "life in the years," but again, the ways of realizing the fulfilment of these needs differ. The results suggest that not only in institutional care but also in homecare, more attention should be paid to offering to older clients support in realizing activities and participation. And it is worth to note that for both client groups, getting outdoors was an important factor improving QoL, and that many had not been out in years. This is a too little discussed, or one may even say a hidden issue in the long-term care of older people, although the consequences of never getting out from home or from care home may be serious for the well-being of these prisoners of their four walls.

Living alone or with a spouse at home, living in an own room, or sharing a room in IC were equally good options, but living with children or siblings at home was not a good situation in our sample. This suggest that in IC, living in an own room is not automatically a quality input, but a good solution for some, while others are satisfied with sharing a room. However, this can be assumed also as being a cultural-sensitive issue, highlighting the importance of clarifying this preference with the client and her close ones before making a decision on accommodation. For homecare, this means that it is not always ideal that the client lives with his children or siblings, and that this should be clarified as a part of the assessment of resources and needs of the old person asking for help.

Regarding the socio-economic factors, economic resources were important QoL factors both for clients in HC and IC, as they are in older and adult populations in general. Additionally, subjective health was important. Age and gender were influential in HC as males had a slightly better QoL than females, and advanced age increased subjective QoL—an effect of adjustment (accommodation) to be expected from previous research. Positive attitude toward own ageing (as measured by the PGCMS; Lawton, 1975) was connected to subjective QoL of clients in HC, indicating higher resilience, and contributing positively to overall subjective QoL. Interestingly, IC seems to eliminate these effects—maybe due to the leveling out of differences by institutionalization. In both client groups, loneliness was associated with decreased subjective QoL, but people in HC (especially in Finland) were lonelier than clients in IC.

The results demonstrated that the effects of (types of) care are differentiating the long-term care clients from older or adult population in general. We assumed satisfaction with care to be an important determinant of crQoL, but that it had most strong direct impact on QoL of the clients in both HC and IC was surprising. And the indicators accounting for the perceived QoC were about the same (client as clean and as well dressed as he likes; client's own home as clean as he likes or care home clean; odour free and cosy; enjoyable meals; care workers who listen to the clients and understand their needs; freedom to get up and go to bed in desired times; satisfaction with help; willingness to recommend the care to other people). We also noticed that satisfaction was dealing not only with quality but also with quantity of care in the sense that clients felt care inputs as appropriate (in kind) and sufficient.

Another important question in Care Keys was what characteristics of care, in terms of professional standards, provide for good outcomes. Our results suggest that in both HC and IC, it is important to assess the clients' competencies and needs comprehensively; to set clear goals to be achieved by care; to plan the care interventions carefully to achieve these goals; to empower the clients and families for participation and use of their own resources in the care processes; as well as to evaluate the care outcomes regularly. Inclusion of informal care was very important both in HC and IC, suggesting that in long-term care of older people, a family orientation should be developed as suggested also, for example, Hellström and Hallberg (2001). Our results suggest that good care documentation is an important prerequisite for long-term care to be efficient, and in IC the relation between good care documentation and good care outcomes was evident. In HC, the results were less pronounced due to the poor documentation in current HC systems, but we were able to show similar connections as in IC.

Although there were a lot of similarities, some items were more highlighted in HC than in IC. First, comprehensive needs-assessment seemed to be critical for HC to be effective. In addition, support for the autonomy of the clients, goal-oriented care interventions, use of (fall) prophylaxes, and adequate management in place were highlighted. Management was assumed to have less impact in HC than in IC, as already stated, and this was confirmed, but somewhat differently than assumed. QoM had more direct impact on client outcomes (perceived QoC and QoL) in HC than in IC, while in IC, management impacted more on quality of documentation of professional care than was the case in HC. In HC, it was important to have management structures and procedures in place to facilitate good care: clear concept of HC as care aiming at supporting the autonomy of the clients; a quality strategy that emphasizes goal-oriented team working and regular evaluation of outcomes; and procedures for involvement of the clients and informal carers. Regarding material resources, HC to be of good quality calls for a sufficient amount of care personnel and utilization of external resources from the wider community. Additionally cooperation with physicians and other coproviders of help and care were important. When these structures and processes were in place, homecare was effective in terms of having a positive connection to the QoL of the clients. In IC, the independent impact of management on QoL was smaller than the importance of structures and processes of professional, often medically oriented care. This probably reflects the different management structures and cultures in these two types of long-term care, and it is an interesting topic for future research whether this result can be repeated and explained.

Finally, when looking at the dimensions of QoL, evaluated by older clients in HC and IC using the WHOQOL-Bref—instruments, we first noticed that the four dimensions (physical, psychological, social, and environment) applied also to our study population, but only some items within the dimensions were important in the sense of being related to care. Second, we noticed that most of these relevant items were common for both client groups, namely subjective health and acute sicknesses, amount of medical treatment needed for daily functioning, enjoying life, feeling alone, having enough energy for everyday life, accepting own bodily appearance, satisfaction with support from fiends, and satisfaction with access to health services. However, there were also some important differences. Our results regarding QoC suggested pain to be poorly managed in HC, which did not appear in IC, and we see that this impacts on the QoL of the clients. Regarding leisure activities, again clients in institutional care were more often better off with having enough things to do, while HC clients were left at home without sufficient support to access leisure activities or outings. Further, access to transportation is not important in IC where all services are close, while people at home need sufficient access to transportation to be able to get things done. To repeat, while the dimensions of the crQoL model were the same for both groups of older persons, on the level of specific indicators there were differences reflecting the different life circumstances associated with different types of care. We ran a number of different statistical analyses with appropriate tests just to find out that the selection of variables from the huge number in Care Keys database varied, but they always loaded on the four dimensions of QoL as defined by the crQoL model and reproduced by WHOQOL-Bref, confirming that a generic model of QoL is relevant and usable also for care-dependent and frail old people.

Reflecting on the Theoretical Models

To summarize, our results confirm the basic theory of Lawton (1991) to be a very important base for understanding the QoL of old care-dependent people. We have discussed and modified the model with reference to social system theory and to an alternative model proposed by Brown, and we indicated an interpretation grounding Brown's model on basic social theory and pragmatic social philosophy, providing also more theoretical depth to our approach. Certainly, the theoretical foundations of the models and the different "patches" worked together in the Care Keys framework need further conceptual elaboration and validation in future empirical research. Many features of the models have been developed in theoretical discussions in the course of the project, and were not yet applied in practice. However, the emerging framework also demonstrated its fruitfulness. We have seen that elements of QoL of old clients could be organized in the four dimensions of Lawton's model (functional competence, psychological well-being, social relations, and environmental support). The value of the model was confirmed by empirical evidence, and the model was differentiated further for different care settings by specific indicators.

In our "meta model" based on the production of welfare approach, we combined client-specific conditions with theories of quality of long-term care and care management, and developed instrumentation for empirical investigation. The value of these attempts consisted in the integration of many elements of crQoL, which so far have been studied separately from different professional perspectives or paradigms. The "meta model" also served to focus our research and to guide the development and design of a practical toolkit for QoM. Although we are aware that we were not able to look at the interactions of different factors in depth, we believe we have contributed to the current theoretical discussion on QoL in care dependent old people, giving stimulus for new research on the topic.

Regarding the theoretical framework for our studies on quality of professional long-term care, we found some important features, which should be of value both for future research and development of long-term care to better meet the needs of older clients. We identified from care theories four central tasks for the professional long-term care of older people, namely: (i) care as sustaining functional competence and autonomy; (ii) care as supporting emotional and existential well-being; (iii) care as supporting social identity, social relations, and social participation; and (iv) care as a service (cf. Bowers et al., 2001). These are in correspondence with the model of "four qualities of life" (Veenhoven), "four dimensions of QoL" (WHO), and with the "four elements of good life" by Lawton, when we understand the environmental support in his terms, that is, as including care. According to our assumption, if all four tasks are fulfilled (and corresponding needs are met), long-term care of older people is regarded as being of good quality (responsive to needs), and our empirical results gave support to this view. Similarly, we found four dimensions of good quality care from the perspective of the clients, namely: (i) ethical standards that respect the client as a valuable person; (ii) responsive interventions; (iv) good interaction quality and socio-psychological support; and (iv) appropriate support services. And finally, we defined the corresponding four dimensions also for care management. They are: (i) concept and vision of quality; (ii) competence and procedures; (iii) conditions and resources; and (iv) cooperation and integration.

Finally, we integrated these findings in a comprehensive structural model ("onion model") of crQoL (see Fig. 4, Chapter 4) with the following "layers":

1. In the heart of the system, there is the client and his life quality, dividing into four dimensions of good life. The client-specific conditions are differentiated in: (1) physical; (2) psychological; (3) social; and (4) socio-demographic and environmental resources and compensation needs.
2. The client preferences and expectations on QoC are differentiated in: (1) responsive interventions; (2) good interaction quality; (3) good ethical standards; and (4) appropriate support services.
3. Professional care inputs are differentiated in four factors: (1) sustaining the functional competence and autonomy of the clients; (2) supporting emotional and existential well-being of clients; (3) supporting social identity, social relations, and social participation of clients; and (4) providing appropriate and sufficient interventions, comfort, and support services.
4. Management inputs are differentiated in: (1) management competence and procedures; (2) cooperation and integration; (3) concept of quality supporting the autonomy and dignity of the clients; and (4) sufficient conditions and resources.
5. The outcomes of care can be further differentiated—measured again in four dimensions of QoL—by identifying the subjective evaluation by the client as the "final outcome" and "inner core of the onion": (1) physical, (2) psychological; (3) social; (4) environmental dimension. (Note: the numbers indicate corresponding dimensions)

The structural model is complemented by a production model and a normative model. In the production model, the elements are rearranged in a production process or causal chain, emphasizing the resilience and the active role of the client in the coproduction process. The normative model addresses the issues of values and "negotiation of order" in care relationships, and introduces the "care triad" as a critical element. And we also developed instrumentation (still to be completed, modified and tested) that is able to measure these dimensions and indicators of crQoL by interviewing the clients, by extracting data from care documentation, and by collecting data from managers and management records.

This type of theoretical and methodological "triangulation"—combining different theoretical approaches and methods—has the potential of finding new solutions when crossing over the borders of different paradigms and professional ways of thinking. By grounding the Care Keys approach in basic social theory and on concepts of practice oriented production of welfare, we tried to achieve the necessary unification of the diverse components and to avoid the dangers of patchwork inherent in multidisciplinary projects. We consider our concept of crQoL, and its integration with concepts of care quality and QoM in long-term care as a theoretical and practical innovation. It will depend on the implementation of the model into concrete care and management practices to achieve the main objective of the Care Keys approach, namely, to make the voice of the clients heard and respected in long-term care, empowering the clients to participate in the coproduction of their life quality. We are aware that the results and instruments need further research and development, and we will continue with exploration and development of our models and instruments, and we hope they offer a stimulus also to other researchers in the field.

References

Baldock, J. C., & Hadlow, J. (2002). Self-talk versus needs-talk: An exploration of the priorities of housebound older people. *Quality in Ageing, 3*(1), 42–48.

Bebbington, A., & Davies, B. (1983). Equity and efficiency in the allocation of the personal social services. *Journal of Social Policy, 12*, 309–330.

Birren, J. E., Lubben, J. E., Rowe, J. C., & Deutschmann, D. E. (Eds.). (1991). *The concept and measurement of QoL in frail elderly.* New York: Academic Press.

Bowers, B. J., Fibich, B., & Jacobson, N. (2001). Care-as-service, care-as-relating, care-as-comfort: Understanding nursing home resident's definition of quality. *The Gerontologist, 41*(4), 539–545.

Brown, I., & Brown, R. I. (2003). *Quality of life and disability. An approach for community practitioners.* New York: Kingsley.

Caris-Verhallen, W., Kerkstra, A., & Bensing, J. (1997). The role of communication in nursing care for elderly people: a review of the literature. *Journal of Advanced Nursing, 25*, 915–933.

Coulon, L., Mok, M., Krause, K.-L., & Anderson, M. (1996). 'The pursuit of excellence in nursing care: what does it mean?' *Journal of Advanced Nursing, 24*, 817–826.

Cummins, R. A. (1997). Assessing QoL. In R. I. Brown (Eds.), *QoL for people with disabilities. Models, research and practice.* Cheltenham: Stanley Thornes.

Davies, B., & Knapp, M. (1981). *Old people's homes and the production of welfare.* London: Routledge & Kegan Paul.

DePorter, C. H. (2005). Regulating food service in North Carolina's long-term care facilities. *North Carolina Medical Journal, 66*(4), 300–303.

Hellström, Y., & Hallberg, I. R. (2001). Perspectives of elderly people receiving home help on health, care and QoL. *Health and Social Care in the Community, 9*(2), 61–71.

Hughes, B. (1990). QoL. In S. M. Peace (Ed.), *Researching social gerontology: Concepts, methods and issues* (pp. 46–58). London: SAGE.

Kavanagh, S., & Stewart, A. (1995). Economic evaluations of mental health care. In M. Knapp (Eds.), *The economic evaluation of mental health care* (pp. 27–60). PSSRU. CEMH. Aldershot: Arena.

Knapp, M. (1984). *The economics of social care. Studies in Social Policy.* Hongkong: MacMillan Education.

Knapp, M. (1995). *The economic evaluation of mental health care.* PSSRU.CEMH, Aldershot: Arena.

Lawton, M. P. (1975). The Philadelphia Geriatric Center Morale Scale: A revision. *Journal of Gerontology, 30*, 85–89.

Lawton, M. P. (1983). Environment and other determinants of well-being in older people. *The Gerontologist, 4*, 349–357.

Lawton, M. P. (1991). A multidimensional view of quality of life in frail elders. In J. E. Birren, J. E. Lubben, J. C. Rowe, & D. E. Deutchman (Eds.), *The concept and measurement of quality of life in frail elders* (pp. 3–27). San Diego, CA: Academic Press.

Øvretveit, J. (1998). *Evaluating health interventions. An introduction to evaluation of health treatments, services, policies and organizational interventions,* Buckingham, Philadelphia, PA: Open University Press.

Power, M., Quinn, K., Schmidt, S., & WHOQOL-OLD Group. (2005). Development of the WHOQOL-old module. *Quality of Life Research, 14,* 2197–2214.

Skevington, S. M., Lofty, M., O'Connell, K., & The WHOQOL Group. (2004). The World Health Organisation's WHOQOL-Bref quality of life assessment: Psychometric properties and the results of the international field trial. A Report from the WHOQOL Group, *Quality of Life Research, 13,* 299–310.

Vaarama, M., Mattila, V., Laaksonen, S., & Valtonen, H. (1997). *Target efficiency— report on development and piloting of the target efficiency indicators and model.* Helsinki: Stakes.

Vaarama, M., Pieper, R., & Sixsmith, A. (2007).*Care related QoL in old age.* Conceptual and Emprical Exploration. In: H. Mollenkopf, & A. Walker (Eds.) (2007). *Quality of Life in Old Age. International and Multi-Disciplinary Perspectives.* Dordrecht, The Netherlands: Springer. pp. 215–232.

Veenhoven, R. (1996). "Happy life-expectancy. A comprehensive measure of quality-of-life in nations", *Social Indicators Research, 39,* 1–58.

Veenhoven, R. (2000). The four qualities of Life. Ordering concept and measures of the good life. *Journal of Happiness Studies, 1,* 1–39.

Subject Index